Handbook of
PEDIATRIC
INTENSIVE CARE

Handbook of
PEDIATRIC
INTENSIVE
CARE

Editor
MARK C. ROGERS, M.D.

Director, Pediatric Intensive Care
Professor of Pediatrics
Professor and Chairman
Department of Anesthesiology/Critical Care Medicine
The Johns Hopkins University School of Medicine
  and
The Johns Hopkins Hospital
Baltimore, Maryland

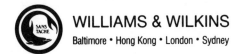

WILLIAMS & WILKINS
Baltimore • Hong Kong • London • Sydney

Editor: Timothy H. Grayson
Associate Editor: Marjorie Kidd Keating
Copy Editor: Bill Cady
Design: Dan Pfisterer
Illustration Planning: Lorraine Wrzosek
Production: Anne G. Seitz

The information in this book is adapted from *Textbook of Pediatric Intensive Care*, edited by Mark C. Rogers, M.D., and published by Williams & Wilkins in 1987. The contributors to the original chapters in the *Textbook* are therefore acknowledged in the table of contents of this work.

Copyright © 1989
Williams & Wilkins
428 East Preston Street
Baltimore, Maryland 21202, USA

The Publishers have made every effort to trace the copyright holders for borrowed material. If they have inadvertantly overlooked any, they will be pleased to make the necessary arrangements at the first opportunity.

Accurate indications, adverse reactions, and dosage schedules for drugs are provided in this book, but it is possible that they may change. The reader is urged to review the package information data of the manufacturers of the medications mentioned.

Printed in the United States of America

Library of Congress Cataloging-in-Publication Data

Handbook of pediatric intensive care.

   Adaptation of: Textbook of pediatric intensive care   /   editor, Mark C. Rogers. c1987.
   Includes index.
   1. Pediatric   intensive   care—Handbooks,   manuals,   etc. I. Rogers,   Mark
C. II. Textbook of pediatric intensive care. [DNLM: 1. Critical Care—in infancy &
childhood—handbooks. 2. Emergencies—in infancy & childhood—handbooks. WS 39
H236]
RJ370.H36   1989   618.92′0028   88-36276
ISBN 0-683-07321-4

90 91 92 93
3 4 5 6 7 8 9 10

Preface

Over a decade ago, we were fortunate enough to be supported in the vision that pediatric intensive care was going to be a new specialty. This required a dedicated pediatric intensive care unit, a devoted group of nurses, a training program with fellows, a major textbook to provide a common body of knowledge, and a handbook for the practical aspects at the bedside.

With the completion of the *Handbook*, which is an adaptation of the *Textbook*, we have made an attempt to reach all of those goals. None of this would have been possible without the enthusiastic help of more than a dozen faculty and nearly three dozen fellows who have made major contributions to our Pediatric Intensive Care Unit and to the field. My gratitude to them, hopefully, will be complemented by their own recognition that they have made a fundamental improvement in the care of critically ill children.

Acknowledgments

The work of compiling the *Handbook* involved a tremendous contribution by Jeannette Sias, Irene Eliou, Peggy Riley, Carol Kearney, Cynthia Sheffield, and Elliott Rice. Without their many hours of dedicated time and effort, this book would not have been published.

Contents

CHAPTER 1

Cardiopulmonary Resuscitation

OVERVIEW OF RESUSCITATION PROCEDURES

The physician must quickly assess whether the child is unconscious, is breathing, or has a heart beat. The steps in the primary survey are: (a) airway, (b) breathing and ventilation, and (c) circulation (see Table 1.1).

Beginning Cardiopulmonary Resuscitation

The beginning steps of cardiopulmonary resuscitation (CPR) include establishing the unresponsiveness of the patient by gently shaking, tapping, and shouting at him or her. The bystander or physician should then call for assistance and place the patient in the supine position.

In cases of the total collapse or unconsciousness of the patient, the absence of adequate ventilation and circulation should be determined im-

TABLE 1.1.
Primary Survey

Airway
Open the airway
   Head tilt
   Head tilt with chin lift
   Head tilt with neck lift
   Jaw thrust
Establish breathlessness

Breathing
Two initial breaths
One-rescuer or two-rescuer CPR
If unsuccessful, check for foreign body in airway

Circulation
Check pulse
Perform chest compressions

mediately. If ventilation alone is absent or inadequate, opening the airway, rescue breathing, or both may be all that is necessary. If the circulation is inadequate, artificial circulation should be started at this time, in addition to rescue breathing.

Positioning—Opening the Airway

The first step in basic CPR is to open the airway and restore breathing. Methods for opening the airway of an unconscious patient are geared to relieving obstruction, usually due to obstruction by the tongue. There are various ways to accomplish this, including neck lift and chin lift.

Head tilt is the initial step in opening the airway (see Fig. 1.1). To accomplish the head tilt, the rescuer's hand is placed on the patient's forehead and firm backward pressure is applied, tipping the victim's head maximally backward.

The head tilt, chin lift method is performed by placing the fingertips of one hand under the mandible near the protuberance of the chin, bringing the chin forward and supporting the jaw, which results in tilting the head back (see Fig. 1.2). Care should be taken not to compress the soft tissues of the chin, which might obstruct the patient's airway.

Jaw thrust without head tilt is the safest technique in opening the airway of a patient with a suspected neck injury, because in most cases it can be accomplished without extending the neck. The head should be carefully supported without turning it from side to side or tilting it backward. If this maneuver is unsuccessful, the head is then tilted back very slightly, and another attempt is made to ventilate.

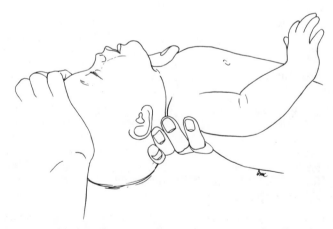

FIGURE 1.1.   Head tilt/neck lift airway position. The rescuer places one hand on the patient's forehead, exerting backward pressure while the other hand is held under the patient's neck.

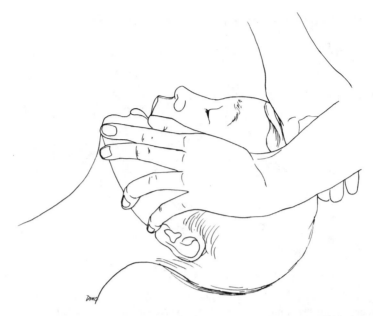

FIGURE 1.2. Head tilt/chin lift airway position. The rescuer places one hand on the patient's forehead, with the other hand supporting the angle of the mandible while pulling the chin upward.

Establishing Breathlessness

After the airway is opened, the rescuer should again check whether the patient is breathing. This is done by placing the ear over the victim's mouth and nose and viewing the patient's chest and abdomen. If the chest and abdomen fall and the rescuer feels air from the mouth and nose and hears air during exhalation, then the patient is breathing. If the patient has respiratory efforts without air exhalation, the airway is still obstructed. Frequently, opening the airway is all that the patient needs in order to breathe effectively. If the patient begins breathing after the above maneuvers, the airway is maintained. If the patient is not breathing after the appropriate maneuvers, rescue breathing is begun. If after opening the airway the patient is gasping or struggling to breathe, the decision to begin rescue breathing depends on the presence or absence of cyanosis, as is discussed above.

Initiating Rescue Breathing

Rescue breathing is initiated once breathlessness is established. In the infant, the rescuer makes a tight seal, covering the infant's mouth and nose with his or her mouth (see Fig. 1.3). If the child is larger, so that the

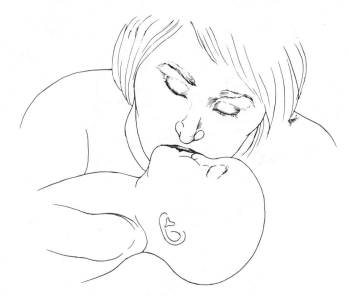

FIGURE 1.3. Artificial ventilation in infants. The rescuer places the patient's head in sniffing position and places his or her mouth over both mouth and nose, making a tight seal.

rescuer's mouth cannot fit over both nose and mouth, the patient's nose is pinched, and the mouth is covered by the rescuer's mouth (see Fig. 1.4).

When an airtight seal has been established by either of the above methods, two slow breaths are delivered in succession without permitting full lung deflation. This is done as a means of checking for airway obstruction as well as opening collapsed alveoli in the lungs. These breaths are limited to the amount of air needed to cause the chest to rise adequately, so this is taken into account especially when ventilating infants.

During single-rescuer CPR, two full, quick breaths, without allowing time for full lung deflation between breaths, are given by the rescuer after each cycle of 15 compressions in adult patients, whereas only one breath is given by the rescuer after each cycle of 5 compressions in children. During two-rescuer CPR, one breath is administered every 5 seconds. This rate would also be performed during single-rescuer respiratory resuscitation for a nonbreathing patient. During two-rescuer CPR, the breath is interposed during the upstroke of the fifth chest compression in adults and children.

Occurrence of Gastric Distention

Gastric distention caused during artificial ventilation interferes with ventilation by elevating the diaphragm and decreasing lung volume. This occurs most often in children but is also seen in adults. The incidence of gastric distention is minimized by limiting ventilation volumes to that which raises the chest, thus avoiding exceeding the esophageal opening pres-

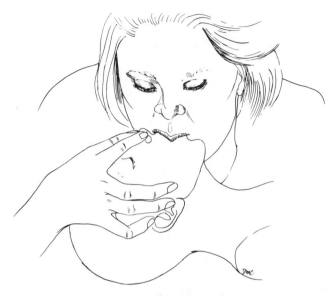

FIGURE 1.4. Mouth-to-mouth ventilation. The rescuer places the patient's head in the sniffing position, pinches the nose, takes a deep breath, and exhales into the patient's mouth.

sure. Gastric distention also commonly occurs when the airway is partially or completely obstructed. Attempts at relieving gastric distention during CPR by pressure on the abdomen should be avoided because of the high risk of aspirating gastric contents into the lungs during this maneuver.

CIRCULATION SUPPORT—TECHNICAL ASPECTS

Assessing Pulse

Once the airway has been opened adequately and two breaths have been delivered, it must be determined whether only breathing has stopped or whether a cardiac arrest has occurred simultaneously. Absence of a pulse in the large arteries in an unconscious victim who is not breathing defines a cardiac arrest.

As in the adult, the pulse of a child can be felt over the carotid artery (see Fig. 1.5). The head tilt should be maintained with one hand on the forehead. While doing this, the tips of the fingers of the other hand locate the patient's larynx, and the fingers are slid into the groove between the trachea and the muscles on that side of the neck. The carotid pulse is then palpated gently and not compressed, so as not to lose the pulsation. Palpation of the carotid pulse is recommended in adults and children for a number of reasons. These include the fact that the patient's head is already accessible to the rescuer while performing artificial ventilation. The neck area can be accessed immediately without the removal of any cloth-

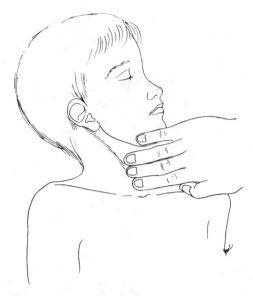

FiGURE 1.5. Feeling the carotid pulse. The fingers are placed laterally into the groove between the trachea and the sternocleidomastoid muscle.

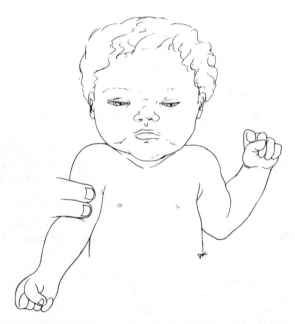

FIGURE 1.6. Feeling the brachial pulse. The brachial pulse is palpated with two finger along the medial aspect of the upper arm above the antecubital region.

ing. In addition, the carotid arteries can frequently still be palpated when more peripheral pulses, such as the radial artery, are no longer palpable in the shock state.

The palpation of the carotid pulse in an infant is more difficult due to the infant's very short and, at times, very fat neck. Precordial activity in the infant is not reliable because it represents an impulse rather than a pulse. Some infants with good cardiac activity may have a quiet precordium, leading to the erroneous diagnosis of cardiac arrest. It is thus recommended that the brachial pulse be palpated in infants for the presence or absence of a cardiac arrest.

The brachial pulse is located on the inside of the upper arm, midway between the elbow and shoulder (see Fig. 1.6). In order to locate the pulse, the rescuer should place his or her thumb on the outside of the arm between the shoulder and elbow. The tips of his or her index and middle finger are then placed on the opposite side of the arm, pressing lightly toward the humerus until the brachial pulse is palpated.

When there is a pulse but no breathing, only breathing has arrested, and rescue breathing must be continued as discussed in the previous section. Absence or questionable presence of a pulse is the indication for starting artificial circulation via external chest compression. Chest compression should never be performed without rescue breathing.

Chest Compression—Pediatrics

The differences in the techniques of external chest compression among infants, children, and adults are related to the position of the heart within the chest, the size of the chest, and the more rapid heart rate of the infant and child as compared with that of the adult (see Table 1.2). As the chest grows, that portion of the chest occupied by the heart diminishes. The

TABLE 1.2.
Guidelines for Chest Compressions in CPR

Patient	Method	Sternal Depression (% of Chest AP[a] Diameter)	Compressions/ Min	Compressions/ Respiration (Two Rescuers)	Compressions/ Respiration (One Rescuer)
Infant	Two fingers or hand encircling	20% (1½ inches)	100	5:1	5:1
Toddler	One hand	20% (1–1½ inches)	80	5:1	5:1
Large child	Two hands	20% (1½–2 inches)	80	5:1	5:1
Adult	Two hands	20% (2 inches)	80	5:1	15:2

[a]AP, anteroposterior.

heart in the infant and child is situated higher in the chest than it is in the adult. One study, however, using radiographic markers, revealed that the heart is actually lower in the chest than was previously believed for infants. Therefore, the recommended area of compression is 2 finger-breadths below the intersection of the intermammary line and the sternum.

The infant's chest is smaller and more compliant than that of the adult. There are two techniques in performing external chest compression on this more compliant chest. One method is to place two or three fingers on the midsternum, halfway between the nipples (see Fig. 1.7). The other method has the hands encircle the chest of the infant, forming a rigid surface on the back, and the thumbs are used at the level of the midsternum to compress the chest (see Fig. 1.8).

The infant's sternum should be compressed approximately 20% of the anteroposterior width of the chest, which would be ½–1 inch in the infant. When the infant becomes large enough so that three fingers cannot adequately depress the sternum or the rescuer's hands cannot reach around the infant's chest, the heel of one hand should be used. As in the adult, the rescuer's fingers should be kept off the chest. If the patient is large

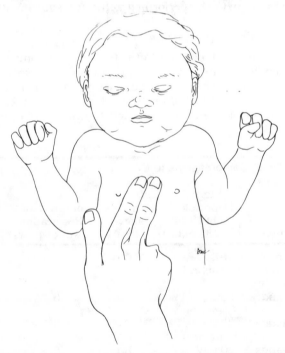

FIGURE 1.7. External chest compression in infants—two-finger method. The rescuer places two fingers over the midsternum and compresses ½–1 inch at a rate of 100/min. For clarity, ventilation is not shown.

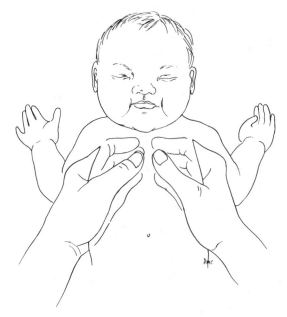

FIGURE 1.8. Hand-encircling technique for external chest compression in infants. The rescuer's hands encircle the infant's chest with thumbs midsternum to compress the chest. For observation of correct placement, the rescuer's hands are seen behind the infant's chest. For clarity, ventilation is not shown.

enough to require the heel of the hand for compression (see Fig. 1.9), the depth of the compression is increased to 1–1½ inches.

The compression rate for external chest CPR is greater in infants and children than in adults. One hundred compressions per minute are used for infants, and 80 compressions/min are used for older children. For two-rescuer CPR, the ratio of compressions to respiration remains 5:1. When only one rescuer is involved, the ratio of 5:1 should also be used. Compressions can easily be counted by the rescuer in order to get the proper rate as follows: in an infant—1, 2, 3, 4, 5, breathe, and in a child—1 and 2 and 3 and 4 and 5 and breathe.

Endotracheal Administration of Drug

During CPR, the rapid establishment of intravenous access, especially in infants or small children, can be very difficult. The endotracheal route for drug administration has been used when vascular access is limited. Absorption rates and physiologic and pharmacologic effects compare favorably with the intravenous route for epinephrine and atropine.

Both the volume of medication and the diluent in which the medication is delivered are important. When a drug is administered in a very large volume, pulmonary surfactant may be altered or destroyed, resulting in

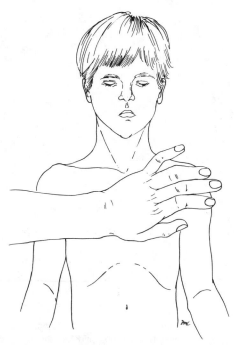

FIGURE 1.9. External chest compression in the young child. The heel of the hand is placed 2 fingerbreadths above the bottom of the sternum for compression. In the older child, the two-hand compression is used as in adults.

atelectasis. As a result, the total volume of fluid delivered into the trachea should not exceed 10 ml in the adult or large child or 5 ml in the infant.

The risks associated with endotracheal or endobronchial administration of drug is the formation of an intrapulmonary depot of drug, which prolongs the effect of that particular drug. Theoretically, this could result in a recurrence of ventricular fibrillation, for example, once the circulation is restored to normal, or in sustained hypertension in the same setting after the administration of epinephrine.

Intracardiac Injection

The intracardiac route of injection is now recommended only if other sites of injection, including intravenous, intraosseus and endotracheal routes, are inaccessible. This is due to the many hazards of the intracardiac injection. The complications cited include coronary artery laceration, cardiac tamponade, pneumothorax, and the need to interrupt external chest compressions and ventilation during the period of injection.

The technique of administering the intracardiac injection is as follows. A large needle, preferably a 22-gauge spinal needle, is placed percutaneously just below the xiphoid process. The needle is aimed toward the left shoulder at an angle of 45° to the body surface. When blood is aspirated, the heart is entered, assuming a hemopericardium is not present, and drugs can then be injected.

Types of Solutions

Intravenous fluids are needed to restore normal circulating blood volume during resuscitation and to expand blood volume after cardiac arrest, because of venous pooling, vasodilation, and capillary leakage.

Controversy still surrounds the choice of fluids given in resuscitation. Some studies have shown no difference; some, an advantage for crystalloid; and others, an advantage for colloid solutions. Electrolyte solutions (isotonic saline or Ringer's lactate solution) spread through both intravascular and interstitial fluid spaces, so that 2 or 3 times the initial blood loss should be replaced with crystalloid. If there is a >20% loss of estimated blood volume, a colloid solution, such as blood, plasma, albumin, dextran, or hydroxyethyl starch, should be administered in volumes equal to the blood loss, because these solutions remain in the intravascular space. If the patient is hypovolemic, a colloid solution is used to prevent a reduction of either the serum albumin concentration to less than one-half of normal or of the colloid osmotic pressure to less than two-thirds of normal (normal value, 25 mm Hg).

Open-Chest Cardiopulmonary Resuscitation

There is an increasing renewal of interest in open-chest CPR. A summary of areas in which it may be useful is shown in Table 1.3.

DRUG THERAPY AND DEFIBRILLATION IN PEDIATRIC CARDIOPULMONARY RESUSCITATION

This section is adapted from the standards and guidelines for CPR and emergency cardiac care of the American Heart Association (1986).*

The first use of drugs is for the correction of hypoxemia, and the primary drug used is oxygen. It should be administered, if possible, as 100% oxygen and should be administered in patients who are hypoxemic, regardless of the cause of hypoxemia, since acute oxygen administration to improve arterial oxygen and tissue perfusion is mandatory in these circumstances.

Drugs Used in Control of Arrhythmias
Atropine

In the presence of bradycardia, atropine sulfate is a very useful drug as a parasympatholytic agent that increases heart rate and atrioventricular conduction. It is useful, particularly in the small infant in whom cardiac

---

*American Heart Association: Pediatric basic life support. *JAMA* 255:2954–2973, 1986.

TABLE 1.3.
Partial List of Indications for Open-Chest CPR as Outlined by Babbs et al.[a]

1. Cardiac arrest precipitated by stab wounds or lacerations of the myocardium.
2. Acute cardiac tamponade precipitating cardiac arrest is usually best treated by directly venting the pericardial sac.
3. Extracardiac intrathoracic hemorrhage causing cardiac arrest.
4. A massive air embolus can be demonstrated by direct visual needle aspiration.
5. A massive pulmonary embolus can be effectively removed by using open-chest CPR.
6. A ruptured abdominal aortic aneurysm is effectively managed by opening the left side of the chest and clamping the aorta proximal to the diaphragm before instituting CPR.
7. During intrathoracic procedures, cardiac arrest is best approached by direct cardiac compression, because the chest is already opened.
8. Sternal malformations including pectus excavatum and pectus carinatum may contradict effective closed-chest CPR.
9. Vertebral abnormalities including marked scoliosis, lordosis, or kyphosis make closed-chest CPR difficult. The difficulty in resuscitating these patients is not clear, especially in view of newer theories of CPR regarding the rise of intrathoracic pressure as the mechanism for blood flow, but may be related to pulmonary hypertension, severe kinking of vascular structures within the chest, or the inability to increase intrathoracic pressure by chest compression due to the deformity itself.
10. When defibrillation is unsuccessful, direct application of electrodes to the pericardium or myocardium may be successful.
11. In the latter two-thirds of pregnancy, a woman in the supine position may have difficulty due to aortocaval compression.
12. A left atrial myxoma or other intracardiac obstruction.
13. In instances when closed-chest CPR is unsuccessful in producing an adequate cardiac output, open-chest CPR may be indicated.
14. Ventricular aneurysms associated with cardiac arrest are best approached by open-chest CPR.

[a]Babbs CF, Winslow EBJ, Ritter G, Redding JS, Stephenson HE, Welborn WS, Weisfeldt, ML, Safar P: Knowledge gaps in CPR: Synopsis of a panel discussion. *Crit. Care Med.* 8:181, 1980.

output is rate dependent and in reflex bradycardia associated with intubation, which occurs in children.

Very small doses of atropine have a paradoxical central nervous system-mediated effect of producing bradycardia, and therefore it is important to give an appropriate dose. Conversely, tachycardia appears to be well tolerated in infants and children and may last for a long time after the administration of the atropine. Finally, prior to the period of agonal heart and respirations following hypoxemia, atropine may be useful for reversing and, occasionally, for masking hypoxemia-induced bradycardia.

The recommended dose is 0.02 mg/kg, with a minimum dose of 0.1 mg and a maximum dose of 1.0 mg. This may be repeated every 5–8 minutes for a total dose of 1.0 mg in a child. In an adult or a big adolescent, a dose of 2.0 mg would be the maximum dose.

Lidocaine

Although atropine is the most useful drug for bradycardia, lidocaine is also frequently used. It is particularly useful for treating ventricular ectopic beats and for stabilizing heart rhythm after defibrillation for ventricular fibrillation or ventricular tachycardia.

The drug is generally given intravenously as a bolus of 1 mg/kg in a patient with ventricular fibrillation or ventricular tachycardia, as well as in patients who have multiple ventricular premature beats. In addition, the use of lidocaine prior to cardioversion may be useful for the patient after the cardioversion is successfully completed, which should never delay the time for the cardioversion to be done. An infusion should follow with a rate of 20–50 μg/kg/min by administering 1–2.5 ml/kg/hr of an infusion of 120 mg lidocaine in 100 ml of 5% dextrose in water.

It should be remembered that the infusion rate of lidocaine should be lowered in the presence of low cardiac output, such as in shock or cardiac arrest, since there is decreased drug clearance. It is standard to give the usual bolus of 1 mg/kg in this circumstance, but it is important not to exceed 20 μg/kg/min in the infusion.

Bretylium Tosylate

Bretylium tosylate is very useful in the treatment of ventricular tachyarrhythmias. It has been particularly useful in the treatment of ventricular fibrillation and is said to produce "spontaneous" chemical defibrillation. It has the property of releasing catecholamines with an increase in the heart rate and in blood pressure, which results in ultimate endogenous catecholamine depletion and hypotension. It should be reserved for use in the setting of ventricular fibrillation and ventricular tachycardia resistant to defibrillation, cardioversion, and lidocaine.

It is generally given as an intravenous infusion of 5 mg/kg immediately prior to defibrillation, and if repeated countershocks are needed, a dose as high as 10 mg/kg may be used. In a conscious patient, a dose of >5 mg/kg should *not* be given because it can induce vomiting, with the potential for aspiration.

Isoproterenol

Isoproterenol is a β-adrenergic agonist that results in an increase in the heart rate and contractility, as well as in peripheral vasodilatation. It is useful in the treatment of bradycardia due to heart block, which is resistant to atropine, and is given as an infusion of 0.1–1.0 μg/kg/min.

In the specific setting of cardiac arrest, the important catecholamine effects are thought to be mediated through α-adrenergic activity; and as a result, isoproterenol is not thought to be as useful. It is for this reason that epinephrine infusion is used more commonly than isoproterenol infusion for atropine-resistant bradycardias in the clinical setting of cardiopulmonary resuscitation.

Drugs Used to Alter Cardiac Output

Epinephrine

Epinephrine has both α- and β-adrenergic properties, and it is the α-adrenergic properties that are important in cardiac arrest. It produces vasoconstriction to improve perfusion pressure, enhances the contractile state of the heart, and has been shown to make the myocardium more likely to terminate ventricular fibrillation following electrical defibrillation.

The commonly used dose in resuscitation is 0.01 mg/kg (0.1 ml/kg of 1:10,000 solution) given intravenously, repeated every 5 minutes as needed.

It can also be used as an infusion, with low-dose infusions ($<0.3\mu g/kg/$min) producing prominent β-adrenergic effects, while higher doses result in α-adrenergic vasoconstriction (Table 1.4) It has the potential to produce profound tachycardia and serious ventricular arrhythmias, as well as profound vasoconstriction which may limit blood flow to the extremities and to the kidney in particular.

Dopamine

Dopamine is an agent that has a variety of effects, depending on its dose. In very low doses (0.5–2 $\mu g/kg/min$), dopamine produces isolated renal and splanchnic vasodilation, said to be the result of dopaminergic receptors (Table 1.5). At rates higher than 5 $\mu g/kg/min$, it produces (a) direct stimulation of the heart through β-adrenergic receptor activity and (b) indirect stimulation through the release of norepinephrine. Infusions at rates higher than 20 $\mu g/kg/min$ result in profound vasoconstriction. Most often, doses in CPR begin at 5–10 $\mu g/kg/min$ and are increased as needed, though care should be taken because at high doses it produces ventricular ectopy.

Dobutamine

The advantage of dobutamine hydrochloride is that it is relatively selective for β_1-adrenergic receptors which increase cardiac contractility. It has a few of the peripheral vascular effects of other catecholamines. It is usually given as 5–15 $\mu g/kg/min$ but may produce ectopy at high doses.

Calcium

Calcium is gradually losing favor for use in CPR, since its beneficial effects are unclear and it has been implicated in vascular spasm. When treatment is needed, it is for hypocalcemia or, possibly, for hyperkalemia, hypermagnesemia, or reversal of calcium channel drug overdose.

The dose is generally given as calcium chloride at 0.2 ml/kg of a solution of 100 mg/ml. This will provide 5.4 mg/kg of elemental calcium. Since bradycardia is a known complication of calcium administration, atropine should be available, and the calcium should be infused very slowly.

TABLE 1.4.
Drugs Used in Pediatric Advanced Life Support

Drug	Dose	How Supplied	Remarks
Atropine sulfate	0.02 mg/kg/dose	0.1 mg/ml	Minimum dose of 0.1 mg (1.0 ml)
Calcium chloride	20 mg/kg/dose	100 mg/ml (10%)	Give slowly
Dopamine hydrochloride	2–20 μg/kg/min	40 mg/ml	α-Adrenergic action dominates at 15–20 μg/kg/min
Dobutamine hydrochloride	5–20 μg/kg/min	250 mg/vial lyophilized	Titrate to desired effect
Epinephrine hydrochloride	0.1 ml/kg (0.01 mg/kg)	1:10,000 (0.1 mg/ml)	1:1,000 must be diluted
Epinephrine infusion	Start at 0.1 μg/kg/min	1:1,000 (1 mg/ml)	Titrate to desired effect (0.1–1.0 μg/kg/min)
Isoproterenol hydrochloride	Start at 0.1 μg/kg/min	1 mg/5 ml	Titrate to desired effect (0.1–1.0 μg/kg/min)
Lidocaine	1 mg/kg/dose	10 mg/ml (1%) 20 mg/ml (2%)	
Lidocaine infusion	20–50 μg/kg/min	40 mg/ml (4%)	
Norepinephrine infusion	Start at 0.1 μg/kg/min	1 mg/ml	Titrate to desired effect (0.1–1.0 μg/kg/min)
Sodium bicarbonate	1 mEq/kg/dose or 0.3 × kg × base deficit	1 mEq/ml (8.4%)	Infuse slowly and only if ventilation is adequate

Sodium Bicarbonate

Although sodium bicarbonate was once very commonly used in cardiac arrest settings, its use now in these settings is controversial. The reasons are that it may aggravate a respiratory arrest cause of CPR, will not improve pH if ventilation is inadequate, may reduce cardiac output, and may produce cerebrospinal fluid acidosis.

In a patient with cardiac arrest who is ventilated, given oxygen, and given epinephrine but who is nonresponsive, a dose of sodium bicarbonate of 1 mEq/kg given intravenously or even intraosseously can be used. In children, it is generally given as 1 ml/kg of 8.4% solution, but it is diluted to 0.5 mEq/ml for administration in infants.

TABLE 1.5. ────────────────────────────────
Preparation of Infusions

Drug	Preparation	Dose
Isoproterenol, epinephrine, norepinephrine	0.6 × body weight (kg) is mg added to diluent[a] to make 100 ml	Then 1 ml/hr delivers 0.1 μg/kg/min; titrate to effect
Dopamine, dobutamine	6 × body weight (kg) is mg added to diluent to make 100 ml	Then 1 ml/hr delivers 1.0 μg/kg/min; titrate to effect
Lidocaine	120 mg (3 ml of 4% solution) into 100 ml of 5% dextrose in water—1,200 μg/ml	Then 1 ml/kg/hr delivers 20 μg/kg/min

[a]Diluent may be 5% dextrose in water or 5% dextrose in half-normal saline, normal saline, or Ringer's lactate.

Defibrillation

The standard infant paddle with electrode paste or saline-soaked gauze pads is used in the asynchronous mode for ventricular fibrillation. A dose of 2 W-sec (J)/kg is generally used but can be doubled, if needed. Rather than increase doses beyond that, attempts should be made to treat hypoglycemia, acidosis, or other metabolic abnormalities while doing manual CPR and before another attempt at defibrillation is made. Lidocaine can be used, as can bretylium tosylate as mentioned above.

Cardioversion of arrhythmias requires the use of the synchronizer to avoid putting a shock on the T wave and producing ventricular defibrillation. Also, a much lower dose is given (0.2–1.0 W-sec/kg).

Emergency Management of the Airway

BASIC AIRWAY MANAGEMENT

In all patients with compromised airways, it is important to clear the mouth and oropharynx of secretions. With the patient in the prone position with head down, the tongue falls forward to relieve obstruction. Also, secretions will be able to drain freely. If the patient must remain supine because of other injuries, a backward tilt of the head will separate the base of the tongue from the posterior pharyngeal wall by stretching the anterior neck and chin.

An oropharyngeal airway may also be used to hold the base of the tongue and epiglottis forward and away from the posterior pharyngeal wall. It is placed to follow the curve of the tongue and must be positioned so as not to push the tongue backward. It may be inserted by placing it in the mouth with curve concave superiorly, to avoid pushing the tongue back, and then rotating it 180° so that the tip is aimed toward the larynx. Complications of placement include trauma to lips and teeth. Laryngospasm or vomiting may occur if the airway is placed in a conscious patient.

A soft nasopharyngeal airway may be useful in a semiconscious patient or if the mouth cannot be opened. It extends to below the base of the tongue and provides an air channel. It should be lubricated and placed in line with the nose. Complications of placement include pushing the epiglottis against the posterior pharyngeal wall, epistaxis, laryngospasm if the airway is pressing on the epiglottis, or ulceration of the nose. Contraindications for placement of a nasopharyngeal airway include (a) nasal bleeding or anticoagulant use, because of possible trauma and further bleeding, and (b) cerebrospinal fluid leak, especially with basilar skull fractures and rupture of the cribriform plate.

When a clear airway has been obtained and the patient is breathing spontaneously, oxygen may be given as needed. Modalities include hood, nasal cannula, and face mask.

If the patient does not spontaneously breathe when the patency of the airway is established, ventilation by mouth to mouth, mouth to nose/mouth in the infant, or bag and mask may be necessary. A tight mask fitted over the nasal, maxillary, and mandibular bones with a seal by the cheeks is

17

needed to ventilate with positive pressure. Several types of masks are available in plastic or rubber and in a variety of colors. Depending on the manufacturer, differing sizes and shapes can be obtained to conform to facial features. Some masks are soft and can be bent, and others have a cushioned edge to mold to the shape of the face to allow the administration of oxygen without a leak. The connector at the top of the mask is used to attach to a bag or breathing system to allow positive pressure ventilation.

Ventilation is accomplished by squeezing the bag and observing for chest movement and breath sounds as evidence of air movement into the chest. The pressure applied from the bag is determined by an effective squeeze and the volume of air displaced from the bag, the resistance of the airway, and the set point of the relief valve of the particular resuscitator bag. In the presence of decreased lung or chest compliance, it may be necessary to bypass the pressure relief valve in order to achieve effective ventilation. The child Puritan manual resuscitator (PMR)2 bag has a volume of 870 ml and a relief valve that opens at 45 cm H_2O. The infant Laerdal resuscitator bag has a 240-ml volume, while the child bag has a 500-ml volume. Both Laerdal bags have a pressure limit of 35 cm H_2O. The infant bag is usually used for infants younger than $1\frac{1}{2}$–2 years of age. The child bag is appropriate for children older than $1\frac{1}{2}$ years of age. Valves are available to adapt the resuscitator bags to provide positive end-expiratory pressure if required for effective oxygenation.

The oxygen concentration delivered is affected by the source of oxygen flow, flow rate, and time allowed for the bag to refill. The PMR 2 is capable of delivering 100% oxygen if the special powered supply value is used or high flow rates of oxygen, with an oxygen accumulator to act as an oxygen reservoir, are present. The Laerdal bags can deliver 100% oxygen if a reservoir assembly is utilized.

ENDOTRACHEAL INTUBATION

Equipment

Equipment that should be available for endotracheal intubation and suggested endotracheal tube sizes are listed in Tables 2.1 and 2.2.

Suction must be available, is possible, and is utilized to clear secretions, vomitus, blood, or debris for better visualization during laryngoscopy. Oxygen is given before laryngoscopy and intubation, to provide a reservoir of oxygen for the apneic period, especially for infants because their resting oxygen consumption is high.

The infant's head is placed in a neutral position. For the older child, if the head is extended at the atlanto-occipital joint and the occiput is elevated to the "sniffing" position, the oropharyngolaryngeal axes are aligned. After evaluation of the mobility of the mouth, temporomandibular joint, and neck, as well as the stability of the teeth, the head is positioned. The mouth is opened by pressure on the mandible. The laryngoscope is held in the left hand, inserted into the right side of the mouth, and moved to the midline while the tongue is pulled to the left. The blade is then advanced

TABLE 2.1.
Equipment for Endotracheal Intubation

Suction—Source, catheters
Oxygen—Source, bag
Mask—For ventilation
Laryngoscope—Blade, handle, bulb, battery
Endotracheal tubes—Appropriate sizes
Forceps
Oropharyngeal airway
Tongue blade
Bite block
Tape—To secure tube
Stylet

slowly over the tongue. Laryngoscope blades are available in multiple lengths according to the size of the child.

With a straight blade laryngoscope, the tip is moved under the laryngeal side of the epiglottis, and with upward pulling along the axis of the handle, the epiglottis and the base of the tongue are raised to expose the glottis. If the larynx is not easily visualized, external pressure on the larynx may help bring the glottis into sight. If the blade has been advanced too deeply, the larynx may be raised and the esophagus may be exposed. With withdrawal of the blade, the glottis should come into view. With a curved blade, the laryngoscope blade is advanced to place the tip between the base of the tongue and valleculae and to rest behind the epiglottis. With an upward pull along the axis of the laryngoscope handle, the glottis should be visualized. The curved blade keeps the tongue out of the line of vision. Diffi-

TABLE 2.2.
Suggested Endotracheal Tube Size

Age	Internal Diameter (mm)
Premature infant	2.5–3.0
Newborn	3.0
Newborn–6 months	3.5
6–12 months	3.5–4.0
12 months–2 yr	4.0–4.5
3–4 yr	4.5–5.0
5–6 yr	5.0–5.5
7–8 yr	5.5–6.0
9–10 yr	6.0–6.5
11–12 yr	6.5–7.0
13–14 yr	7.0–7.5

culties with visualization occur if the laryngoscope is rotated onto the maxillary teeth, because the larynx is pushed farther anteriorly.

Endotracheal tubes used in infants and young children usually are uncuffed because the airway lumen is small, with the cricoid ring as the narrowest portion. For children over 8 years of age, cuffed tubes may be used. The cuffs currently recommended have a high residual volume and inflate symmetrically to seal air leaks at a low pressure. As pressure equilibrates across the cuff wall, the intracuff pressure approximates that of the lateral tracheal wall. Problems arise because prestretched cuffs may not inflate symmetrically. Temperature changes may also change cuff pressure. Also, the cuff may herniate over the end of the tube, causing partial obstruction. Cuff filling is confirmed by distention of the pilot balloon. The cuff should be inflated to the minimal pressure required to seal an air leak and allow effective ventilation. Cuff pressure should be monitored; it is recommended to keep the pressure at <20 mm Hg.

Use of a stylet has the potential for trauma, from the stylet itself or from stiffening of the tube. However, it should be available to change the position of the tip of the tube for difficult intubation in patients with anatomic abnormalities.

Drugs for Facilitation of Intubation

Neuromuscular Blocking Agents (Table 2.3)

Muscle relaxants are either depolarizing (succinylcholine) or nondepolarizing (curare, pancuronium, etc.). Most individuals should restrict themselves to succinylcholine unless they are knowledgeable about the other drugs. In all patients, serum potassium increases 30 seconds after administration of succinylcholine, with a peak by 5 minutes and a gradual decrease by 15 minutes. Marked hyperkalemia has been noted after the use of succinylcholine in patients with burns, spinal cord section, cerebrovascular accident, multiple sclerosis, encephalitis with motor involvement, muscle trauma, and denervated muscle. Pretreatment with a small, partial dose of nondepolarizing blocking agents may prevent the hyperkalemic response.

Nondepolarizing agents include pancuronium, d-tubocurarine, metocurine, atracurium, and vecuronium. Although these drugs can be very useful in specific intubation sequences, they should be restricted to individuals knowledgeable about them.

Sedatives (Table 2.4)

Useful agents to aid initial placement of an artificial airway in patients who are not comatose or stuporous from the underlying disease include short-acting barbiturates, such as thiopental and methohexital; the phencyclidine derivative, ketamine; or other short-acting hypnotic agents. Potentially, the use of sedation in hemodynamically unstable patients is dangerous and, in patients who have eaten in the past 6–8 hours, requires knowledge of the "rapid sequence" technique described below.

TABLE 2.3.
Neuromuscular Blocking Agents
to Facilitate Intubation

Depolarizing
Succinylcholine
Infants	2 mg/kg i.v.
Children	1 mg/kg i.v.

Nondepolarizing
Pancuronium
Neonate	
0–1 week	30 μg/kg i.v.
1–2 weeks	60 μg/kg i.v.
2–4 weeks	90 μg/kg i.v.
Children	0.1–0.15 mg/kg i.v.
Defasciculating dose	0.01 mg/kg i.v.

d-Tubocurarine
Neonate	0.2–0.4 mg/kg i.v.
Children	0.6 mg/kg i.v.
Defasciculating dose	0.03 mg/kg i.v.
Metocurine	0.5 mg/kg i.v.
Atracurium	400 μg/kg i.v.
Vecuronium	70 μg/kg i.v.

Sequence

An outline of a suggested sequence for intubation is shown in Table 2.5. Adequate oxygen reserves may be provided by preoxygenation with 100% oxygen for 4–5 minutes before paralysis, laryngoscopy, and intubation or by hyperventilation with 100% oxygen for 1 minute after sedation/paralysis and before laryngoscopy and intubation.

In an awake patient, sedation with a rapidly acting agent such as thiopental, methohexital, diazepam, or ketamine is often suitable to provide loss of consciousness and amnesia. If initial attempts at placement of the endotracheal tube are unsuccessful, the child should be ventilated with a bag and mask prior to further attempts.

Muscle relaxants should be avoided if there is a compromised upper air-

TABLE 2.4.
Sedatives to Facilitate
Endotracheal Intubation

Thiopental	2–4 mg/kg i.v.
Methohexital	1.5–2 mg/kg i.v.
Ketamine	0.5–2 mg/kg i.v.
Diazepam	0.1–0.2 mg/kg i.v.

TABLE 2.5. ————————————————————————————
Sequence for Intubation

Equipment available, including suction
Preoxygenate with 100% oxygen
Intravenous sedation
Mask ventilate with 100% oxygen
Intravenous muscle relaxant
Laryngoscopy and intubation with full relaxation

way from diseases such as acute supraglottitis or in situations in which upper airway anatomy is unclear. In an awake, struggling, or anxious child with possible difficult laryngoscopy due to a compromised upper airway, paralysis is contraindicated. General inhalation anesthesia should be utilized for evaluation of the upper airway and intubation.

Nasotracheal Intubation

Nasotracheal intubation provides protection to the tube from biting, allows easy fixation to the nose and upper lip, is associated with less movement from the tongue pushing than occurs with an orotracheal tube, has less curvature along the posterior oropharynx than occurs with an orotracheal tube and therefore produces less pressure on the posterior larynx, and allows for easier suctioning of the mouth. Problems associated with a nasotracheal tube include epistaxis, trauma to adenoids, pressure necrosis of the nares, trauma to the mucosa and posterior dissection of the posterior pharyngeal wall at the area of the sphenoid prominence, obstruction of the Eustachian tube, and possible otitis or maxillary sinusitis if long-term intubation is used. Contraindications to nasal intubation include: a fracture of the cribriform plate with cerebrospinal fluid leak, because of the risk of infection and meningitis or intracranial passage of the tube; bleeding disorders or the use of anticoagulants, because of the risk of active hemorrhage necessitating nasal packing; or deformity of the nose, obstructing passage of the tube.

Rapid Sequence Intubation

In a patient with a "full stomach," abolition of pharyngolaryngeal reflexes by general anesthesia or by muscle relaxants given with sedation may allow for regurgitation and aspiration. Patients with a full stomach include those with: recent oral intake; decreased gastric emptying from bowel obstruction; swallowed blood from orofacial trauma; abnormal esophageal peristalsis due to scleroderma; and delayed gastric emptying, as is often seen with ascites, pain, peritonitis, shock, or increased intraabdominal pressure from large masses. Intubation may be accomplished in these patients under "awake" conditions to preserve pharyngolaryngeal reflexes or by "crash induction" of a rapid sequence infusion of medica-

TABLE 2.6.
Rapid Sequence Intubation

Equipment available, including suction with large-bore catheter
Nasogastric tube to suction
Preoxygenate with 100% oxygen
Cricoid pressure
Rapid intravenous infusion of sedative and muscle relaxant
Laryngoscopy and intubation with full relaxation

tions and by utilization of cricoid pressure. Cricoid pressure has been shown to effectively occlude the esophagus in infant cadavers, even with the presence of a nasogastric tube in the esophageal lumen. It has been suggested that the presence of the nasogastric tube can serve as an outlet for stomach contents, while the cricoid pressure can effectively prevent regurgitation to the pharynx during elevated intraesophageal pressure. Positive pressure ventilation is not applied to avoid gastric insufflation and distention. For the "crash induction" (see Table 2.6.), the patient is preoxygenated with 100% oxygen, and the head is placed in the optimal "sniffing" position. Suction must be available. Some intensivists believe that a nasogastric tube should be passed and suctioned. The sedative and muscle relaxant drugs (see Table 2.7) are given by rapid sequence intravenous infusion as external pressure is applied to the cricoid cartilage to compress the esophagus.

EMERGENCY ESTABLISHMENT OF ARTIFICIAL AIRWAY—CRICOTHYROTOMY

When intubation is not possible or is contraindicated, surgical establishment of an airway is indicated. Cricothyrotomy is faster and requires fewer instruments and less skill than does an emergency tracheostomy. This procedure is indicated if intubation is not possible due to: lack of equipment; anatomic problems, such as oropharyngeal edema due to burns, infection, or allergy; foreign body causing obstruction; trauma to the face

TABLE 2.7.
Suggested Drugs for Rapid Sequence Intubation in Children

Thiopental	2–4 mg/kg i.v.
or ketamine	0.5–2 mg/kg i.v.
Pancuronium	0.01 mg/kg i.v.
+ succinylcholine	1–2 mg/kg i.v.
or *d*-tubocurarine	0.03 mg/kg i.v.
+ succinylcholine	1–2 mg/kg i.v.
or pancuronium	0.1–0.15 mg/kg i.v.
or *d*-tubocurarine	0.6 mg/kg i.v.

or larynx, causing distortion or obstruction; cervical spine injury impeding positioning and head tilt; or inexperience. The cricothyroid membrane is located between the inferior edge of the thyroid cartilage and the upper edge of the cricoid cartilage. If there is no injury to the cervical spine, the head may be tilted back, and the larynx may be stabilized with the finger while the cricothyroid membrane is palpated. The membrane can be punctured in the anterior midline of the neck. An angiocath, as is frequently used for intravenous infusions, is suitable for this technique. The needle should be inserted at a caudad angle to avoid injury to the vocal cords, which are located cephalad. It will be necessary to penetrate skin, subcutaneous tissue, cervical fascia, and then the cricothyroid membrane. Confirmation of the location of the tip of the needle in the trachea is obtained by aspirating air. If an angiocath is used, a 3.0 endotracheal adapter (15 mm) can be used to connect to an oxygen source.

CHAPTER 3

Upper Airway Disease

NOSE—NASAL OBSTRUCTION

Although not generally appreciated, the nose and mouth account for 50% of respiratory resistance. Causes of nasal obstruction are of significant importance (Table 3.1). Choanal atresia has been reported to occur in 1 of 8000 live births, and approximately 90% of these (those with choanal atresia) have bony obstruction and 10% have membranous obstruction. Girls seem to be affected more than boys. Infants with bilateral occlusion present with severe respiratory distress at birth because the newborn is an obligate nose-breather. Clinically, a cyclical cyanosis will be noted with respiratory distress, and the cyanosis will be relieved by crying. Cyanosis recurs when the mouth is closed. This causes a true medical emergency, and immediate treatment of the infant with bilateral posterior choanal atresia is placement of an oral airway to provide an opening for airflow.

Diagnosis is confirmed by attempting to pass 5- or 6-French catheter

TABLE 3.1.
Causes of Nasal Obstruction

Posterior choanal atresia
Posterior choanal stenosis
Congenital nasal atresia
Midface hypoplasia—Apert's syndrome, Crouzon's syndrome
Dermoid cyst
Nasal encephalocele
Nasal glioma
Nasal tumor—Teratoma, hemangioma, lipoma, lymphoma, neurofibroma,
    nasopharyngeal angiofibroma, rhabdomyosarcoma, chordoma, chondroma
Foreign body
Trauma
Scar tissue
Inflammation
Adenoid hypertrophy
Nasogastric tube with tape occluding other nostril

through the nose, by taking an X-ray with contrast or a computed tomography (CT) scan of the nasal cavity, and by placing gentian violet or methylene blue dye into the nares and observing for dye in the oropharynx. The final therapy is surgical, and restenosis is not common.

Posterior choanal stenosis or hypoplastic nasopharynx may present as symptoms similar to choanal atresia. These infants may have adequate airflow until feeding and have symptoms of obstruction during feeding. They may have chronic mucus discharge. Diagnosis is confirmed by contrast, X-ray studies or CT scan of the nasal cavity. Therapy is symptomatic, as the nasal cavity increases with growth.

Nasal encephalocele occurs in approximately 1 of 4000 live births and usually communicates with the subarachnoid space. Nasal obstruction is seen when the mass is located at the base of the skull. It may be seen as a nasofrontal or nasoethmoid swelling and may be located intranasally and/or over the bridge of the nose. This swelling is often soft and compressible and may be pulsatile. The mass may be located and confirmed by CT scan. Biopsy is contraindicated because of the risk of cerebrospinal fluid rhinorrhea or meningitis. Treatment is full surgical excision.

Nasal tumors are uncommon in children. Papular hemangioma masses usually undergo spontaneous resolution. A cavernous hemangioma may increase in size rapidly and cause nasal obstruction and/or epistaxis. Treatment is surgical excision. Juvenile nasopharyngeal angiofibroma may extend to the nasal cavity and cause nasal obstruction, epistaxis, or rhinorrhea. Symptoms are more common at puberty, when these lesions have been noted to increase in size. Treatment is radiation therapy or surgery. Lymphoma may also cause nasal obstruction and is usually responsive to radiation therapy or chemotherapy. Rhabdomyosarcoma may also be located in the nasopharynx or nasal cavity and therefore cause obstruction. Therapy usually involves surgery, chemotherapy, and radiation treatment. Other uncommon tumors that may be located in the nose or nasopharynx include craniopharyngioma, chordoma, lipoma, chondroma, and neurofibroma. All cause problems by mechanical obstruction to nasal overflow. Nasal polyps may also cause nasal obstruction. These are usually seen in patients with a history of allergy or cystic fibrosis. Relief of obstruction is obtained by surgical removal.

Respiratory distress and nasal obstruction secondary to trauma are usually due to dislocation of the nasal bones and septum. It is common in patients with maxillary fractures who have "black eyes" and is associated with rhinorrhea. Nasotracheal intubation and nasogastric (NG) tubes are to be avoided in these patients.

LARYNX AND TRACHEA

Structure

In the infant, the larynx is located opposite C3–C4. The infant larynx is funnel shaped and soft, and the elastic cartilage is easily collapsed or compressed by airway pressures. The narrowest portion of the infant airway is the area of the cricoid ring, where the cartilage diameter is approximately 5.5 mm, with a lumen of 4.5 mm.

With growth, the larynx descends caudally, and the hyoid and thyroid cartilages separate. By 12 years of age, it has assumed the adult location C6.

Function

If Poiseuille's law is utilized, it can be seen that the radius of the airway is an important determinant of pressure and, therefore, resistance. Poiseuille's law assuming laminar flow is expressed as

$$R = \frac{8 \times l \times n}{r^4}$$

where l is the length of the conducting tube; n is the viscosity of the gas; r is the radius of the conducting tube; and R is the resistance to airflow. A marked increase in resistance to airflow can occur in the infant as a result of any decrease in the radius of the airway. If the diameter of the airway is 4 mm, the cross-sectional area will be decreased by 75% when there is a 1-mm uniform decrease in size, as may occur with uniform edema. This causes a 16-fold increase in resistance, as noted from Poiseuille's law. An 8-mm airway with 1-mm uniform edema will have a 43% decrease in the cross-sectional area. Edema of obstructing lesions may not be uniform but will, nevertheless, add to resistance to airflow.

Airway Obstruction
Location and Symptoms

In the presence of an extrathoracic airway lesion, airway narrowing and turbulent flow result from the pressure gradient of extraluminal pressure being greater than the intraluminal pressure generated during inspiration. Airway dilatation, and therefore less effect on maximal flow, occurs during expiration because the intraluminal pressure generated is relatively greater than the extraluminal pressure. On the other hand, extraluminal pressure (intrapleural pressure) is relatively less than intraluminal pressure during inspiratory efforts in the presence of an intrathoracic lesion. This pressure gradient produces dilation of the airway. The reverse is noted on expiration, because the extraluminal pressure becomes positive and greater than the intraluminal pressure, thereby resulting in airway narrowing.

With partial airway obstruction, airflow is noisy. Stridor is "noisy" breathing caused by rapid, turbulent flow through an obstructed or narrowed portion of the airway. Clinical observation of the phase of stridor can aid in location of the obstruction. Inspiratory stridor is common with lesions at the supraglottic or glottic area, because the negative pressure generated during inspiration favors inward collapse of the structures. Expiratory stridor is more often noted with lesions below the level of the true vocal cords.

The degree of airway obstruction determines symptoms other than stridor. Moderate airway obstruction usually causes retractions, which will not be seen with central nervous system or cardiac anomalies. Other signs of airway obstruction are nonspecific, with tachypnea, tachycardia, hypertension, restlessness, and confusion occurring due to hypoventilation. Cyanosis is a late sign of airway obstruction.

Evaluation of Child with Stridor

Children with stridor may have symptoms so severe that they require an emergency airway prior to any diagnostic tests other than a brief history or physical examination. Some children may not even have time for this. On the other hand, in some children it is possible and necessary to evaluate the cause of their airway obstruction in order to know how properly to treat them. A list of these tests is shown in Table 3.2.

Causes of Airway Obstruction

A full list of the causes of upper airway obstruction is shown in Table 3.3. Some of the more important lesions are described below.

Laryngomalacia

The most common congenital laryngeal anomaly is laryngomalacia. No gross anatomic abnormality has been described. However, the laryngeal cartilage is flaccid, and the aryepiglottic folds are reported to fall into the glottis on inspiration. Stridor is usually inspiratory and high pitched, may be intermittent, may decrease when the patient is placed prone with the neck extended, may increase with agitation, and is present from birth or the first few weeks of life. The infant's cry is usually normal. Feeding problems associated with increased respiratory distress and stridor may be present. Accurate diagnosis is important because laryngomalacia resolves spontaneously by 1½–2 years of age. Evaluation may include fluoroscopy

---

TABLE 3.2.
Useful Diagnostic Studies (Time Permitting) in Children with Upper Airway Disease

Chest X-ray—Anteroposterior and lateral, inspiratory and expiratory
Cinefluoroscopy
Barium swallow
Bronchoscopy
Xeroradiography
Magnetic resonance imaging
Flow volume loops
Angiography for vascular abnormalities

TABLE 3.3. _____
Causes of Upper Airway Obstruction

Congenital Lesions
Intrinsic lesions—Subglottic stenosis, web, cyst, laryngocele, tumor, laryngo-
    malacia, laryngotracheoesophageal cleft, tracheomalacia, tracheoesophageal
    fistula
Extrinsic lesions—Vascular ring, cystic hygroma
Birth trauma
Neurologic lesion
Craniofacial anomalies
Metabolic disorders—Hypocalcemia

Acquired Lesions
Infections—Retropharyngeal abscess, Ludwig's angina, laryngotracheobron-
    chitis (croup), supraglottitis, epiglottitis, fungal infections, peritonsillar ab-
    scess, diphtheria, bacterial tracheitis
Trauma—Internal (postextubation croup, posttracheostomy removal), external
Burns—Thermal, chemical
Foreign body aspiration
Systemic disorders
Neoplasms—Internal, external
Neurologic lesions
Chronic upper airway obstruction
Hypertrophic tonsils, adenoids
Tight surgical neck dressing

_____

and cineradiography to view the laryngeal airway and, with inspiration,
possible collapse. Laryngoscopy confirms the clinical diagnosis. Treatment
is supportive, because symptoms usually clear by 2 years of age. A tracheostomy may be required if respiratory distress is prominent enough to interfere with feeding and growth.

Laryngeal Webs

Laryngeal webs account for 2–4% of laryngeal anomalies and may be
located at different levels. Laryngeal webs are probably related to failure of
absorption of epithelial plugs during recanalization of the laryngotracheal
groove at the tenth week of embryonic development. Symptoms are frequently noted at birth, with inspiratory stridor. Diagnosis is confirmed at
laryngoscopy. The treatment involves lysis if the web is composed of a thin
membrane. Tracheostomy and laryngofissure may be required for treatment of a thick web.

Laryngeal Cysts

Laryngeal cysts may also cause stridor and respiratory distress. Laryngeal cysts do not connect with the pharynx or interior of the larynx. These
lesions are soft, mucus filled, compressible, and often pedunculated. Glot-

tic cysts usually extend from the true or false vocal cords and present as stridor and varying degrees of respiratory distress. Diagnosis is confirmed at endoscopy.

Congenital Subglottic Stenosis

The most common symptom in a patient with congenital subglottic stenosis is stridor, which is usually noticed several weeks after birth or only after an upper respiratory infection (URI) causes further luminal narrowing due to edema. A lateral neck X-ray may suggest the diagnosis by funnel-shaped subglottic narrowing with little change in size with respiration. Most children who require tracheostomy as infants are decannulated successfully by 3–4 years of age.

Tracheomalacia

Tracheomalacia involves malformed tracheal cartilage rings with lack of rigidity and an oval shape to the lumen. Wheezing or stridor are usually noticed on expiration, with the tendency of the tracheal lumen to collapse due to decreased luminal pressure. Tracheomalacia is commonly seen in children with tracheoesophageal fistula or external tracheal compression, as with vascular ring. The diagnosis is confirmed by fluoroscopy and bronchoscopy, which show tracheal collapse on expiration. Cartilaginous development eventually improves airway support.

Tracheoesophageal Fistula

Patients with tracheoesophageal fistula usually exhibit episodes of feeding difficulty and cyanosis. Several types of fistula have been described (Fig. 3.1).

The diagnosis is suggested by a chest X-ray with NG tube in place. The diagnosis is confirmed by barium swallow and endoscopy to exhibit the communication between the trachea and the esophagus. Treatment is gas-

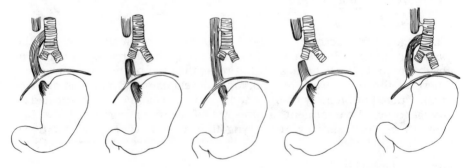

FIGURE 3.1. Schematic representations of tracheoesophageal fistula and atresia. From *left* to *right:* The most common type with a blind upper esophageal pouch and fistulous connection of trachea to distal esophagus, esophageal atresia without fistula, H-type fistula without atresia, fistula from trachea to proximal esophageal pouch, and fistulous connections to both proximal pouch and distal esophagus.

trostomy, to decompress the stomach to lessen the chance of gastroesophageal reflux, and then surgical repair of the fistula itself.

Vascular Ring

The airway may be narrowed by external pressure from congenital malformations of the intrathhoracic great vessels (Fig. 3.2). Infants with airway compression due to vascular anomalies usually present with stridor at
birth or within the first few weeks of life. Other symptoms include wheezing, dry cough, cyanosis, recurrent bronchopulmonary infections, and
dysphagia. Respiratory symptoms may be intermittent and may vary with
position changes. The physical examination may be unremarkable except
for the variable signs of airway obstruction.

Diagnosis can be confirmed by contrast esophagogram and endoscopy,
which reveal indentations secondary to extrinsic compressure (Fig. 3.3).
The anatomy of the vascular malformation is determined by angiography.

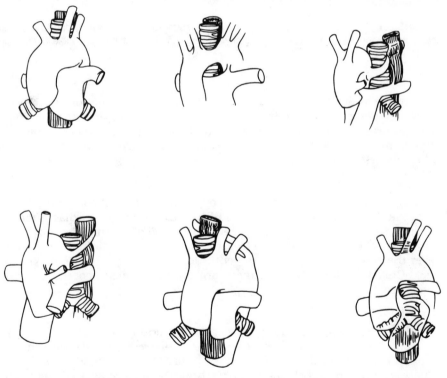

FIGURE 3.2. Schematic representations of various anomalies of the great vessels. *Top:* Normal vascular arrangement, double aortic arch, and right-sided aortic arch with left ductus arter-
iosum. *Bottom:* Right-sided aortic arch with aberrant left subclavian artery, left-sided arch with
aberrant right subclavian artery, and anomalous origin of left pulmonary artery from right pulmonary artery.

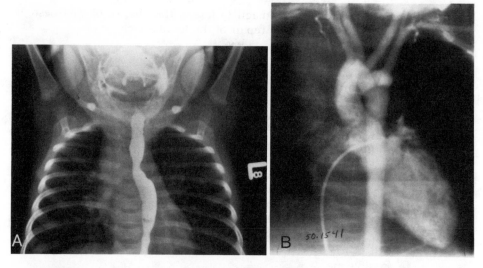

FIGURE 3.3. *A:* The diagnosis of vascular ring is suggested by narrowing, due to extrinsic compression, on the contrast esophagogram. *B:* Angiography confirmed a double aortic arch anomaly.

Treatment is surgical correction of the vascular malformation. Postoperatively, symptoms improve in most patients with vascular rings; however, respiratory problems may persist due to distortion of the tracheobronchial tree from prolonged compression, even after surgical removal of the anomalous vessel.

Neurologic Abnormalities

Congenital vocal cord paralysis accounts for 6–10% of congenital laryngeal anomalies. It may be related to birth trauma or to cardiac anomaly affecting the left recurrent laryngeal nerve or be of unknown etiology. Bilateral vocal cord paralysis may be seen with stretching of the vagus nerves over the edge of the jugular foramen in infants with hydrocephalus or Arnold-Chiari malformation, intracerebral bleeding, meningocele, or encephalocele.

Craniofacial Anomalies

Infants with a wide variety of congenital craniofacial anomalies may present with varying degrees of respiratory distress. Infants with macroglossia may have oral obstruction due to the enlarged tongue mass. Micrognathia may cause obstruction by pushing the tongue against the posterior pharyngeal wall, resulting in a ball-valve obstruction.

The incidence of cleft lip and palate is approximately 1.5 of 1000 live births, with 50% of these having combined cleft lip and palate. Cleft lip and/or cleft palate is often associated with other facial developmental defects. Problems may occur if the infant's tongue becomes impacted in the cleft palate.

Retropharyngeal Abscess

The retropharyngeal space is a midline area formed by cervical fascia, extending from the base of the skull to the level of T2. Bounded by the posterior pharyngeal wall and the prevertebral deep cervical fascia, this area contains nodes draining the nasopharynx, sinuses, and Eustachian tubes. Suppuration of the lymphoid tissue may cause pus accumulation in the retropharyngeal space. Retropharyngeal abscess is usually seen in infants or children under 3 years of age. Presenting symptoms and signs include a history of a preceding URI or sore throat, fever, toxic appearance, meningismus, stridor, dysphagia, and difficulty handling secretions. The child often positions himself or herself with the neck extended.

Evaluation may be difficult, but the diagnosis is usually suggested by a widening in the soft tissues between the air column and cervical vertebrae on a lateral neck X-ray (Fig. 3.4). The chest X-rays should also be obtained to evaluate possible mediastinal extension. Treatment involves surgical incision and drainage and antibiotic coverage. The usual organisms involved are staphylococci, group A β-hemolytic streptococci, and anaerobes.

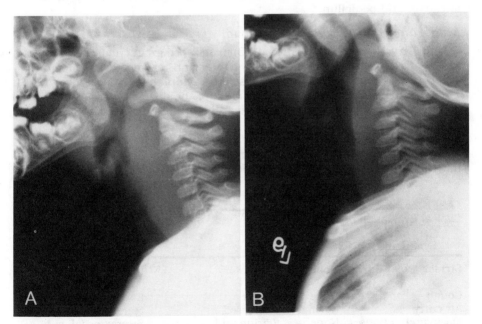

FIGURE 3.4. *A:* Lateral neck X-ray of toddler with fever and drooling shows a widened soft tissue area between the air column and cervical vertebrae. *B:* Follow-up film after surgical drainage of retropharyngeal abscess.

Ludwig's Angina

Ludwig's angina involves rapidly spreading inflammation of the sublingular, submandibular, and submaxillary spaces with inflammation of fascia, muscle, and connective tissue. Symptoms are caused by an edematous tongue and induration of the suprahyoid area, causing the tongue to be pushed upward and posteriorly, promoting airway obstruction. Infection is associated with cellulitis and is not purulent in drainage.

Peritonsillar Abscess

Peritonsillar abscess may cause airway obstruction, due to the size of the lesion. It is usually noted between the base of the tonsil and lateral pharyngeal wall. It is uncommon in young children. The usual symptoms include trismus, pain with talking, muffled voice, drooling, and dysphagia.

Diphtheria

Uncommon in recent times, although increasing in occurrence due to problems with assuring vaccination, diphtheritic pharyngitis is associated with a thick pharyngeal membrane that, when removed, may leave a bleeding area. Muscle involvement may be associated with problems with palatal movement and competence. The child usually complains of a sore throat and has a low-grade fever and cervical adenopathy. The patient should be isolated until the cultures are evaluated. Treatment involves diphtheritic antitoxin and penicillin.

Acute Laryngotracheobronchitis (Croup)

Acute laryngotracheobronchitis (LTB) usually occurs in children 6 months to 3 years of age. It is often noted in winter and may occur in epidemics. The course is slow with a gradual onset and symptoms of a preceding URI. The "croup score" is a clinical assessment of the degree of respiratory distress. It involves evaluation of airflow and work of breathing, as noted in Table 3.4.

The diagnosis of acute LTB is confirmed by a funnel-shaped narrowing of the glottic and subglottic airway on an inspiratory X-ray. It is best evaluated on frontal view of the airway (Fig. 3.5).

TABLE 3.4.
Clinical Evaluation of Croup

Symptom	0	1	2
Stridor	None	Inspiratory	Inspiratory and expiratory
Cough	None	Hoarse	Bark
Air entry	Normal	Decreased	Markedly decreased
Flaring/retractions	None	Flaring and suprasternal	Suprasternal, subcostal, intercostal
Color	Normal	Cyanosis in room air	Cyanosis in 40% O_2

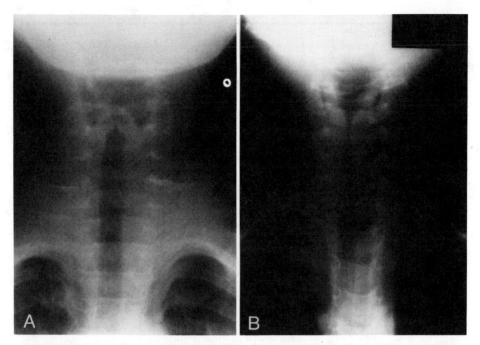

FIGURE 3.5. Narrowing of the subglottic airway, as occurs with acute LTB, may be noted on an anteroposterior film of the airway *A:* High-kilovolt film of the neck in a 5-year-old child with a normal airway. *B:* Subglottic swelling in a 5-year-old child with clinical diagnosis of croup.

The etiology of acute LTB is usually viral, most commonly respiratory syncytial virus, parainfluenza A, and adenovirus. Occasionally, a bacterial source may be identified, most commonly *Haemophilus influenzae* or *Strepococcus* species. Membranous croup resulting from *Staphylococcus aureus* infection involves formation of an inflammatory exudate attached to the tracheal wall. Spasmodic or allergic croup is different from acute LTB. It is usually self-limited, occurring at night with sudden onset and mild upper respiratory signs and recurring episodes. The child is usually afebrile, and the symptoms clear rapidly.

The aims of therapy (see Table 3.5) are to relieve the airway obstruction and to decrease the work of breathing. Humidification and good hydration are utilized to liquefy secretions. Oxygen is given by hood or face mask, because of the hypoxemia reported with croup and the correlation of respiratory rate with arterial oxygenation. Antibiotics have no proven benefit in the treatment of patients with viral LTB. Observation of the degree of respiratory distress is the mainstay of therapy. For moderate respiratory distress (croup score, ≥7), the child should be observed in the intensive care unit (ICU), and racemic epinephrine may be of benefit. The action of racemic epinephrine is unknown but may involve topical vasoconstriction

TABLE 3.5. ——————————————————————————————
Treatment of Croup

Treatment	Comment
Oxygen	Humidified by hood or face mask
Racemic epinephrine	2.25% (1:8 dilution)—see text
Steroids	Not clearly indicated—see text
Intubation	Nasotracheal intubation vs. tracheostomy— see text
Helium	May be useful in acute emergency—see text

and temporary decrease in swelling. It has also been suggested that nebulized moisture rather than epinephrine gives clinical improvement. Although improvement in symptoms occurs with racemic epinephrine, no effect has been noted on the P_aO_2 or natural history of LTB, as the incidence of ultimate establishment of an artificial airway is unchanged. The authors presently use racemic epinephrine 2.25% diluted 1:6 or 1:8 in water or saline, respectively, nebulized or delivered by intermittent positive pressure breathing for children with moderate respiratory distress. This treatment is repeated as needed, with a minimum internal of 30 minutes.

Controversy exists over the use of steroids in patients with acute LTB. A review of early studies on the topic outlined faults in designs, while another review noted that there may be some dose-related benefits due to steroids. Indications for the establishment of an artificial airway include cyanosis, fatigue, and more frequent need for racemic epinephrine at shorter intervals. The use of racemic epinephrine at less than half-hour intervals is tiring and indicates significant respiratory distress. The airway may be supported by endotracheal intubation or tracheostomy. Nasotracheal intubation has been recommended as safer than tracheostomy with lower mortality and few complications. The delayed complications were noted in approximately 3% of patients and did not significantly affect respiratory function.

Most patients require only several days' intubation. Once intubation is accomplished, special care should be maintained to secure the airway properly as well as to prevent inadvertent extubation by restraining the child. Once the child is intubated, sedation is also useful. Nursing observation should be continuous, since the child is still dependent on an artificial airway.

Helium therapy may be used to gain time to carry a patient through a period of acute respiratory distress while awaiting personnel and the operating room setup to establish the airway. Helium is an inert gas with low density. Therefore, use of helium-oxygen gas mixture would decrease the work of breathing and lessen fatigue. A mask or headbox is needed to deliver high concentrations, because helium concentrations of >60% are needed to improve the gas flow rate. Clinical improvement in patients with croup has been noted with 70–80% helium-in-oxygen mixtures.

Acute Supraglottitis (Epiglottitis)

Acute supraglottitis usually occurs in children 2–6 years of age but may occur at any age, including adulthood. The child will normally be extubated when breathing spontaneously with a leak around the endotracheal tube. The child should have nothing by mouth (liquids or NG feeds) for 6 or more hours, and all facilities for emergency intubation as well as appropriate personnel should be available.

The pathology involves a thickened epiglottis and aryepiglottic folds. The course is rapidly progressive, and total obstruction of the laryngeal opening may result. A protocol should be established for evaluation and establishment of an airway as soon as the diagnosis is suspected. At the author's institution, the protocol indicates immediate notification of senior personnel from the departments of ear, nose, and throat (ENT), anesthesiology, and pediatrics, as well as from the pediatric ICU. The epiglottitis team accompanies the patient to the operating room when the diagnosis is strongly suspected. The child is disturbed as little as possible to avoid agitation. In the operating room, an airway is established. If the patient is moribund, awake intubation should be performed rapidly. If the patient is stable, general inhalation anesthesia with assisted respiration will allow time for intravenous insertion and direct laryngoscopy to confirm the diagnosis and establish an artificial airway.

At the authors' institution, direct laryngoscopy is performed under general inhalation anesthesia to confirm the diagnosis. The patient is maintained in a comfortable position in a quiet atmosphere with little stimulation, to avoid agitation. A senior ENT surgeon is present at an opened tracheostomy and rigid bronchoscopy setup. General inhalation anesthesia is provided with halothane and 100% oxygen to improve the oxygen reserves of the patient's functional residual capacity. Spontaneous ventilation is maintained with gentle assisted respiration as needed. Sedatives and muscle relaxants are avoided. Laryngoscopy is performed under deep inhalation anesthesia. An orotracheal intubation is accomplished with a tube smaller than that recommended for the patient's age, to decrease the pressure on the swollen tissues and allow breathing around the tube. If the attempted intubation is unsuccessful, rigid bronchoscopy is attempted. If this is unsuccessful, the ENT surgeon establishes the airway by emergency cricothyrotomy, followed by controlled tracheostomy. If orotracheal intubation is achieved, nasotracheal intubation then proceeds, with the nasal tube passed alongside the oral tube under direct visualization of the larynx.

The usual etiology is *H. influenzae* type B. Other organisms have included β-hemolytic strepococci, *S. aureus*, *Diplococcus pneumoniae*, and *Neisseria catarrhalis*. Intravenous antibiotic coverage is started after obtaining the cultures. Ampicillin and chloramphenicol are initiated until sensitivities are available.

The patient is transferred to the pediatric ICU where sedation and arm restraints to prevent reaching the artificial airway are continued to decrease movement of the tube in the larynx. Nursing observation is continuous, since the patient is dependent on an artificial airway. Respiratory and electrocardiographic monitoring are standard as well. Humidified oxygen is continued. Tracheobronchial suctioning is important to avoid blockage of the tube by secretions. Blood pressure and cardiac monitoring should continue after return to the ICU.

Manifestations of acute infection usually resolve within 24–72 hours. Criteria for extubation vary among institutions and include resolution of fever, breathing around the artificial airway, and direct examination of the epiglottis. Extubation is accomplished when the child has awakened from the sedation and has had nothing by mouth for 6 or more hours. The child is then maintained without oral fluids for 4–6 hours, until it is evident that reintubation will not be required. The child is then observed for at least 24 hours in the pediatric ICU.

Table 3.6 provides a summary of the clinical characteristics differentiating LTB from supraglottitis. Frequently, the clinical presentation dictates further work-up and management.

Acquired Subglottic Stenosis

The incidence of prior intubation in patients with acquired subglottic stenosis has been reported to be as high as 86%. Other possible etiologies are external neck trauma, burns, high tracheostomy sites, and tumors. The pathology has been described as a circumferential narrowing due to web, band, or stenosis. The etiologies suggested for the development of

TABLE 3.6. ─────────────────────────────────
Clinical Characteristics Differentiating LTB from Supraglottitis

Characteristic	LTB	Supraglottitis
Age	6 months–3 yr	2–6 yr
Onset	Gradual	Rapid
Etiology	Viral	Bacterial
Swelling site	Subglottic	Supraglottic
Symptoms		
Cough-voice	Hoarse cough	No cough
		Muffled voice
Posture	Any position	Sitting
Mouth	Closed; nasal flaring	Open chin forward
		Drooling
Fever	Absent to high	High
Appearance	Often not acutely ill	Anxious, acutely ill
X-ray	Narrow subglottic area	Swollen epiglottis
		and supraglottic
		structures
Palpation larynx	Nontender	Tender
Recurrence	May recur	Rarely recurs
Seasonal incidence	Winter	None

subglottic stenosis have included size of tube, material of tube, trauma during intubation, and movement of tube in the larynx.

Aspiration of a Foreign Body

Aspiration of a foreign body usually occurs in toddlers 1–3 years of age and is more common in boys than in girls. The initial episode is frequently associated with choking and coughing. A radiopaque density confirms the presence of a foreign body in the airway (Fig. 3.6). Fluoroscopy or inspiratory/expiratory chest X-rays may aid evaluation. With partial bronchial occlusion, there may be mediastinal shifts *to* the affected side on inspiration and *away from* the affected side on expiration, or air trapping may be noted. With complete bronchial occlusion by a large foreign body, distal atelectasis is more common on the affected side. The right bronchus is more often the site of the foreign body than is the left bronchus. The diagnosis of a foreign body aspiration is confirmed at endoscopy.

Systemic Disorders

Angioneurotic edema involves localized skin swellings as well as edema of the face, hands, feet, and genitals. It is common for the edema to involve

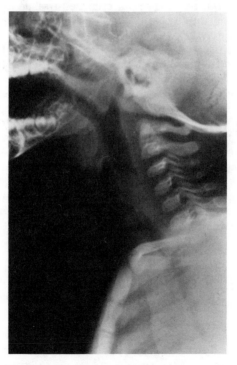

FIGURE 3.6. Diagnosis of subglottic foreign body is confirmed by radiopaque object on airway film.

the mucous membranes of the lips, tongue, and pharynx, and these patients may have evidence of upper airway obstruction. Some episodes have been provoked by local trauma or extremes of temperature. Treatment involves supportive measures and maintenance of an adequate airway. If an allergic etiology is suspected, medical therapy is indicated and epinephrine may be particularly useful.

Neoplasms

Papillomas are the most common airway tumor in children, with the symptoms usually appearing before the age of 7 years. The papillomatous lesions are frequently multiple and are most commonly located on the vocal cords, but they may also be seen on the palate, uvula, pharynx, and lower respiratory tract.

The goal of therapy is to remove all lesions to decrease the source of virus while preventing trauma and further seeding of the lesions. The current treatment involves repeated endoscopy with forceps removal of the exophytic portion and CO_2 laser therapy for the base of the lesion.

Chronic Upper Airway Obstruction

Chronic upper airway obstruction, as occurs with micrognathia, facial anomalies, hypotonia, macroglossia, enlarged tonsils and adenoids, nasal masses, obstructing tongue, and other lesions causing partial airway obstructions. It also may be associated with obstructive sleep apnea.

Problems in evaluation occur because frequently the child is normal while awake. Children with sleep apnea syndrome frequently have snoring, restless sleep, unusual sleeping positions, nocturnal enuresis, nightmares, behavior disturbances, easy fatigability, daytime sleepiness, abnormal head positions, mouth-breathing, irritability, and morning headaches. The child with sleep apnea syndrome is evaluated by polysomnography, electroencephalography, oximeter oxygen saturations, measurements of chest and abdominal movement while sleeping, awake pulmonary function tests, chest X-ray, neck airway films, and electrocardiography. The underlying cause of obstruction is usually determined at endoscopy. Complicating factors of chronic airway obstruction include developmental delay and failure to thrive, as well as pulmonary hypertension and cor pulmonale, probably associated with chronic hypoxemia.

CHAPTER 4

Bronchiolitis

Bronchiolitis is an acute inflammatory disease of the lower respiratory tract, resulting in obstruction of small airways. It commonly is stated that bronchiolitis is the wheezing disease of infants up to 2 years of age, while asthma begins at that age. This approach is too simplistic.

ETIOLOGY

Respiratory syncytial virus (RSV) accounts for the majority of cases of bronchiolitis in which a specific agent can be identified. It is estimated that between 40 and 75% of infants admitted to hospitals with bronchiolitis have RSV as the cause. Other viruses that cause bronchiolitis are rhinovirus, parainfluenza virus type 3, adenovirus types 3, 7, and 21, influenza virus, and occasionally mumps.

EPIDEMIOLOGY

If a broad clinical definition such as "wheezing associated with respiratory infection" is used, the highest incidence of this disease is in the first year of life. The incidence falls during the second year of life. Over 80% of those infants hospitalized are younger than 6 months of age. Those young infants who contract severe bronchiolitis may be at higher risk because of low levels of maternally transmitted neutralizing antibody.

RSV epidemics develop yearly in the winter, while parainfluenza virus outbreaks occur in the fall. This disease (RSV) is highly contagious. Once the virus is introduced in a day care setting, virtually all exposed children become infected. Transmission of RSV within families is also significant.

The rate of nosocomial spread is also high. Hospital staff members are probably the major carrier source during nosocomial spread of RSV infection through contamination with secretions from infected infants.

CLINICAL MANIFESTATIONS

The affected infant is typically exposed to an older child or an adult with an upper respiratory infection. Cough, sneeze, and rhinorrhea develop first. Subsequently, the patient suffers marked respiratory distress, with tach-

41

ypnea, retractions, wheezing, and irritability. A low-grade fever may be present, and marked dyspnea makes feeding difficult. Physical examination reveals all the signs of acute respiratory distress: tachypnea, cyanosis, flaring of alae nasi, and chest wall retractions. The lungs are hyperinflated, and the liver may be palpable several fingerbreadths below the costal margin. Auscultation of the lungs reveals diffuse wheezes, prolonged expiration, and rales.

Appropriate laboratory tests for the infant with severe bronchiolitis include: chest X-ray, complete blood count, arterial blood gases, immunologic tests for RSV, and bacterial cultures in cases in which bacterial pneumonia cannot be ruled out. Radiologic examination of infants with acute bronchiolitis demonstrates air trapping in the majority of patients (Fig. 4.1). About half the patients will have evidence of peribronchial thickening. Consolidation and collapse are seen less commonly on chest X-ray.

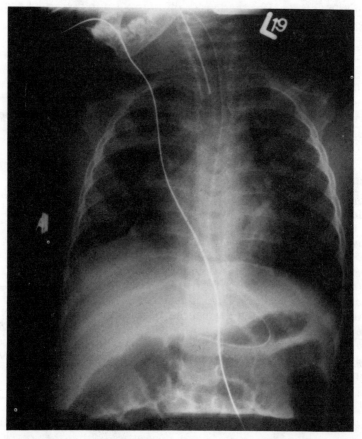

FIGURE 4.1. Chest X-ray of infant with bronchiolitis and respiratory failure, showing air trapping and peribronchial thickening.

Bacterial pneumonia cannot be excluded on radiologic grounds alone. The complete blood count is generally normal. RSV may be identified by complement fixation or indirect immunofluorescent antibody testing on nasal wash specimens.

In order to make the diagnosis of respiratory failure in bronchiolitis, arterial blood gas measurements are necessary. All infants are hypoxemic, and hypoxemia is persistent, lasting 3–7 weeks, even after clinical improvement has occurred. Nearly all patients are hypoxic in room air. A significant percentage of these patients reveal a severe uncompensated respiratory acidosis with P_aCO_2 levels above 65 mm Hg.

PATHOPHYSIOLOGY

The results of pulmonary function studies follow predictably from the small airway obstruction and hyperinflation in bronchiolitis. The thoracic volume at end expiration is increased almost twofold above normal. Most studies demonstrate an increase in inspiratory and expiratory resistance. The expiratory resistance is generally increased to a greater extent than is the inspiratory resistance.

The principal abnormality in gas exchange is hypoxemia. It is believed that ventilation/perfusion mismatching accounts for arterial desaturation. Most infants are able to maintain normocarbia in spite of an increased physiologic dead space-to-tidal volume ratio (V_D/V_T) by increasing minute ventilation significantly. Hypercarbia and respiratory failure develop when the infant becomes fatigued. Apnea in RSV bronchiolitis is not due to upper airway obstruction but rather is due to a complete absence of respiratory effort.

MANAGEMENT (TABLE 4.1)

The infant with acute bronchiolitis and respiratory distress should be hospitalized, particularly if his or her respiratory rate is increased and he or she is younger than 6 months of age. Pediatric intensive care unit admission should be considered for younger infants and particularly those

TABLE 4.1.
Management in Bronchiolitis

Therapy	Comment
Oxygen	Normal humidification required
Steroids	No proven value
Bronchodilators	No convincing evidence of efficacy
Antibiotics	No proven use
Nasal CPAP[a]	Can be useful prior to intubation
Riboviran	Antiviral agent of potential interest
Intubation	$P_aCO_2 > 60$ torr

[a]CPAP, continuous positive airway pressure.

patients showing signs of impending respiratory failure. Given the high risk of nosocomial spread of the disease, these infants should be cohorted, and staff members involved in their care should employ strict hand-washing procedures.

Supplemental oxygen administration is the mainstay of therapy. Humidified oxygen may be administered in a croup tent; however, there is no evidence that a mist tent adds any benefit over normally humidified supplemental oxygen alone, and there are major concerns about observing children inside these tents. Because expiratory resistance in particular is increased in bronchiolitis, aerosolized isoproterenol and salbutamol have been tried as bronchodilators. No beneficial effect could be demonstrated in these studies. A large, controlled, multi-institutional study showed corticosteroids to be of no value in the treatment of bronchiolitis. Steroid therapy in adenovirus-induced bronchiolitis obliterans has not been studied. As expected in a viral infection, antibacterial agents are useless. Occasionally, bacterial pneumonia cannot be excluded on clinical and radiologic grounds. In such circumstances, antibiotics may be started until appropriate cultures are negative. Antiviral chemotherapy with ribavirin aerosol, a nucleoside analog, has been used with moderate success in clinical trials.

Prematurely born infants younger than 3 months postnatal age are at risk for RSV-associated apnea, particularly if they have a history of apnea of prematurity. Therefore, these patients should receive cardiorespiratory monitoring on admission to the hospital.

When the P_aCO_2 rises above the normal 40–45 torr in a patient with tachypnea and respiratory distress, impending respiratory failure is present. Infants in respiratory failure from bronchiolitis who have been managed with continuous positive airway pressure have sometimes improved without need of intubation. These results strengthen the argument for a trial of nasal continuous positive airway pressure before endotracheal intubation and mechanical ventilation are instituted. In general, when P_aCO_2 reaches 60–65 torr, positive pressure ventilation is begun.

Fluid Administration

When impending respiratory failure is diagnosed, fluid administration must be tightly controlled in order to ensure euvolemia with risking overhydration. It is reasonable to assume that patients with lower airway obstruction from bronchiolitis are at risk of pulmonary edema due to negative pleural pressures with airway obstruction. Furthermore, severe bronchiolitis may include a necrotizing injury to bronchiolar and alveolar walls, which would favor transudation of fluid into air spaces.

Monitoring

During the period of impending respiratory failure, the patient requires meticulous surveillance and monitoring in the pediatric intensive care unit. Nursing observations include a frequent notation of vital signs, sensorium, breathing pattern, and skin color, as well as fluid intake and output. A continuous record of heart rate and respiratory rate is mandatory, particularly in view of the high incidence of apnea, especially in the very young or prematurely born infant.

The arterial blood gas remains the standard means of measuring oxygenation and ventilation. However, care of these infants is now facilitated greatly by the noninvasive measurement of cutaneous oxygen saturation ("pulse oximetry").

Central venous and pulmonary artery catheter placements are generally unnecessary in bronchiolitis patients with respiratory failure, because the critical phase of the disease is not associated with major hemodynamic changes.

OUTCOME

Respiratory failure in bronchiolitis generally resolves after 48–72 hours. However, impaired oxygenation may exist for several weeks after apparent clinical recovery. The relationship between acute bronchiolitis in infancy and the subsequent development of asthma remains confusing. It is unclear whether bronchiolitis leads to subsequent development of asthma or whether atopic individuals are predisposed to bronchiolitis.

Adenovirus-induced bronchiolitis obliterans produces a far more severe acute lung injury and a more debilitating chronic lung disease in survivors. As a result of some of these more severe infections, a small percentage of patients may develop a more severe and prolonged respiratory failure than the general 2–3-day need for respiratory support needed in most patients.

CHAPTER 5

Status Asthmaticus

DEFINITION

Status asthmaticus is a life-threatening form of asthma that accounts for most deaths that result from this disease. It is defined as a condition of progressively severe attack that is unresponsive to usual appropriate therapy with adrenergic drugs and theophylline and that leads to totally disabling acute pulmonary insufficiency.

DIAGNOSIS AND EVALUATION

Cough, dyspnea, and wheezing are the major clinical features in status asthmaticus, but the presentation varies with age. The degree of wheezing does not correlate well with the severity of the attacks, but the relative absence of wheezing in the presence of respiratory distress and poor air entry on auscultation of the lungs is indicative of severe obstruction. The use of accessory muscles of respiration and the presence of pulsus paradoxus usually signify severe compromise of respiratory function.

DIFFERENTIAL DIAGNOSIS

Congenital Malformations

Congenital anomalies of the respiratory, cardiovascular, and gastrointestinal systems can cause varying degrees of airway obstruction that mimic asthma. Among those common malformations are larynogotracheomalacia, vocal cord paralysis, tracheal or bronchial stenosis, lobar emphysema, lung cysts, vascular ring, and gastroesophageal reflux.

Foreign Bodies

Sudden onset of dyspnea, cough, and respiratory distress in previously healthy children without a history of recurrent attack favors the diagnosis of foreign bodies, in either the trachea or the bronchi.

Infections

Any respiratory tract infection in infants and young children can cause signs and symptoms of either upper or lower airway obstruction. Common problems include croup, bronchiolitis, and pneumonia.

EVALUATION AND PREDICTION OF NEED FOR HOSPITALIZATION AND FOR INTENSIVE CARE

When the following features of a severe acute attack are noted, hospitalization and intensive care may be warranted:

1. History of frequent repeated attacks, previous severe asthma that needed hospitalization, excessive daily use of bronchodilator and corticosteroids for control of symptoms, and failure to respond to previous effective therapy
2. Use of accessory respiratory muscles
3. Pulsus paradoxus of >18 mm Hg in teenagers and >10 mm Hg in children
4. Change in consciousness and/or obvious exhaustion
5. Cyanosis
6. Pneumothorax and pneumomediastinum
7. $FEV_{1.0}$ of <20% predicted value, with little or no response to acute therapy
8. Hypoxemia, with a P_aO_2 of <60mm Hg
9. Hypercapnia, with a P_aCO_2 of >40 mm Hg in the presence of dyspnea and wheezing
10. Metabolic acidosis
11. Electrocardiographic abnormalities

In pediatric patients, there is a clinical scoring system to detect an impending or existing respiratory failure in status asthmaticus patients, based on the signs and symptoms of airway obstruction, use of accessory respiratory muscles, oxygenation, and cerebral function. This may add another guideline for the physician in the emergency room and enable him or her to feel more comfortable with the plan of management. It seems also to be correlated well with both an increase in P_aCO_2 and a decrease in P_aO_2 (Table 5.1). Patients who have the following clinical signs and therapeutic requirements that suggest respiratory failure should be admitted to the intensive care units.

1. Impending and/or existing respiratory failure as assessed by an asthma score of >5
2. Isoproterenol infusion
3. Respiratory arrest and/or cardiac arrest
4. Mechanical ventilation
5. Tendency to develop theophylline toxicity, i.e, congestive heart failure or hepatic cirrhosis

THERAPY

Usual Forms of Treatment

A summary of the various drug regimens used in severe asthma is given in Table 5.2.

TABLE 5.1. ─────────────────────────────────
Clinical Asthma Evaluation Score[a]

Variables	0	1	2
P_aO_2	70–100 in air	≤70 in air	≤70 in 40% O_2
Cyanosis	None	In air	In 40% O_2
Inspiratory breath sounds	Normal	Unequal	Decreased to absent
Accessory muscles used	None	Moderate	Maximal
Expiratory wheezing	None	Moderate	Marked
Cerebral function	Normal	Depressed or agitated	Coma

[a]Clinical asthma score for children with status asthmaticus: a score of ≥5 = impending respiratory failure; and a score of ≥7 plus a P_aCO_2 of ≥65 mm Hg = existing respiratory failure. (From Wood DW, Downes JJ, Lecks HI: A clinical scoring system for the diagnosis of respiratory failure. *Am J Dis Child* 123:227, 1972.)

Theophylline

Theophylline is a xanthine derivative that has a structure similar to caffeine. The mechanism of action was thought to be the inhibition of phosphodiesterase enzymes. This mechanism has been questioned, however, because other phosphodiesterase inhibitors are not bronchodilators and the degree of inhibition of this enzyme is minimal in therapeutic concentrations of theophylline. It has been suggested that the bronchodilating effect of theophylline may occur by one or more of the following mechanisms: prostaglandin antagonism, increased binding of cyclic adenosine monophosphate to cyclic adenosine monophosphate-binding protein, and adenosine receptor antagonism.

The bronchodilator effect of theophylline is well correlated with increasing serum concentration within the range of 5–20 μg/ml, whereas the optimal response usually occurs at a serum concentration of >10 μg/ml. Because of the narrow effective therapeutic range, the efficacy and toxicity of theophylline are correlated more closely with plasma level than with the administered dosage. If the patient has not received a theophylline preparation within the previous 24 hours, the loading dose of 5 mg/kg should be given slowly over 20 minutes, followed by a continuous infusion dose, which depends on the age and other underlying diseases of the patient (Table 5.3). If the patient has taken theophylline recently, a serum theophylline level should be obtained. Clinical evidence of theophylline toxicity must be considered before the lower loading dose of 2.5 mg/kg is administered and followed by the same continuous infusion dose as above. Further adjustment of the theophylline infusion rate depends on the clinical response and serum theophylline concentration.

Aside from the variation in elimination of theophylline from the body,

TABLE 5.2. ————————————————————————————
General Pharmacologic Agents for Treatment of Acute and Severe Asthma in Children

Agent	Parenteral	Aerosol Inhalation
Adrenergic drugs		
Epinephrine hydrochloride	Subcutaneous (1:1000) solution, 1 mg/ml, 0.01 ml/kg/dose (maximum, 0.5 ml) every 15–20 min; repeat 3 times, as necessary	Not indicated
Sus-Phrine	Subcutaneous (1:200) solution, 5 mg/ml, 0.005 ml/kg/dose (maximum, 0.15 ml) every 6 hr	Not indicated
Terbutaline	Subcutaneous (0.05%) solution, 0.5 mg/ml, 0.01 mg/kg/dose (maximum, 0.25 mg) every 20–30 min for 3 doses, as necessary	1% solution, 10 mg/ml, 0.03 ml/kg (maximum, 1 ml); diluted with 1.5 ml saline every 4–6 hr
Albuterol (salbutamol)	Intravenous (0.1%) solution, 1 mg/ml, 0.2 μg/kg/min (maximum, 2 μg/kg/min or 10 μg/kg diluted and given over 10 min)	0.5% solution, 5 mg/ml, 0.01–0.03 ml/kg (maximum, 1 ml); diluted with 1.5 ml saline every 4–6 hr
Isoproterenol	Intravenous (0.02%) solution, 0.2 mg/ml, 0.05–0.1 μg/kg/min; increase by 0.05–0.1 μg/kg/min every 15–20 min	0.5% solution, 5 mg/ml, 0.01–0.02 ml/kg (maximum, 0.5 ml), diluted with 1.5 ml saline every 2–6 hr
Isoetharine	Not available	1% solution, 10 mg/ml, 0.01 ml/kg (maximum, 0.5 ml); diluted with 1.5 ml saline every 2–6 hr
Metaproterenol	Subcutaneous (0.10%) solution, 1.0 mg/ml, 0.01 ml/kg every 20–30 min for 3 doses, as necessary	5% solution, 50 mg/ml, 0.005–0.010 ml/kg (maximum, 0.4 ml); diluted with 1.5 ml saline every 4–6 hr
Theophylline	Intravenous aminophylline (USP[a]), 25 mg/ml, with a load-	No

TABLE 5.2.—*continued*

Agent	Parenteral	Aerosol Inhalation
	ing dose of 6–7.5 mg/kg over 20 min, given by constant infusion pump; modify loading dose on basis of (*a*) previous medication history or initial serum theophylline level or (*b*) 1 mg/kg for each 2 μg/ml increased, if desired in previous serum theophylline level; continuous infusion (monitor serum levels) at <10 kg body weight, 0.65 mg/kg/hr; and at >10 kg body weight, 0.9 mg/kg/hr	
Anticholinergic drugs		
Atropine		0.03–0.05 mg/kg nebulized
Ipratropium bromide		20–40 μg metered dose every 6 hr for those over 6 yr old; 250 μg nebulized dose for those under 6 yr old
Corticosteroid drugs		
Hydrocortisone	Intravenous loading dose, 5–7 mg/kg; maintenance, 5 mg/kg every 6 hr	No
Methylprednisolone	Intravenous loading dose, 1 mg/kg; maintenance, 0.8 mg/kg every 4–6 hr	No
Beclomethasone dipropionate	No	50–100 μg inhaler dose every 6 hr, provided 42 μg metered dose
Cromolyn sodium (useful for prevention of attacks)	No	1% solution, 10 mg/ml, 2 ml every 6 hr

[a]USP, United States Pharmacopeia.

TABLE 5.3.

Guidelines for Continuous Infusion Rate of Theophylline after Loading Dose for Target Concentration of Theophylline of 10 μg/ml[a]

Patient	Theophylline (mg/kg/hr)	Aminophylline[b] (mg/kg/hr)
Neonates	0.13	0.16
Infant	0.4	0.5
Infants 6–11 months	0.7	0.85
Children 1–9 yr	0.8	1.0
Children over 9 yr and otherwise healthy adults who smoke	0.6	0.75
Otherwise healthy nonsmoking adults	0.4	0.5
Cardiac decompensation and liver dysfunction	0.2	0.25

[a]Modified from Weinberger M, Hendeles L, Ahrens R: Clinical pharmacology of drugs used for asthma. *Pediatr Clin North Am* 28:47, 1983.
[b]Aminophylline = theophylline dose ÷ 0.8.

many concomitant drugs that have been given in the asthmatic patient can alter the theophylline metabolism. These are summarized in Table 5.4.

Adrenergic Drugs

Epinephrine

Although epinephrine was introduced as a bronchodilator drug in 1910, it is still the drug of choice for the treatment of acute asthmatic attacks. It has both α- and β-adrenergic agonist effects, has short action, and is effective when given by inhalation or subcutaneous injection. It is ineffective when given orally, because it is susceptible to inactivation by cathecol-o-methyltransferase (COMT), an enzyme that is present in the gastrointestinal tract. Because epinephrine effects both β_1- and β_2-adrenergic receptors, it also effects the cardiovascular system, in addition to its effect as a bronchodilator. Recent research has shown that drugs that have predominantly β_2-adrenergic or bronchodilator effects have a longer duration of action and are not susceptible to inactivation by the enzyme COMT, so they can be given by mouth. However, the use of epinephrine is likely only in the emergency room setting and is rarely given in the intensive care unit.

Isoetharine

Isoetharine (e.g., Bronkometer or Bronkosol) is a bronchoselective catecholamine that has a longer duration of action than epinephrine and is still susceptible to COMT enzymes, so that it is ineffective by mouth. Its peak activity is 15 minutes following inhalation, and the duration of bronchodilation is <2 hours. Some cardiovascular side effects still exist.

TABLE 5.4. ───────────────────────
Medications That Alter Theophylline Clearance

Increased theophylline metabolism

Barbiturate	Increased theophylline clearance by 25% on average when phenobarbital was used for at least 1 month and had a serum concentration over 10 μg/ml
Phenytoin	Increased theophylline clearance by 75% on average when phenytoin was used for more than 10 days and serum levels of phenytoin ranged between 10 and 20 μg/ml; phenytoin level also was reduced
Isoproterenol	Increased theophylline clearance by 15–20% during the concomitant intravenous therapy; clearance resumed to previous level after cessation of isoproterenol infusion

Decreased theophylline metabolism

Allopurinol	Decreased theophylline clearance by 25% on average when allopurinol was administered in high dose (600 mg/day); theophylline clearance decreased after 2 weeks of therapy
Cimetidine	Decreased theophylline clearance (23–100%) results in a twofold to threefold increase in serum theophylline concentration
Erythromycin (base and salts)	Decreased theophylline clearance by 25% on average; effect appeared after 7–10 days of erythromycin therapy and was dose related; erythromycin level also was reduced
Troleandomycin	Decreased theophylline clearance by 50%; serum theophylline concentration increased twofold
Propranolol	Decreased theophylline clearance by 40% in cigarette smokers and by 20% in nonsmokers
Oral contraceptives	Decreased theophylline clearance by 34% in chronic contraceptive users for 6 months or longer

Metaproterenol

Metaproterenol (e.g., Alupent) is a noncatecholamine adrenergic bronchodilator that is resistant to inactivation by COMT and is effective orally and parenterally as well as by aerosol. It has a longer duration of action and equivalent action to isoprotererol in its relative cardiac and brochodilator potency. Tremor is a common adverse effect of the drug, particularly after oral administration.

Terbutaline and Albuterol

The noncatecholamine, β_2-selective adrenergic bronchodilators terbutaline and albuterol (e.g., salbutamol) have been shown to stimulate β_2-adrenergic receptors in the bronchial trees more than β_1-adrenergic receptors in the heart. These drugs are effective orally and parenterally (subcutaneously for terbutaline; intravenously for albuterol), as well as by inhalation, and have a longer duration of action than has epinephrine. Both drugs are equally effective when given orally or by aerosol in equivalent doses. The bronchodilator response to parenteral administration of albuterol is no different from that for aerosol administration of the drug, but the relief of pulsus paradoxus has been shown to be significantly better with the aerosol treatment. The subcutaneous dose of terbutaline is widely used as an alternative to epinephrine in the treatment of acute asthmatic attacks, with the equal effectiveness in bronchodilation. The dose response of terbutaline by various routes of administration has been clearly demonstrated (Fig. 5.1). In comparison to parenteral aminophylline, the brochodilator response of parenteral albuterol seems to be greater, but the differences are not statistically significant, and the side effects seem to be fewer.

Isoproterenol

Isoproterenol is a nonselective β-adrenergic agonist that has both β_1- and β_2-adrenergic receptor stimulation. It is a potent bronchodilator when administered by inhalation, with a peak bronchodilation attained within 5 minutes and a progressive decline in bronchodilator effect by 2 hours. Intravenous isoproterenol has been shown to be effective in managing children with respiratory failure and carbon dioxide retention from asthma. In addition, intravenous isoproterenol has been said to prevent the need for mechanical ventilation in approximately 80–90% of these patients, thereby reducing the considerable numbers of complications from positive pressure ventilation. The isoproterenol infusion is generally started at a rate of 0.05–0.1 μ/kg/min via a constant infusion pump and is increased every 15 minutes by 0.05 μg/kg/min until the patient responds (P_aCO_2 of ≤ 40 torr) or until the attempt is stopped because of marked tachycardia (heart rate increase of $>20\%$ or heart rate of >200/min) or because an arrhythmia has developed. As the patient improves, the isoproterenol infusion is slowly tapered off. The issue of concomitant aminophylline infusion is controversial. Great care must be taken with those combinations of drugs.

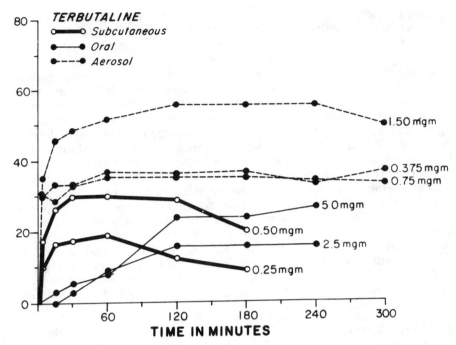

FIGURE 5.1. Effect of three different routes of administration of terbutaline on $FEV_{1.0}$. (From Dulfano MJ, Glass P: The bronchodilator effects of terbutaline: Route of administration and pattern of response. *Ann Allergy* 37:357, 1976.)

Anticholinergic Drugs—Atropine

Atropine is the prototype of anticholinergic drugs. It has been used since the beginning of the 19th century for the treatment of reversible airway obstruction. The bronchodilating response depends on the dose and route of administration. The predominant effect on large and central airways is obtained by aerosol administration, whereas the generalized bronchodilating response occurs after intravenous administration. Atropine sulfate inhalation is accepted widely at the dose of 0.05–0.10 mg/kg, producing maximal bronchodilatation and consistently reducing airflow obstruction. This mode of treatment seems to be especially useful for patients with bronchospasm associated with chronic bronchitis.

Corticosteroids

There is general agreement that corticosteroids are of great value in reducing morbidity in acute severe asthmatic attacks that are refractory to standard bronchodilator therapy. However, the precise mechanisms are still uncertain.

The guideline for initiating steroid therapy in asthma depends upon the severity of the disease, the history of the patient's requirement for gluco-corticoid, and his or her response to previous therapy. The initial improvement usually occurs within 6 hours after steroid administration, but in more severe cases, a longer time is usually required for the effect of steroids to become fully manifest. The recommended dose of steroids varies, and it has been suggested that plasma steroid concentration be maintained in a range of 100–150 μg cortisol per 100 ml. This can be achieved by giving hydrocortisone hemisuccinate intravenously at a dose of 4–8 mg/kg (or an equivalent) every 4–6 hours or methylprednisolone at a dose of 2–3 mg/kg/day in four divided doses, which produces less sodium retention than does hydrocortisone. This may be tapered after 48 hours as the patient improves. The aerosolized steroids are useful only in chronic maintenance therapy and are not recommended in the treatment of acute asthma. The side effects of long-term steroid therapy include increased susceptibility to infection, hypothalamic-pituitary-adrenal axis suppression, Cushingoid appearance, growth retardation, bone demineralization, hyperglycemia and glycosuria, myopathy, sodium retention, and secondary hypertension. However, there is no evidence that a short period of therapy (<2 weeks) is associated with a significant risk of serious adverse reactions. In addition, steroids may help to reverse a potentially life-threatening episode of severe asthma.

Antibiotic Therapy

Antibiotic therapy should be reserved for asthmatic patients who have signs and symptoms suggesting bacterial infection, which can be assessed by correlating clinical and laboratory findings including fever, leukocytosis, and intracellar bacterial organisms on Gram stain of sputum. Furthermore, both the presence of lobular infiltration on a chest X-ray and the evidence of sinusitis by physical or radiographic examination support the diagnosis of bacterial infection. An appropriate antibiotic should be initiated promptly in these children in order to eliminate the source that precipitates bronchospasm and, therefore, to reduce the morbidity from asthma.

Hydration and Correction of Acidosis

In asthmatics, secretions become viscid and contribute to a worsening degree of airway obstruction. The correction of dehydration, if present, is the rule for treatment of children with status asthmaticus. Once adequate urinary output is established, careful monitoring of fluid intake, urine output, serum electrolytes, and osmolarity is necessary to prevent excessive fluid administration and allow early detection of hyponatremia and evidence of water intoxication due to an increase in antidiuretic hormone secretion. Furthermore, the more negative intrapleural pressure during severe asthmatic attacks favors fluid accumulation in the interstitial space around the bronchiole. This effect, if combined with the overhydration, can facilitate the development of pulmonary edema. Hence, the guideline for hydration in asthmatic patients is to maintain the patient at near-normal water balance and avoid excessive fluid administration.

Mechanical Ventilation

Despite the understanding of pathophysiologic consequences of acute severe asthmatic attacks and recent advances in the pharmacologic management of status asthmaticus with inhalation adrenergic compounds and isoproterenol infusion, a small number of children still develop rapidly progressive respiratory failure, resulting in coma and death. The most effective treatment of respiratory failure in these children is ventilatory support via mechanical ventilation in order to reduce the work of breathing and allow bronchodilator drugs to reverse the basic pathology of status asthmaticus.

There are no absolute guidelines for initiating mechanical ventilation in status asthmaticus, except cardiopulmonary arrest and coma; however, the criteria that should be considered include:

1. A decrease in respiratory effort due to progressive exhaustion
2. Deterioration in mental status
3. Absence of breath sounds and wheezing
4. Cyanosis in 40% oxygen
5. Hypoxemia with a P_aO_2 of <60 torr on O_2 at 6 liters/min
6. Hypercapnia with a P_aCO_2 of >50 torr, increasing by more than 5 torr/hr

Choice of Ventilator

Because of the severe bronchoconstriction as well as mucosal edema and thick secretions that contribute to high airway resistance, a volume-cycled ventilator is preferred in patients with status asthmaticus in order to maintain the more uniform alveolar ventilation, despite high airway resistance. The appropriate respiratory rate depends upon the patient's age and usually ranges from 15 to 20/min with an inspiratory/expiratory ratio of 1:2.

Monitoring

Monitoring should include:

1. Continuous arterial pressure measurement via an indwelling catheter that permits determination of arterial blood gases and the degree of pulsus paradoxus
2. Electrocardiogram which is helpful in the early detection of cardiotoxic effects of theophylline and isoproterenol
3. Chest X-ray after intubation and then daily, as dictated by the clinician when complications are suspected
4. Peak-inspiratory pressure which is directly related to increased airway resistance and to the risk of pneumothorax

5. Hourly intake and output to keep patient at near-normal water balance and not overhydrated
6. Serum electrolytes, especially in patients receiving steroids

Weaning

Criteria used for weaning status asthmaticus patients from mechanical ventilation should be based on reliable physiologic criteria and evidence of clinical improvement of reversible airway obstruction. These include:

1. Decreased bronchospasm
2. Normal arterial blood gases in 40% oxygen
3. Inspiratory pressure of ≤ 35 cm H_2O
4. Pulsus paradoxus of <10 torr
5. Chest X-ray showing reduced hyperaeration with minimal or no atelectasis

Unusual Forms of Treatment
Halothane

Historically, inhalation anesthetic agents such as diethyl ether and cyclopropane have been used in the operating room as therapeutic bronchodilators in patients with severe asthma. More recently, halothane has been described as a useful bronchodilator in pediatric and adult patients with status asthmaticus.

Calcium Antagonists

The beneficial effects of calcium antagonists in preventing spontaneously occurring asthmatic attacks are not yet established. Based on the basic pathophysiologic consequences of asthma, in addition to the absence of adverse effects of calcium antagonists on resting airway tone, the concept of calcium channel blockade remains as an important investigative avenue for the development of newer drugs that will have more specific effects on airway smooth muscle tone and mast cell secretion.

CHAPTER 6

Adult Respiratory Distress Syndrome

DEFINITION

The diagnosis of adult respiratory distress syndrome (ARDS) requires that a number of elements be present. Among these are *(a)* a catastrophic pulmonary or nonpulmonary event in the patient with previously normal lungs that is associated with respiratory distress with hypoxemia as well as decreased pulmonary compliance and *(b)* increased shunt ($\dot{Q}_S/\dot{Q}_T$) fraction. In addition, generally there is radiologic evidence of diffuse pulmonary infiltrates. Furthermore, there must be exclusion of left heart disease and congestive heart failure.

ETIOLOGIES

Because ARDS is a clinical syndrome for which no specific marker exists, it is unclear whether the precipitating events are truly causative or merely associated phenomena. Nevertheless, a list of suspected causes is given in Table 6.1. Shock, sepsis, and near-drowning are the most common causes in published pediatric series.

PATHOPHYSIOLOGY

Mechanism of Pulmonary Edema

Ultrastructural evidence supports the notion that disruption of the alveolar capillary membrane is responsible for pulmonary edema in ARDS. The high protein content of edema fluid in ARDS patients suggests that the restrictive properties of the membrane have been disrupted.

Mechanisms of Microvascular Injury

Several lines of evidence suggest that the activated granulocyte is the principal mediator of microvascular injury in ARDS (see Fig. 6.1).

Role of Arachidonic Acid Metabolites in Acute Lung Injury

Pulmonary artery hypertension occurs in experimental animals and patients with ARDS. Cyclo-oxygenase pathway products may act as media-

TABLE 6.1. _____
Disorders Associated with (Causing) ARDS

Common	Uncommon
Trauma	Drug overdose (e.g., narcotic)—
Sepsis	Idiosyncratic reaction
Near-drowning	Cardiopulmonary bypass
Shock	Hemodialysis
Surface burns	Fat embolism
Smoke inhalation	High altitude
Infectious pneumonia	Strangulation
Gram-negative bacteria	Toxic gas inhalation
Viral	Pancreatitis
Pneumocystis	Massive transfusion
Aspiration pneumonia	
Disseminated intravascular	
coagulopathy	

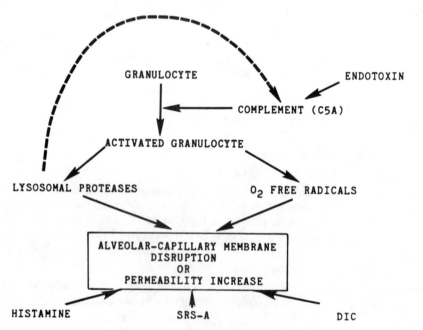

FIGURE 6.1. Proposed mechanisms of microvascular injury in ARDS. *SRS-A,* slow-reacting substance of anaphylaxis; and *DIC,* disseminated intravascular coagulopathy products.

tors of this pulmonary vascular response because the prostaglandins 6-keto-PGF and $PGF_{2\alpha}$ and thromboxane B_2 are found in significantly increased concentrations in lung lymph after endotoxin-induced ARDS.

Diminished Surfactant Activity and Airway Collapse

Surfactant is a surface-active material that lines alveoli and promotes alveolar stability. The physiologic importance of sufactant is appreciated from the Laplace equation:

$$P = \frac{2T}{r}$$

In the absence of surfactant, the surface tension (T) would remain constant, despite changes in alveolar size. The end result would be that alveoli of small radius (r) would require greater transpulmonary pressure (P) to stay open. Small alveoli would regularly empty into larger ones, leading to collapse of the smaller alveoli and overdistention of larger alveoli.

In ARDS, alveoli are unstable, and it is postulated that hypovolemia and increased pulmonary vascular resistance lead to decreased perfusion of type II alveolar pneumocytes and subsequent disruption of surfactant synthesis.

Lung Volumes and Mechanics

Patients with ARDS consistently exhibit reduced lung volumes, especially a reduction in functional residual capacity (FRC). The low FRC is associated with a large intrapulmonary shunt fraction ($\dot{Q}_S/\dot{Q}_T$) and hypoxemia. Because raising FRC with positive end-expiratory pressure (PEEP) greatly improves arterial oxygen tension, it is assumed that low FRC reflects closure of many terminal gas-exchanging units and is a major cause of hypoxemia in this disease.

Gas Exchange Abnormalities

Venous Admixture

Arterial hypoxemia with a large venous admixture ($\dot{Q}_S/\dot{Q}_T$) is a consistent finding in ARDS, which could be explained by either ventilation/perfusion ($\dot{V}/\dot{Q}$) mismatching or right-to-left intrapulmonary shunting. It has become clear in both patients and experimental animals with ARDS that the venous admixture results from distribution of a portion of the pulmonary circulation to both shunt units and low $\dot{V}/\dot{Q}$ units. Intrapulmonary shunt is clearly the predominant cause of venous admixture, particularly in patients with the most severe ARDS.

Dead Space in Adult Respiratory Distress Syndrome

Hypercarbia is seldom found early in the course of ARDS. The pulmonary lesions of early ARDS do not result in an increase in dead space.

Furthermore, hypoxemia and pulmonary reflexes stimulate the patient to hyperventilate, so that P_aCO_2 is normal or low. After days or weeks, fibrosis and pulmonary capillary obliteration may occur, and if the patient is unable to hyperventilate sufficiently, P_aCO_2 will rise.

Cardiovascular Alterations—Pulmonary Hemodynamics

In the initial stage of ARDS not triggered by hypovolemic shock, the pulmonary artery pressure is thought to be normal or minimally elevated. Nevertheless, a large number of clinical reports have documented sometimes severe pulmonary artery hypertension in ARDS patients. The duration and severity of ARDS are factors that influence the development of pulmonary artery hypertension. Other factors include pulmonary hypertension with low lung volumes, generalized hypoxic pulmonary vasoconstrictions, and circulating mediators.

CLINICAL MANIFESTATIONS

The history of the patient with ARDS will vary, depending upon the inciting event. In some cases, the time of onset and the nature of the previous injury are unknown. Once direct or indirect lung injury takes place, there is usually a latent period in which the patient seems to be in little respiratory distress except for hyperventilation. Auscultation and X-ray of the chest may be normal. During the next several hours to days, hypoxemia gradually progresses, and unequivocal respiratory distress becomes evident. The patient appears cyanotic, dyspneic, and tachypneic.

Arterial blood gas measurements reveal profound hypoxemia refractory to the use of supplemental oxygen alone. The P_aO_2 is often <50 torr on an F_IO_2 of >0.6. The ratio of P_aO_2 to F_IO_2 (P_aO_2/F_IO_2) is significantly reduced. A P_aO_2/F_IO_2 ratio of <200 correlates with a $\dot{Q}_S/\dot{Q}_T$ of >20%. Other physiologic measurements reveal stiff lungs with decreased total compliance.

The radiographic picture of ARDS is nonspecific. Immediately after the inciting event, the X-ray may show an entirely normal chest. Subsequently, pulmonary edema without cardiomegaly becomes apparent (Fig. 6.2). After the first 24 hours, an interstitial pattern becomes more prominent and ultimately evolves into a picture suggestive of diffuse interstitial fibrosis (see Fig. 6.3) If the patient survives, the complications of therapy with PEEP may appear on X-ray. These include pulmonary hyperinflation with interstitial gas, pneumothorax, pneumomediastinum, and subcutaneous emphysema (Fig. 6.3). During convalescence, the chest X-ray may return to normal.

MANAGEMENT

Oxygen Therapy

All patients with acute respiratory failure require supplemental oxygen; however, the dose and duration of use of supplemental oxygen must be

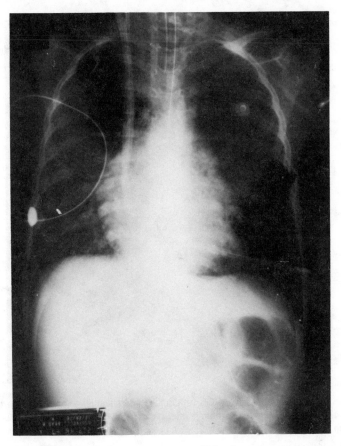

FIGURE 6.2.   Chest X-ray of early ARDS, showing mild pulmonary edema with normal heart size.

titrated carefully. As discussed previously, increased inspired concentrations of oxygen denitrogenate the lungs and result in areas of increased atelectasis which, in turn, worsens right-to-left shunting. This absorption atelectasis cannot be prevented by the application of end-expiratory pressure. Furthermore, prolonged exposure to high inspired concentrations of oxygen is directly toxic to long tissue. In the initial stages of the disease process, oxygen may be delivered successfully with nasal prongs or face mask. However, most patients with ARDS progress rapidly to a stage in which an inspired oxygen concentration of up to 50% delivered by face mask is no longer sufficient to prevent hypoxemia. At that point, endotracheal intubation is usually required in order to improve oxygenation by the addition of PEEP without incurring the risks of oxygen toxicity.

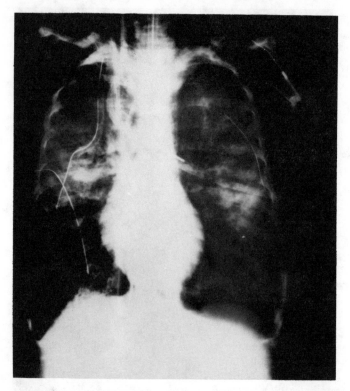

FIGURE 6.3.   Chest X-ray of late ARDS with diffuse interstitial fibrosis and severe barotrauma consisting of pulmonary interstitial emphysema, left pneumothorax, and marked subcutaneous emphysema.

Positive End-Expiratory Pressure
Respiratory Effects

It is rational therapy to attempt to increase the volume of ventilated lung, particularly during expiration, in an effort to improve gas exchange in patients with low FRC. Numerous studies have shown that PEEP clearly succeeds in increasing FRC.

Two mechanisms have been proposed to explain the increase in FRC with PEEP:

1. Recruitment of terminal air spaces may occur if PEEP is able to reopen otherwise closed terminal airways and alveoli. PEEP is known to prevent inactivation or depletion of surfactant in the lung, which may facilitate opening terminal air spaces. If recruitment of new terminal air space is the major reason for expansion of FRC, increased compliance of the lung and improved oxygenation would be predicted.

2. Overdistention of already patent alveoli could likewise account for an increase in FRC. However, overdistention of alveoli should not improve compliance and, in fact, carries the risk of barotrauma and decreased pulmonary blood flow from compression of alveolar vessels.

These mechanisms are not mutually exclusive. Whether recruitment or overdistention predominate in a given patient depends on the disease process and on the level of PEEP

Effect on Distribution of Pulmonary Blood Flow and V̇/Q̇ Matching in ARDS

In addition to improving lung volumes, a second mechanism responsible for better oxygenation with PEEP seems to be the ability of PEEP to redistribute pulmonary blood flow to better ventilated lung units. With PEEP, pulmonary blood flow is redistributed to nondependent regions. Under these circumstances, PEEP improves V̇/Q̇ matching by shifting pulmonary blood flow from nondependent lung regions to dependent regions.

Effect on Pulmonary Hemodynamics

Even though there are profound effects of PEEP on lung volume and mechanics, the beneficial effects of PEEP in improving gas exchange cannot be appreciated fully without understanding the effects of PEEP on the pulmonary circulation. During the past decade, a large body of research has been devoted to determining the effects of PEEP on thoracic intravascular pressures and resistances that, in turn, determine the regional distribution of pulmonary blood flow. Furthermore, it has become clear that PEEP-induced changes in pulmonary hemodynamics affect the production of extra.ascular lung water as well as the total cardiac output and oxygen transport to peripheral tissues. A schematic representation of the effect of PEEP on pulmonary hemodynamics and extravascular lung watch is shown in Figure 6.4.

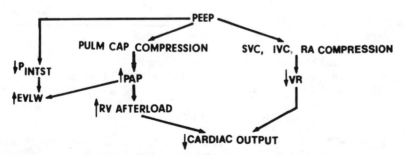

FIGURE 6.4. Effect of PEEP on pulmonary hemodynamics and extravascular lung water *(EVLW)* production. *Pulm* cap, pulmonary capillary; *PAP*, pulmonary artery pressure; *SVC*, superior vena cava; *IVC*, inferior vena cava; *RA*, right atrium; *VR*, venous return; P_{INTST}, pulmonary interstitial pressure; and *RV*, right ventricle.

Clinical Application

In general, endotracheal intubation and application of PEEP are appropriate in the ARDS patient when:

1. Clinical and radiographic evidence suggest worsening lung disease.
2. F_IO_2 of >0.5 by face mask is required to prevent hypoxemia.

Considerable debate has focused on the question of how much PEEP to apply. When PEEP was first introduced into widespread clinical use, many reports recommended limiting PEEP to an upper level of 15 cm H_2O. Although the benefits of increasing FRC and compliance and decreasing $\dot{Q}_S/\dot{Q}_T$ were clearly recognized, the negative side effects of falling cardiac output and pulmonary barotrauma were believed to restrict the upper limit of PEEP.

Subsequently, it has become apparent that PEEP can be used to its optimal potential by targeting therapy to improve oxygen delivery (OD) and to decrease $\dot{Q}_S/\dot{Q}_T$ to <12−15%. A comprehensive guideline for determining optimal PEEP is shown in Table 6.2.

Respiratory Modes

Various inspiratory modes may be combined with PEEP. For example, the combination of intermittent positive pressure ventilation and PEEP is termed "CPPV." There are a number of theoretical objections to this mode of ventilation. If the patient's P_aCO_2 is above apneic threshold, he or she will attempt to breathe spontaneously out of phase with ventilator breaths. This frequently leads to hyperventilation and alkalemia. In addition, there seems to be a higher incidence of barotrauma when CPPV is employed. Some of these problems are reduced via intermittent mandatory ventilation (IMV) and continuous positive airway pressure. This mode allows the patient to breathe spontaneously through the ventilator circuit. The otherwise spontaneous breathing pattern is interrupted by intermittent me-

TABLE 6.2. ————————————————————————————————
Guidelines for Determination of Optimal PEEP Level

1. Ensure normal blood volume prior to starting PEEP.
2. Increase PEEP in increments of 3−5 cm H_2O every 30 minutes.
3. Continue PEEP increase until
   (a) $\dot{Q}_S/\dot{Q}_T$ is <2−15%,
   (b) OD is optimal (usually >650 ml/min/m^2), and
   (c) $\dot{V}O_2$ is optimal (usually >160 ml/min/in^2).
4. If decreased cardiac output is encountered, expand volume until wedge pressure equals 18 mm Hg (referenced to atmosphere).
5. Start inotropic agents if cardiac output remains depressed after volume expansion.
6. If cardiac output remains depressed, begin decreasing PEEP in increments until cardiac output is restored.

chanical breaths. The use of spontaneous ventilation with this mode allows better distribution of gas, which, in turn, lowers physiologic dead space compared to CPPV. With this technique, it is easier to maintain a normal alveolar ventilation ($\dot{V}_A$) and pH. The frequency of IMV is adjusted such that pH remains between 7.35 and 7.40. The initial tidal volume for IMV may be set at 15 ml/kg.

Weaning

Weaning from respiratory support begins when the following criteria have been met. The patient should be hemodynamically stable. The effects of narcotics, sedatives, and muscle relaxants should have dissipated. There should be clinical, radiologic, and arterial blood gas evidence of stable or improving lung disease. The weaning process begins with a stepwise reduction in IMV rate while normal arterial pH is maintained. F_IO_2 is decreased to nontoxic levels consistent with adequate oxygen delivery. Finally, PEEP is reduced in small increments (e.g., 2 cm) to prevent sudden decreases in FRC or compliance.

Blood and Fluid Therapy

There is continuing controversy over crystalloid and colloid support in ARDS. At this time, only volume expansion with blood seems to be clearly preferable to crystalloid, because oxygen delivery (OD) is improved both by the increased hemoglobin concentration and by the augmented cardiac output. Several lines of evidence suggest that the hematocrit should be maintained between 40 and 49%. OD per unit cardiac work expended is greatest when hematocrit is kept in this range. Likewise, cerebral OD is optimal with hematocrits in this range. As blood viscosity rises with higher hematocrits, cerebral oxygen delivery is reduced. Asmundson showed that the survival rate is doubled in adult acute respiratory failure patients with hematocrits of 40–49%.

Monitoring

All patients with acute respiratory failure require meticulous routine care that includes: an hourly record of vital signs; frequent observations of sensorium, breathing pattern, and perfusion; and a summary of intake and output after every nursing shift. The patient's weight should be measured daily.

Hemodynamic monitoring requires a continuous record of the electrocardiogram. Arterial lines permit beat-to-beat measurement of blood pressure, which may fluctuate widely, secondary to the underlying disease or PEEP therapy. As suggested previously, knowledge of oxygen delivery and consumption, in addition to $\dot{Q}_S/\dot{Q}_T$ and P_aO_2, should guide therapy in ARDS. This requires placement of a pulmonary artery catheter. The information obtained from a pulmonary artery catheter must be interpreted critically. Although determination of cardiac output by thermodilution and mixed venous oxygen content from a pulmonary artery blood sample is likely to be accurate, measurement of pulmonary capillary wedge pressure as an indication of left ventricular preload should be approached cautiously. The reason is that PEEP may raise alveolar and pleural pressure above atmospheric pressure, so the effective filling pressure is different from that in normal circumstances.

Respiratory monitoring principally involves the evaluation of gas exchange and lung mechanics. The arterial blood gas forms the foundation for monitoring gas exchange. Samples are obtained via an indwelling arterial line. End-tidal CO_2 is analyzed with infrared photometry or mass spectrometry. In the normal lung, end-tidal CO_2 closely approximates arterial PCO_2. When ventilation is poorly matched to perfusion, a gradient develops between end-tidal CO_2 and arterial P_aCO_2. However, end-tidal CO_2 analysis remains useful as a trend monitor and as an additional ventilator disconnect alarm.

Drug Therapy
Steroids

There is no specific drug therapy for ARDS. The use of steroids in ARDS remains controversial. The preponderance of evidence indicates that steroids are of no benefit and, possibly, are harmful in interfering with metabolism.

Vasodilators

Successful pulmonary vasodilator therapy in ARDS would require that pulmonary vascular resistance be lowered more than systemic vascular resistance and that vasodilation of pulmonary vasculature occur in well-ventilated lung regions in order to improve $\dot{V}/\dot{Q}$ matching. Most vasodilators cannot do this. As a result, although occasionally helpful, vasodilators have a limited role in ARDS.

Inotropic Agents

Increased pulmonary vascular resistance in ARDS significantly raises the work load placed on the right ventricle. Maintenance of adequate cardiac output depends on the ability of the right ventricle to increase stroke work. When inotropic agents are needed to augment ventricular contractility to maintain cardiac output, dobutamine is the preferred agent because it raises cardiac output without producing significant pulmonary vasoconstriction.

Nutrition

Although nutritional repletion is vital in patients with ARDS just as in other critically ill patients, the source of nonprotein calories may have profound effects on respiration. If excessive carbohydrate in the form of hypertonic dextrose is used, CO_2 production may increase dramatically. This occurs because excess glucose is metabolized to fat in the liver. The respiratory quotient for this lipogenesis pathway is 8, resulting in large amounts of CO_2 production. Patients with respiratory failure may not be able to increase minute ventilation sufficiently in order to excrete this excess CO_2 load.

Extraordinary Management

High-frequency ventilation has been used in the treatment of patients with severe ARDS. Although this modality achieves adequate gas exchange, there is no improvement in outcome over conventional ventilation. In certain circumstances, such as bronchopleural fistula, high-frequency jet ventilation may have distinct advantages over conventional volume-cycled ventilation.

Extracorporeal membrane oxygenation (ECMO) through venoarterial bypass is technically feasible in children. In most cases, adequate gas exchange can be achieved in patients with ARDS who have previously failed conventional therapy. However, because ECMO remains only supportive therapy, if the underlying disease process continues unchecked, the mortality rate remains high. Thus, the role for ECMO remains limited unless the patients with reversible lung disease can be identified early in their course.

OUTCOME

Interpretation of mortality rates and clinical status of survivors of ARDS is complicated because of the wide variety of triggering insults, severity of the acute illness, and differences in premorbid pulmonary function. Nevertheless, it is quite apparent that ARDS is associated with a high mortality rate, and preliminary data suggest that pediatric survivors are left with worse pulmonary function than are adults who recover from ARDS.

Mortality rates range from 28 to 64% in recent adult series in which patients received aggressive intensive care including the use of PEEP.

Children seem to suffer approximately the same mortality rates as adults; however, the reported series are smaller. The average mortality rate of the five published pediatric series combined is 52%, with a range of 28.5–90% (Table 6.3).

TABLE 6.3.
Mortality Rates for Published Pediatric ARDS Series

Author	Mortality	Years
Holbrook et al.	17/18 (90%)	1975–1980
Lyrene and Truog	9/16 (60%)	1976–1979
Pfenninger et al.	8/20 (40%)	1978–1981
Katz et al.	8/23 (35%)	1979–1981
Nussbaum	2/7 (28.5%)	1979–1982
Overall	44/84 (52%)	

COMPLICATIONS

Oxygen Toxicity

Despite this fairly detailed biochemical understanding of pulmonary oxygen toxicity and of the free radical problem, the clinician has no specific therapy to offer the patient at risk. Therefore, prevention of pulmonary oxygen toxicity is the major goal, and the following guidelines are appropriate:

1. Use the lower F_1O_2 consistent with adequate tissue oxygenation.
2. Consider the use of PEEP in order to permit a lower F_1O_2.
3. Never deny a patient 100% O_2 if this is necessary to prevent hypoxemia.

Barotrauma

Pulmonary barotrauma develops in ARDS as a function of both the lung pathology and the therapeutic use of PEEP. With increased transpulmonary pressure exerted by PEEP, some alveoli become overdistended while the interstitial space is compressed. Partial airway obstruction exaggerates this tendency. Mechanical forces on the alveolar wall produce rupture when a critical traction force is exceeded, particularly in the face of lung tissue that is already damaged and noncompliant. Gas dissects along a perivascular sheath into the mediastinum and from there through the visceral pleura into the pleural space. Less commonly, the escaping gas may rupture directly from interstitial space into the pleural cavity. Air may also dissect along fascial planes into the neck and chest wall if the PEEP level is sufficiently high.

Pneumothorax should be suspected whenever the ARDS patient exhibits an unexplained sudden deterioration in clinical appearance, arterial oxygen tension, or hemodynamic stability. Chest X-ray will confirm the diagnosis.

Successful management of the pneumothorax almost always requires closed-chest thoracostomy tube evacuation of air to an underwater seal system, because a continuing leak is virtually inevitable as long as the patient is breathing against positive pressure. Provided this complication is recognized promptly and the chest tube is inserted correctly with strict sterile technique, barotrauma should not contribute to mortality in ARDS.

CHAPTER 7

Neuromuscular Disease and Respiratory Failure

Although the term "respiratory failure" usually connotes profound pulmonary pathology, it is just as applicable to situations characterized by normal lung mechanics and diminished respiratory muscle function. A number of disorders affecting the neuromuscular system impact significantly on ventilatory gas exchange by impairing central control of breathing, patency of the proximal airway, or respiratory muscle function primarily. These are shown schematically in Figure 7.1.

CENTRAL HYPOVENTILATION SYNDROME

Clinical Features

Prior to pursuing a discussion of central hypoventilation syndrome, it is important to consider the definitions of various types of apnea encountered in the pediatric critical care setting. Central apnea is characterized by the cessation of all respiratory efforts, resulting in the arrest of ventilatory gas flow. Obstructive apnea, as previously noted, can also lead to alveolar hypoventilation and asphyxia. In this case, apnea is characterized by continued spontaneous respiratory efforts that fail to generate respiratory gas flow. Mixed apnea, as the name implies, has characteristics of central and obstructive apnea. In this case, a central apneic episode is usually followed by inspiratory efforts that, due to superimposed airway obstruction, do not generate respiratory gas flow.

The clinical presentation of congenital central hypoventilation syndrome usually takes the form at birth of cyanosis that responds readily to mechanical ventilatory support. Frequently, efforts directed at weaning respiratory support are met with repeated failure. In less severe cases, abnormalities in respiratory pattern during sleep are noted, leading to a presumptive diagnosis of near-miss sudden infant death syndrome (SIDS).

Central hypoventilation syndrome must be differentiated from primary reversible disorders that can be associated with apnea or hypoventilation. In infants, other considerations include sepsis, hypothermia, electrolyte abnormalities, hypocalcemia, hypoglycemia, and seizures. Also, virtually

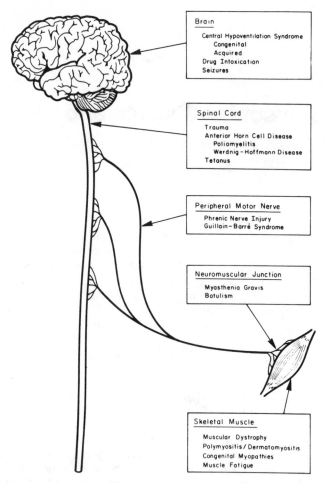

Brain

Central Hypoventilation Syndrome
    Congenital
    Acquired
Drug Intoxication
Seizures

Spinal Cord

Trauma
Anterior Horn Cell Disease
    Poliomyelitis
    Werdnig-Hoffmann Disease
Tetanus

Peripheral Motor Nerve

Phrenic Nerve Injury
Guillain-Barré Syndrome

Neuromuscular Junction

Myasthenia Gravis
Botulism

Skeletal Muscle

Muscular Dystrophy
Polymyositis/Dermatomyositis
Congenital Myopathies
Muscle Fatigue

FIGURE 7.1. Anatomical representation of selected neuromuscular disorders associated with respiratory failure in children.

any cardiorespiratory disease resulting in severe hypoxemia or respiratory muscle fatigue can culminate in cessation of breathing. Viral or bacterial infections of the central nervous system (CNS), intracranial hemorrhage, acute hydrocephalus, or other conditions associated with acute intracranial hypertension can trigger hypoventilation or apnea. The precise role of gastroesophageal reflux in pathogenesis of apnea is controversial.

In order to evaluate central hypoventilation syndrome definitively, monitoring of respiratory patterns during sleep is necessary. Continuous recording of the following physiologic variables is recommended: (a) heart rate and respiratory rate; (b) chest and/or abdominal excursions with techniques such as impedance pneumography; (c) arterial oxygenation, with transcutaneous oximetry or comparable monitoring used; (d) respiratory gas flow at the airway opening, via tidal CO_2 thermal recording; and (e) sleep state, with electroencephalography and/or electronystagmography used.

Management

Management of patients with central hypoventilation syndrome include several therapeutic approaches (Table 7.1). Pharmacologic agents directed at stimulating respiratory drive have generated mixed results. Generally, drugs that act by increasing the sensitivity of medullary centers of respiration to the effects of blood carbon dioxide tension have yielded inconsistent results in congenital forms of central hypoventilation, although the salutary effects of agents such as theophylline and progesterone have been noted in some trials.

Agents that stimulate peripheral chemoreceptor sensitivity may be more effective. Intravenous doxapram has improved respiratory drive in some cases, although severe gastrointestinal side effects have been reported. Recently, almitrine has been employed on a limited basis with some success. However, the role of these agents in the long-term management of central hypoventilation syndrome requires further investigation.

Chronic mechanical ventilatory support with positive or negative pressure devices has been used successfully in the management of central hypoventilation syndrome. The need for mechanical ventilatory assistance is frequently permanent in genital forms of the disease, although recovery of adequate respiratory function has been reported.

Radiofrequency bilateral phrenic nerve pacing has been performed in children suffering from central hypoventilation, including infants with congenital forms of the disorder. Despite the short-term success of the technique in recent trials, however, it should be stressed that radiofrequency phrenic nerve pacing currently is a highly specialized procedure that is confined to several centers with expertise in the area.

Finally, regardless of the therapeutic approach in central hypoventilation syndrome, particular attention must be directed at the maintenance of adequate oxygenation and carbon dioxide clearance. Otherwise, chronic hypoxemia and hypercapnea may lead to severe, irreversible pulmonary hypertension and death.

TABLE 7.1. ————————————————————————————————
Management of Central Hypoventilation

Pharmacologic CNS stimulation of respiratory drive—Theophylline, progesterone
Pharmacologic peripheral chemoreceptor stimulation—Doxapram, almitrine
Chronic ventilatory support
Phrenic nerve pacing

SPINAL CORD TRAUMA

Fortunately, spinal cord injuries are unusual in children. Although spinal cord injury is associated with multiple medical complications, those attributable to the respiratory system are particularly important.

Pathogenesis

The pathogenesis of acute respiratory failure associated with spinal cord injury is usually multifactorial. Respiratory motor deficits are directly related to the level of spinal injury. High cervical injuries (C1–C2) usually result in early death. Injury to the upper cervical cord at the level of C3–C5 occurs in approximately one-third of children with spinal trauma. These injuries result in loss of diaphragmatic, intercostal, and abdominal muscle function. Accessory muscles of inspiration located in the neck and shoulders remain intact by virtue of their cranial innervation. However, activity of these muscles alone is inadequate to maintain gas exchange, resulting in acute hypoventilation shortly after injury. In younger children, effective spontaneous ventilatory function is virtually absent.

In an equal number of children, injury is sustained at the level of the lower cervical spine, below the origin of the phrenic motor fibers. Lesions in this area result in sparing of the diaphragm with loss of intercostal and abdominal muscle function. Lack of intercostal muscle function results in chest wall instability, a problem that is magnified in younger children with increased compliance of the chest. Thus, diaphragmatic contraction is accompanied by paradoxical chest wall retraction and diminished efficacy of inspiratory efforts.

Acute respiratory failure during the intensive care course of patients with spinal injury can arise as a result of factors unrelated to respiratory muscle deficits. Pulmonary edema is noted occasionally and has been attributed to excessive fluid resuscitation of spinal shock. Frequently, spinal injuries are associated with severe head and/or thoracoabdominal injuries that exacerbate hypoventilation or present as a source of superimposed pulmonary parenchymal disease. Patients with spinal cord injury are also at high risk for aspiration of gastric contents.

Management

The airway should be secured by endotracheal intubation in cases complicated by severe coma, diminished airway reflexes, inability to clear pulmonary or pharyngeal secretions, or frank hypoventilation. After the acute injury, use of depolarizing muscle relaxants such as succinylcholine can cause severe hyperkalemia and acute life-threatening cardiac arrhythmias; therefore, these agents should be avoided beyond the immediate period of resuscitation.

As noted previously, frequently patients with spinal cord injury suffer from associated ventilation/perfusion mismatching. Therefore, supplemental oxygen is frequently required to avoid hypoxemia. The application of continuous positive airway pressure is helpful in reversing the decrease in functional residual capacity and the associated ventilation/perfusion mismatching. Intermittent positive pressure ventilation should be applied in any patient exhibiting difficulty in maintaining adequate alveolar ventilation and normal P_aCO_2. It should be noted that patients who breathe spontaneously and maintain normal blood gases while awake can develop hypoventilation during sleep, presumably due to abnormalities in central respiratory drive. Under these circumstances, positive pressure ventilatory support is required during periods of sleep.

An aggressive regimen of chest physical therapy is necessary to avoid retention of pulmonary secretions. Position changes can be performed by using a mobile-frame bed. However, placement of the patient in the head-down position may result in regurgitation and aspiration of stomach contents. Also, if the diaphragm is flaccid, abdominal loading associated with this position may result in impaired ventilation. Augmentation of the patient's cough with manual abdominal compression can improve tracheal mucus clearance. Suctioning, in patients with spinal cord trauma, occasionally induces exaggerated vagal responses such as bradycardia. These episodes are usually aborted by pretreatment with atropine.

TETANUS

Clinical Features

Tetanus is characterized by severe, painful muscle rigidity and spasms caused by the toxic product of the bacterium *Clostridium tetani*. Involvement of the laryngeal or respiratory muscles can give rise to acute respiratory insufficiency, requiring urgent intervention. Early symptoms are usually attributable to muscle rigidity and spasm. In 50–75% of patients, trismus is noted at the time of clinical presentation. This may be accompanied by nuchal rigidity, generalized body stiffness, irritability, or dysphagia due to pharyngeal and facial muscle dysfunction.

Management

In addition to acute emergencies arising from sympathetic dysfunction, the major focus of intensive care in tetanus is directed at the management of respiratory complications. Several situations that can arise during the course of the disease are associated with respiratory failure. Spasms of the laryngeal muscles can precipitate acute airway obstruction and asphyxia. In addition, muscle spasms of the chest wall and respiratory muscles may interfere with ventilation, either primarily or secondarily, due to retained secretions, atelectasis, and pneumonia. Newborn infants afflicted with tetanus seem to be particularly prone to the development of aspiration pneumonitis.

Tetanic contractions of the laryngeal muscles can result in acute upper airway obstruction. These so-called "respiratory convulsions" often arise unexpectedly and may be associated with severe hypoxemia. Episodes of laryngeal spasm require the prompt cessation of muscle contraction. Succinylcholine is recommended in the setting. Muscle relaxation should be followed immediately by endotracheal intubation. Continued muscle relaxation following intubation is advised to avoid vocal cord damage from recurrent laryngeal spasms. Severe cases of tetanus are characterized by progression of respiratory muscle spasms that ultimately interfere with ventilatory gas exchange. Under these circumstances, the preferred method of management includes the administration of a nondepolarizing muscle relaxant, such as pancuronium or vecuronium, and the provision of controlled positive pressure ventilatory support. Duration of mechanical ventilation varies considerably but generally ranges from 3 to 5 weeks. Because this period is complicated by a high incidence of atelectasis and pneumonia, considerable attention must be directed toward chest physical therapy, frequent postural changes, and tracheal toilet.

Weaning from positive pressure ventilatory support is attempted when heavy sedation and muscle relaxants are no longer required to control severe spasms. This generally occurs 2–4 weeks following the initiation of mechanical ventilation.

Survival following tetanus has improved considerably over the past decade. Once associated with an average death rate of 45–55%, tetanus now carries a fatality rate of 10–20%. The improvement in mortality is particularly gratifying, in that long-term complications following acute convalescence are uncommon.

POLIOMYELITIS

Clinical Features

Poliomyelitis represents an acute viral infection of the CNS that in its severest form results in widespread muscle paralysis and secondary respiratory failure. Sporadic cases still are reported in the United States in immunocompromised patients exposed to live attenuated virus used for active immunization.

The clinical expression of the disease is variable. Depending upon the locality of nervous system involvement, respiratory failure can arise from deficiencies in airway control, clearance of secretions, central control of ventilation, and inspiratory muscle weakness. In acute paralytic poliomyelitis, muscle weakness often progresses with alarming rapidity following the onset of neurologic symptoms. Therefore, patients can initially present to the intensive care unit (ICU) with acute respiratory collapse of unknown etiology. In addition to the acute disease, the paralytic residua of polimyelitis can result in chronic respiratory disability. The first expression of disease usually takes the form of a minor febrile illness lasting 1–2 days. This prodromal illness generally involves symptoms of an upper respiratory infection or gastroenteritis. In less than a week following the onset of the prodromal phase, the patient typically experiences the onset of severe muscle pain, accompanied by fever, headache, irritability, and paresthesia. Patients usually display muscle fasciculations and diminished deep tendon reflexes in affected muscles at the time of presentation. In some cases, this picture progresses to one of total paralysis in as little as several hours.

Several studies are useful in supporting the diagnosis of poliomyelitis. Examination of the cerebrospinal fluid (CSF) shows an elevated protein level and mild pleocytosis with a predominance of polymorphonuclear leukocytes early in the course of the disease; later, mononuclear inflammatory cells are usually found. The causative virus can be isolated from fecal and oropharyngeal specimens. Serologic confirmation of the infection is made by identifying specific antibodies to the poliovirus.

Management

Abnormalities in the control of breathing during acute paralytic poliomyelitis have been well described and have been incriminated as a cause of SIDS in isolated instances. Bulbar palsy can result in loss of airway control due to pharyngeal muscle paralysis and can lead to airway obstruction or aspiration of oropharyngeal secretions. At a minimum, pharyngeal muscle weakness requires meticulous nursing care and feeding precautions to avoid aspiration. With severe bulbar involvement resulting in loss of airway protective reflexes, endotracheal intubation is required. Loss of abdominal muscle function results in severely impaired coughing, difficulty in clearing the airway, and predilection for pneumonia. All of these respiratory complications require endotracheal intubation, mechanical ventilatory support, and chest physical therapy.

Historically, respiratory support in acute paralytic poliomyelitis was provided with a tank respirator or so-called "iron lung." More recently, positive pressure ventilatory techniques have been used. Provision of controlled positive pressure ventilatory support should be maintained in any patient displaying hypoventilation from central or peripheral neurologic manifestations of the disease. Despite the customary prolonged need for airway care and positive pressure ventilatory support, some patients with paralytic disease recover rapidly over the course of a few weeks, precluding the need for tracheostomy. Tracheostomy can be performed electively during the course of the disease in more protracted cases.

Survival in acute paralytic poliomyelitis is the rule, although mortality in pediatric patients can surpass 30%. Also, as note previously, persistent residua of the disease can result in a variety of chronic respiratory difficulties. These include: persistent respiratory insufficiency; vocal cord paralysis; scoliosis and secondary respiratory restriction; and persistent abnormalities in the central control of breathing, resulting in central hypoventilation.

Clearly, selected groups in the United States and other industrialized nations remain susceptible to poliovirus infection, and concern has been expressed over the decreasing prevalence of widespread immunity in certain populations. For these reasons, poliomyelitis should be considered in any child with acute onset of respiratory failure associated with bulbar or respiratory muscle weakness.

GUILLAIN-BARRÉ SYNDROME

Clinical Features

Guillain-Barré syndrome, also known as "acute postinfective neuritis," "acute inflammatory polyradiculoneuropathy," and other eponyms, is an acute inflammatory peripheral neuropathy that affects both adults and children. Although other associated conditions, such as autonomic nervous dysfunction, can produce life-threatening complications during the disease course, mortality associated with Guillain-Barré syndrome is largely attributable to respiratory muscle weakness and secondary respiratory failure.

Classically, the earliest neurologic sign of Guillain-Barré syndrome is weakness in the lower extremities, involving the distal musculature to a greater degree than the proximal musculature. This is followed by progressive ascending paralysis. Sensory symptoms, such as numbness or paresthesias, frequently accompany the early onset of weakness and are distributed distally.

It should be stressed that deviation from the classical presentation and characteristic ascending progression of weakness is not uncommon. For example, a well-described variant involves findings dominated by cranial nerve palsy and/or cerebellar ataxia. Also, >10% of patients present with weakness predominantly in the upper extremities.

Certain diagnostic studies provide supportive evidence for the diagnosis. Particularly noteworthy is the finding of an elevated CSF protein level (>45 mg/100 ml) in the absence of pleocytosis—so-called "albumino-cytologic dissociation." However, although the CSF cell count is generally normal, pleocytosis is encountered in approximately 55% of patients. The majority of patients demonstrate delayed motor conduction 2–3 weeks following onset of the disease, and electromyography is consistent with lower motor neuron disease.

Management

Specific indications for admission to the ICU in patients without frank respiratory failure have not been defined firmly.

In the ICU, management consists, first, of general supportive care directed at preventing complications of immobilization and decreased motor activity. Second, meticulous attention to monitoring the progression of motor weakness, particularly as it affects respiratory muscle function, and appropriate intervention in the event of respiratory failure are imperative. Third, careful observation and intervention for other complicating conditions, such as autonomic dysfunction, are imperative. Finally, consideration should be given to specific therapeutic interventions directed at speeding the onset of recovery and reversing muscle weakness.

The most important aspect of the management of patients with Guillain-Barré syndrome in the ICU involves the care of acute respiratory failure secondary to atelectasis and/or respiratory muscle fatigue. As previously

noted, approximately 20% of children with Guillain-Barré syndrome ultimately progress to frank respiratory failure, requiring mechanical ventilatory assistance. Therefore, frequent assessment of respiratory reserve is
imperative. Recommended techniques for the bedside assessment of respiratory muscle strength in children include determination of forced, or crying,
vital capacity and maximum negative inspiratory pressure. Provision of
mechanical ventilatory assistance should be considered if: (a) forced vital
capacity falls below 15–20 ml/kg, (b) maximum negative inspiratory pressure falls below 20–30 cm H_2O, or (c) alveolar hypoventilation (P_aCO_2 of >
50 torr) ensues. In addition, endotracheal intubation should be performed
whenever there is evidence of retention of pulmonary secretions refractory
to chest physical therapy, weakness of protective reflexes of the airway (i.e.,
cough and gag), or atelectasis.

Previously, tracheostomy was recommended as the preferred method of
airway management in patients with acute respiratory failure requiring
mechanical ventilatory support. More recently, reports of prolonged nasotracheal intubation in children with Guillain-Barré syndrome have suggested that this technique of airway management can be used safely for
several weeks.

Certain complications of Guillain-Barré syndrome are attributable to autonomic dysfunction manifested by swings in peripheral vasomotor tone
and abnormalities in cardiac rhythm. Specific abnormalities include sinus
tachycardia (50%), bradycardia (20%), S-T segment and T wave abnormalities (64%), hypertension (61%), and postural hypotension (43%).

Specific therapy for Guillain-Barré syndrome remains a topic of controversy. Because of the inflammatory nature of the disease, corticosteroids
and adrenal corticotropin have been used in an attempt to improve the
clinical course. However, most of these trials have been performed in an
uncontrolled fashion.

More recently, clinical trials using plasma exchange techniques have been
conducted in the hopes of removing autoimmune factors that have been
incriminated in the pathogenesis of Guillain-Barré syndrome. Early trials
with plasmapheresis have led to anecdotal reports of clinical improvement
in motor function in cases of acute Guillain-Barré syndrome and chronic
relapsing inflammatory neuropathy. Beneficial effects of plasmapheresis were
noted, particularly in patients treated within 7 days of the onset of disease
and in those who subsequently required mechanical ventilation.

MYASTHENIA GRAVIS

Clinical Features

The functional deficiency in muscle strength encountered in patients with
myasthenia gravis is attributed to immunologic interference with neuromuscular transmission associated with acetylcholine receptor antibodies.

Myasthenia gravis takes several forms in the pediatric population; each
is associated with a unique clinical picture, disease course, and pathogenesis. Classical or juvenile myasthenia gravis represents an extension of the

disorder encountered in adults. Onset of disease generally occurs during adolescence, although symptoms have been described in patients as young as 2 years of age.

In the congenital form of myasthenia gravis, onset of symptoms occurs within the first few days of life. Historically, mothers of these patients do not have myasthenia gravis, although a history of the disorder in siblings is common. Respiratory failure associated with this form of the disease is unusual.

On the other hand, neonatal myasthenia gravis can be associated with severe generalized muscle weakness in two-thirds of patients. In this form of childhood myasthenia gravis, involved infants are uniformly born to mothers with myasthenia gravis; indeed, transplacental transmission of antibodies to acetylcholine receptor protein in the neuromuscular junction is believed to account for this disorder.

Management

Although the patient with myasthenia gravis may require intensive care under a variety of circumstances, critical care services are usually needed under two conditions. First, with the introduction of thymectomy as a surgical mode of therapy for juvenile myasthenia gravis, patients may require postoperative intensive care including mechanical ventilatory support. Second, in particularly refractory cases or in cases complicated by progression of muscle weakness or excessive treatment with anticholinesterase therapy, severe respiratory muscle weakness can be encountered, necessitating frequent monitoring of respiratory muscle strength, vigorous chest physical therapy for clearance of pulmonary secretions, or mechanical ventilatory support.

Indications for mechanical ventilatory support in patients with myasthenia gravis include apnea, hypoventilation, or evidence of severe respiratory muscle fatigue. Therefore, frequent assessment of respiratory muscle strength is necessary. Nonspecific indices of respiratory muscle weakness can signal impending respiratory failure and include decreased forced, or crying, vital capacity (<15 mg/kg) and decreased maximum negative inspiratory pressure (<30 cm H_2O). It should be recalled that muscle strength typically deteriorates with repetitive contractions in the myasthenic patient. Therefore, a single, isolated assessment of respiratory muscle strength may not be adequate for detecting impending ventilatory fatigue.

In addition to providing necessary supportive care, management of patients with myasthenia gravis in the ICU should be concerned with specific therapeutic interventions directed at reversing muscle weakness. This is complicated by the fact that respiratory fatigue in the myasthenic patient can be encountered because of excessive or inadequate cholinergic activity at the neuromuscular junction. Specifically, in myasthenic crisis, acute deterioration in muscle strength is attributable to diminished neuromuscular transmission. On the other hand, excessive treatment with anticholinesterase medications can also produce progressive muscle weakness or cholinergic crisis.

Clearly, the management of these two forms of crisis encountered in patients with myasthenia gravis differs markedly. Myasthenic crisis is generally associated with a recent viral illness, surgery, or other systemic stress in a known or previously asymptomatic myasthenic patient. In cases of myasthenic crisis and in newly diagnosed cases of myasthenia, administration of anticholinesterase agents is the primary mode of therapy. Use of the short-acting anticholinesterase, edrophonium, is generally reserved for establishing the diagnosis at the time of initial presentation. Ongoing therapy with longer acting anticholinesterases, such as neostigmine or pyridostigmine, is necessary. Dosage of specific anticholinesterase agents is determined largely by patient response. Administration of anticholinesterase agents usually results in prompt improvement in muscle strength and effort-dependent respiratory functions. Administration of anticholinesterase agents can be associated with bronchoconstriction, and patients should be monitored carefully for this potential complication.

Cholinergic crisis can usually be differentiated from myasthenic crisis by the presence of signs of excessive parasympathetic activity. These include lacrimation, salivation, diarrhea, and bradycardia. Symptoms attributed to excessive parasympathetic activity are usually responsive to atropine administration. Weakness associated with cholinergic crisis frequently responds to the temporary withdrawal of anticholinesterase medications.

Plasmapheresis has been used on a limited basis in adult patients with advanced disease who have severe refractory respiratory failure prior to thymectomy. Preliminary trials with plasmapheresis indicate that the technique is highly effective in improving muscle strength and decreasing the duration of postoperative mechanical ventilatory support in severely affected patients. Definition of the precise role of plasma exchange techniques in the management of myasthenia gravis requires further study.

BOTULISM
Clinical Features

Botulism is an acute paralytic disorder characterized by disruption of neuromuscular transmission by the neurotoxin elaborated by *Clostridium botulinum*. This bacterial toxin causes diffuse muscle weakness that often culminates in loss of protective airway reflexes and respiratory muscle function. Botulism can be encountered in the pediatric population in several settings defined by the specific portal of entry of the botulinum toxin. In all forms, a prolonged course of respiratory failure characteristically ensues, requiring mechanical ventilatory support in addition to general supportive care.

Botulism is classified clinically into several categories, based on the portal of entry of the botulinum toxin. In classical food-borne botulism, toxin is ingested with food that has been contaminated by the organism and processed under anaerobic conditions. In older children and adults, ingestion of the ubiquitous organism itself does not cause disease. Approximately 75% of cases are associated with the ingestion of home-canned foods. Symptoms usually appear within 36 hours of ingestion of the toxin. Anticholinergic effects of the toxin on the gastrointestinal tract account for the early symptoms of nausea, vomiting, colicky abdominal pain, and constipation. Generalized motor weakness progresses in a descending, symmetrical fashion, which, in severe cases, ultimately affects the respiratory musculature, resulting in hypoventilation and acute respiratory failure. In patients with respiratory failure, the need for mechanical ventilatory support generally lasts from 2 weeks to 3 months. Significantly longer periods are required for total recovery; indeed, persistent motor abnormalities occurring up to 13 months after initial presentation have been reported.

As the name implies, wound botulism is caused by contamination of a wound by clostridial organisms, followed by elaboration of the neurotoxin at the wound site. In this rare form of botulism, toxin is transported to the target sites in the peripheral nervous system from the wound; therefore, early gastrointestinal symptoms are not encountered. The usual incubation period from the time of the initial wound is approximately 7 days but ranges from 4 to 14 days. In this form of botulism, early symptoms arise from bulbar palsy; complaints of diplopia, ptosis, and dysphagia are common. Nearly all cases have been reported following injury to an extremity.

Infant botulism represents a form of the disease that is unique to the pediatric population. Presently, it accounts for the majority of cases reported in children. Initially recognized in 1976, infant botulism has received considerable attention both as a cause of respiratory insufficiency in infants and as a consideration in SIDS. As previously noted, a unique feature of infant botulism is the intestinal portal of entry of the toxin formed in vivo by ingested organisms. Consumption of contaminated honey has been implicated in some cases.

Constipation caused by the parasympatholytic effects of the toxin is the most frequent early symptom; presentation usually occurs several days after its onset. By this time, evidence of neuromuscular dysfunction characteristically has appeared, resulting in poor feeding, lethargy, and generalized hypotonia. In very severe cases, infant botulism can mimic SIDS.

The diagnosis of all forms of botulism is primarily based on clinical recognition of the signs and symptoms in conjunction with appropriate confirmatory testing. An acute motor disorder with early bulbar involvement followed by descending symmetrical muscle weakness should suggest botulism. Serum electrolytes and CSF examination typically are normal. Electrophysiologic studies can be particularly helpful in diagnosing botulism; electromyography shows the typical pattern of "brief, small amplitude, overly abundant motor unit action potentials."

ICU care includes the careful delivery of general supportive care. Oral feedings should be avoided because of the high risk of aspiration pneumonia. The anticholinergic effects of botulinum toxin on the urinary bladder may cause urinary retention and require bladder decompression.

Recommendations for the treatment of botulism with equine antitoxin vary. In cases of wound and food-borne botulism, administration of trivalent botulinum antitoxin is usually recommended. However, use of the horse-serum antitoxin in infant botulism has been avoided because of its lack of proven efficacy and the relatively high incidence of anaphylactic complications.

Respiratory Management

Indications for the initiation of mechanical ventilatory support in botulism are the same as those in other cases of respiratory failure associated with peripheral neuromuscular disease. Specifically, alveolar hypoventilation and hypercarbia are absolute indications for mechanical ventilatory support. Signs of severe third cranial nerve dysfunction have been linked to the eventual development of respiratory muscle failure.

In older patients, monitoring of forced vital capacity and maximum negative inspiratory pressure provides a means for assessing respiratory muscle strength at the bedside. Deterioration in these parameters serves as an early indication of impending respiratory failure and the need to institute mechanical ventilatory support.

Given appropriate respiratory support, recovery from all forms of botulism is the rule. Mortality in this disease currently stands at <10%, largely due to the timely institution and maintenance of appropriate respiratory support. As previously noted, the duration of assisted ventilation varies considerably, ranging from several days to months. Aggressive physical therapy during the period of support is mandatory to avoid respiratory complications, such as atelectasis and pneumonia.

CHAPTER 8

Myocardial Ischemia and Cyanosis

MYOCARDIAL ISCHEMIA IN CHILDREN

Classically, the pediatrician tends to ignore myocardial ischemia as a pathophysiologic process in critically ill children. Recently, it has been increasingly recognized that myocardial ischemia, angina, myocardial infarction, and ischemic coronary artery disease occur in children of all ages. Although the leading causes of ischemic heart disease (IHD) in children (Table 8.1) are different from those in adults (which is, of course, atherosclerotic coronary artery disease), the physiologic factors underlying myocardial oxygen consumption and oxygen delivery are the same.

Determinants of Myocardial Oxygen Consumption

Hemodynamic function is determined by cardiac output and vascular resistance. Cardiac output, in turn, depends on the product of heart rate and stroke volume, which is determined by preload, afterload, and myocardial contractility. Not surprisingly, all of the determinants of overall hemodynamic function also have distinct effects on myocardial oxygen consumption ($M\dot{V}O_2$). Simplistically, $M\dot{V}O_2$ depends on how much work the myocardium must perform; however, not all myocardial "work" is as expensive in terms of metabolic demand. Understanding the underlying determinants of $M\dot{V}O_2$ is the basis for avoiding and treating myocardial ischemia.

In summary, the major factors that influence $M\dot{V}O_2$ are:

1. Myocardial wall tension
2. Contractile state of the heart
3. Heart rate
4. External work load

Of course, these are interdependent and alterations in one can have complex effects on overall $M\dot{V}O_2$ by altering these other factors. In children, increases in $M\dot{V}O_2$ may cause myocardial ischemia, which may be significant during tachydysrhythmias, or during increased work load, as in valvular heart disease or pulmonary hypertension.

TABLE 8.1. ————————————————————————
Causes of Myocardial Ischemia in Children

Neonatal IHD
Asphyxia neonatorum
Increased demand
   Persistent transitional circulation
   Pulmonary hypertension, i.e., respiratory distress syndrome, meconium
     aspiration

Congenital heart disease
Cyanotic heart disease
   Total anomalous pulmonary veins
   Transposition of great vessels
Obstructive disease
   Aortic or pulmonary stenosis
Anomalous coronary arteries

Increased demand
Catecholamine-induced ischemia, i.e., isoproterenol treatment of asthma
Head injury

Vascular disease
Kawasaki disease
Infantile periartereitis nodosa
Embolism
Atheroma (rare)
Trauma
Trauma and head injury

Myocardial Oxygen Supply

If myocardial oxygen supply were infinite, increases in $M\dot{V}O_2$ would be irrelevant. Occasionally, even in the infant's and child's heart, myocardial oxygen supply may be compromised or even a normal supply may be inadequate to meet an increased need. In order to understand oxygen balance, the factors regulating oxygen delivery must be understood. These factors are:

1. Arterial oxygen content
2. Coronary perfusion pressure
3. Coronary artery patency

In any vascular bed, perfusion is determined by perfusion pressure (inflow pressure minus outflow pressure) and vascular resistance. The vascular resistance is, in turn, determined by intrinsic factors (e.g., vascular tone, blood viscosity) and extrinsic factors (e.g., external compression). In the heart, perfusion pressure for the left ventricle is usually defined as aortic pressure minus ventricular pressure. Clearly, both of these pressures vary throughout the cardiac cycle, and thus, phasic flow variation would be expected. The coronary vascular resistance is, as in all vascular beds, autoregulated and subject to metabolic demand but, in addition, is subjected to dramatic external compression due to cardiac contraction.

Neonatal Ischemic Heart Disease

Previously, myocardial ischemia and infarction were believed to be a rare occurrence in neonates and infants and then to occur only in those children with congenital heart disease. Recently, it has become increasingly evident that in stressed neonates, even with normal coronaries and in the absence of congenital anomalies, myocardial ischemia and necrosis are not uncommon and may even be a significant factor in the mortality of acutely ill infants. The occurrence of myocardial ischemia and necrosis in these infants is perhaps less surprising than expected when the underlying pathophysiology is considered. the unusual stresses imposed on the transitional circulation perinatally can lead to both increased myocardial oxygen demand and impaired oxygen delivery. Superimposition of hypoxia, hypovolemia, sepsis, and respiratory distress during this period can severely impair myocardial perfusion.

Unfortunately, the clinical picture of IHD in neonates is not sharply delineated from other causes of neonatal respiratory distress. The picture is one of hypoxemia with heart failure characterized by cardiomegaly, tricuspid or mitral insufficiency, and cardiogenic shock. Frequently, there is electrocardiographic evidence of ischemia with right ventricular hypertrophy, S-T segment depression, T wave inversion, and even frank myocardial infarction (Fig. 8.1). In addition, creatine phosphokinase (CK-MB) may be

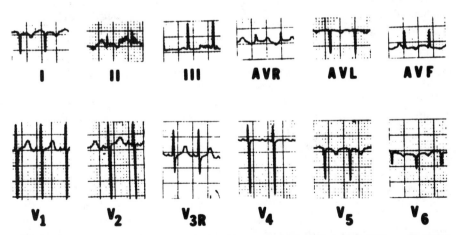

FIGURE 8.1. Electrocardiogram of a 13-day-old neonate. Note Qs in I, V_5, and V_6, and inverted T waves in I, II, AVL, AVF, V_5, and V_6, which are consistent with inferolateral myocardial infarction. (From Kilbride H, Way GL, Merenstein GB, Winfield JM: Myocardial infarction in the neonate with normal heart and coronary arteries. *Am J Dis Child* 134:759, 1980, ©1980, American Medical Association.)

elevated, although this is a less reliable indicator in children than in adults. The differential diagnosis includes structural heart diseases such as total anomalous pulmonary venous drainage, hypoplastic left heart syndromes, and anomalous origin of the coronary arteries. Angiography and radionuclide imaging may be helpful.

Myocardial Ischemia Associated with Congenital Heart Disease

It is unusual to consider myocardial ischemia in managing children with congenital heart disease, although, logically, hypertrophy, cyanosis, increased hematocrit (Hct), and the fequency of the postoperative state would suggest that ischemia would frequently occur. This is supported by the occurrence of right ventricular infarction in total anomalous pulmonary venous drainage, left ventricular infarction in aortic stenosis, and biventricular infarction in transposition of the greater arteries. In patients with aortic stenosis and pulmonary stenosis, almost certainly another contributing factor is increased intraventricular pressures and, thus, decreased coronary perfusion pressure. Hyperviscosity and hypoxemia due to cyanotic heart disease are also probable contributing factors. Although electrocardiographic evidence of myocardial infarction is only present in half of the patients, it is clear that significant myocardial ischemia and, possibly, fatal myocardial occurs in many patients with congenital heart disease.

Anomalous Origin of Coronary Arteries from the Pulmonary Artery

The anomalous origin of a coronary artery results developmentally from abnormal formation of the bulbospiral septum in the truncus arteriosus. The origin of one or both of the coronary arteries may, therefore, be included in the pulmonary artery. Anomalous origin of the right coronary artery is generally benign, as the low-pressure right ventricle appears to be adequately supplied by this right coronary artery with additional left coronary artery collaterals. Anomalous origin of both coronary arteries is very rare and uniformly rapidly fatal. It is the chance for prolonged survival, surgical correction, and early recognition that focuses the majority of interest on the anomalous origin of the left coronary artery.

Clinical Features

In the first few months of life, the infants seem normal. The symptoms fall into three categories: (a) recurrent respiratory infections, (b) discomfort, and (c) heart failure. Although failure may be the first presenting symptom, there is frequently a history of irritability, screaming (especially with feeds), drawing up of the legs, apparent anxiety, pain, pallor, and sweating—all most likely due to anginal symptoms.

The most useful diagnostic tool is the electrocardiogram (ECG), which usually reveals a pattern that is consistent with an anterior myocardial infarction pattern characterized by a Q-R pattern and inverted T waves in I and aVL. Frequently, a left ventricular hypertrophy pattern is seen with deep Qs in V_5 and V_6 and S-T changes in the precordial leads. Radio-nuclide imaging will reveal myocardial hypoperfusion, and angiography will define the anatomy.

In addition to this classic presentation, older children may also present to the intensive care unit (ICU). The authors have seen several children with acute onset of chest pain (often during exercise) and electrocardiographic evidence of ischemia who, despite no previous symptoms, have had an anomalous origin of a coronary artery. This condition must be considered for children with chest pain, ischemia, or infarction and potentially in every child with the acute onset of a dysrhythmia.

Therapy

Medical management directed at initial resuscitation and stabilization traditionally includes oxygen, digoxin, fluids, and diuretics. Logical extension of the therapy in adults would indicate that optimizing fluid balance, afterload reduction, and nitrates could be useful. The definitive therapy requires surgical intervention.

Catecholamine-Induced Ischemia

Whereas the previous examples of myocardial ischemia have largely dealt with defects in substrate delivery, theoretically, increased myocarial oxygen demand also could lead to ischemia. Clinical experience and reports have supported the existence, in fact, of myocardial ischemia in asthmatic children receiving isoproterenol (Fig. 8.2).

The underlying cause for this is almost certainly multifactorial. In untreated status asthmaticus, desaturation and acidosis occur and may adversely affect myocardial oxygen balance. In addition, quite negative intrapleural pressures occur and are associated with profound cardiorespiratory interactions, the overall effect of which is to increase ventricular afterload and, thus, oxygen consumption. The addition of isoproterenol to this picture has several effects. Increased heart rate and enhanced myocardial contractility may dramatically increase $M\dot{V}O_2$ while they may compromise delivery by a direct β_2-adrenergic vascular effect, lowering diastolic pressure.

The use of epinephrine and norepinephrone also poses a threat to myocardial oxygen balance. Isoproterenol's marked salutary effects in status asthmaticus need to be balanced against the possibility of induced myocardial ischemia. Furthermore, theophylline also increases $M\dot{V}O_2$ and, in animals, can lead to myocardial necrosis. It is conceivable that theophylline and isoproterenol present an additive challenge to the myocardium in these patients.

Kawasaki Disease

Clinical Picture

The clinical picture of Kawasaki disease consists of three well-defined phases: (a) the acute febrile stage, which usually lasts 1–2 weeks; (b) a subacute phase, and (c) a convalescent phase occurring usually after 6

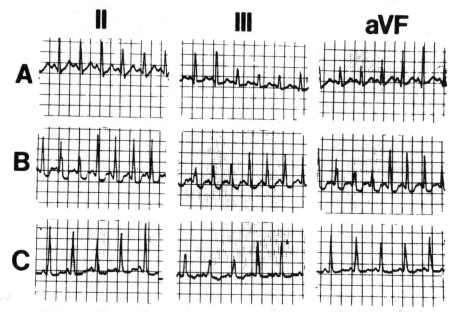

FIGURE 8.2.   Three ECG leads at different times in the child described in the text. *A:* Before intravenous isoproterenol but 25 minutes after chest pain during isoproterenol aerosol. *B:* During isoproterenol infusion. *C:* 20 minutes after discontinuing infusion. Note profound S-T depression and T wave changes during isoproterenol administration. (From Matson JR, Loughlin GM, Strunk RC: Myocardial ischemia complicating the use of isoproterenol in asthmatic children. *J Pediatr* 92:776, 1978.)

weeks. The diagnosis of Kawasaki disease rests on identification of the following six criteria, at least five of which are required for diagnosis:

1. Cervical lymphadenopathy, with a hard tender lymph node mass of >1.5 cm that frequently may be unilateral
2. Mucosal changes in the oropharynx, often with bleeding, cracked lips, fissuring, pharyngeal hyperemia, and a strawberry tongue
3. A spiking remittent fever of 101–104°F, lasting for more than 5 days and usually for approximately 2 weeks
4. Conjunctival involvement with edema and injection of both the bulbar and palpebral conjunctiva
5. Deep red erythema of the palms and soles, accompanied by induration and edema of the hands and feet, which often limit the ability to walk; frequently followed by periungual desquamation approximately 2 weeks after the onset of the illness
6. An erythematous rash that is polymorphous, nonvesiculated, generally pruritic, migratory, occasionally urticarial, and usually truncal

Other manifestations of Kawasaki disease include aseptic meningitis (25%), diarrhea (40%), meatal ulceration (20%), urethritis (25%), arthralgia (30%), and sporadic central nervous system (CNS) involvement with symptoms of lethargy and emotional irritability. Much more rarely, hydrops of the gall-bladder, jaundice, uveitis, hepatitis, pleural and pericardial effusions, and pneumonia occur.

Cardiac Involvement

The most serious feature of Kawasaki disease is, by far, myocardial and coronary artery involvement. Although, as mentioned previously, only 20% of children affected by Kawasaki disease clinically demonstrate cardiac involvement, the heart is affected in an least 40% of all cases, and cardiac involvement is the primary cause of death in 2% of all children with Kawasaki disease. Autopsy studies invariably demonstrate coronary artery involvement. Unfortunately, fatal cardiac complications can arise in patients initially free of clinical cardiac symptomatology. These considerations mandate careful observation and ECG monitoring, best performed in a pediatric ICU.

The chest X-ray is frequently normal, although pneumonitis has been reported in a few patients. Cardiomegaly, due to either left ventricular failure or hypertrophy, and pericardial effusions may occasionally occur during the second or third week. Other noninvasive diagnostic tests designed specifically to detect underlying cardiac abnormalities and an ECG are essential and may show the abnormalities mentioned previously. M-mode echocardiography has been reported to detect a subset of children who develop coronary aneurysms; it probably should be serially performed in children with Kawasaki disease. In addition, echocardiographic abnormalities of ventricular wall motion appear to be sensitive indicators of cardiac involvement in Kawasaki disease.

Pathology

The pathologic evolution of Kawasaki disease seems to undergo four distinct stages. *Stage 1* (<10 days) shows a panvasculitis of the microcirculation and includes the coronary arteries. Acute myocarditis, pericarditis, and endocarditis with valvulitis are evident. In *stage 2* (11–28 days), aneurysm formation and coronary artery stenosis with persistence of pancarditis are found. In *stage 3* (28–45 days), global evidence of myocardial ischemia with thrombosis and intimal proliferation is obvious. The pancarditis is resolving and the vasculitis is absent. During *stage 4* (>50 days), resolution of the ravages of the first three stages in the coronary circulation is seen with calcifications, stenosis, scarring, recannulization, and chronic aneurysm formation. Endocardial fibroelastosis and ischemic myocardial changes are prominent.

Treatment

Without question, the therapy for Kawasaki disease includes prompt treatment with aspirin at a dose of 100 mg/kg/day at the earliest possible time, followed by prolonged treatment with 30 mg/kg/day during the convalescent stage. Recently, in a multicenter study it was concluded that high-dose intravenous γ-globulin is safe and effective in reducing the prevalence of coronary artery abnormalities when given early in the course of this syndrome. Steroids are no longer recommended.

Trauma

Several forms of injury can accompany chest injuries, including myocardial contusions, myocardial concussions (commotio cordis), valvular damage, rupture, and coronary vascular occlusion, and frequently the diagnosis is missed. The long-term results include myocardial scarring, arrhythmias, and ventricular aneurysms. Although direct myocardial injury occurs, some have speculated that coronary vascular lesions result in trauma-associated damage. Certainly, traumatic coronary artery aneurysm occurs, and the authors have seen acute coronary occlusion following trauma. In the setting of trauma, unexplained hemodynamic compromise should suggest the possibility of myocardial damage or ischemia. ECG, enzymes, and echocardiography may provide useful diagnostic information, but it seems that radionuclide angiography is the most sensitive test to discover traumatic myocardial dysfunction.

CYANOSIS

Cyanosis is "a bluish purple discoloration of the mucous membranes and skin, due to excess amounts of reduced hemoglobin in capillaries, or less frequently to the presence of methemoglobin." The presence of 4–5 g of reduced hemoglobin per 100 ml of blood is necessary to produce the cyanosis. "Any state where a physiologically inadequate amount of oxygen is available to, or utilized by, tissue without respect to cause or degree" is referred to as hypoxia. The presence of cyanosis is clinically significant because it implies severely decreased oxygen content of blood (hypoxemia), an important consequence of which is inadequate oxygen delivery to tissues for metabolic needs (hypoxia). A review of the physiologic causes of cyanosis is presented in Table 8.2.

Evaluation

The variety of clinical situations that can lead to cyanosis requires a methodical approach for efficiently evaluating the affected patient. That is one of the purposes of the entire book. An extremely shortened conceptual approach is all that can be presented here.

History

A history is important not only for detection of congenital defects but also for beginning the process by which a decision is made as to whether the current episode is an acute problem, a chronic problem, or both. A history of cyanotic congenital heart disease does not ensure that the current episode of cyanosis is solely due to that heart disease and not to an episode of aspiration. Even cyanotic children ingest poisons, for example. The history in a patient with obvious cyanosis from pulmonary disease

TABLE 8.2. _____
Physiologic Causes of Cyanosis

Environmental decreased availability of oxygen
Altitude
Inhalation of nonphysiologic gas mixtures

Alveolar hypoventilation
CNS depression (e.g., trauma, drugs, infection)
Upper airway obstruction (e.g., tracheal rings, epiglottitis, etc.)
Hypotonia (e.g., CNS insults, spinal cord insults, drugs)
Restricted lung movement (e.g., diaphragmatic hernia, tension pneumothorax)

Major diffusion abnormalities
Interstitial fibrosis
Oxygen toxicity
Adult respiratory distress syndrome
Pulmonary edema

Abnormalities of hemoglobin and oxygen-carrying capacity
Abnormal hemoglobin (e.g., methemoglobin, carboxyhemoglobin, sulfhemoglobin)
Alterations in oxyhemoglobin affinity (e.g., changes in 2,3-diphosphoglycerate content, pH, temperature)
Too much reduced hemoglobin (e.g., hyperviscosity)

Abnormalities of pulmonary blood flow
Congenital obstruction to heart disease with pulmonary blood flow (and/or right-to-left shunting, e.g., tetralogy of Fallot, pulmonary atresia)
Primary pulmonary hypertension
Persistent fetal circulation
Intracardiac chronic heart disease with right-to-left shunts
Hypotension
Abnormalities of ventilation/perfusion matching
Pharmacologic effects, e.g., sodium nitroprusside

Poor tissue perfusion
Shock with inadequate compensation for tissue perfusion (e.g., septic, hemorrhagic, cardiac etiology)
Impaired rheology (hyperviscosity)

_____

may seem irrelevant if the patient looks as if he or she has pneumonia, but a history may reveal an underlying immune deficiency or other additional cause of the cyanosis.

Physical Examination

The physical examination also can often clarify the reason for the cyanosis. The presence of gastric contents in the nostrils or pharynx suggests aspiration. This may be the primary cause of the cyanosis or secondary to it. Cyanosis with hypotonia, apnea, or bradypnea is commonly associated with CNS disorders caused by asphyxia or infection, with neuromuscular disease, or with effects of pharmacologic agents. Clubbing of the digits indicates hypoxia of several months' duration. Signs of progressive hyperviscosity include plethora, lethargy, tachycardia, tachypnea, grunting, and retractions. More dramatic evidence of the polycythemia-hyperviscosity syndrome is the presence of nonspecific neurologic abnormalities as well as arterial or venous thromboses, including those in intracranial sites.

The respiratory pattern may be helpful in diagnosing the cause of cyanosis. Tachypnea, use of accessory muscles, retractions, stridor, and grunting are usually mainfestations of pulmonary pathology. Nasal obstruction can produce a snorty respiratory sound; laryngeal obstruction is frequently associated with inspiratory stridor; and bronchial and lower airway obstruction can produce expiratory wheezing. However, localization of the obstruction is sometimes difficult in the neonate, who may show similar signs in the presence of many causes of airway obstruction. Asymmetrical chest movements may occur because of bronchial obstruction, pneumothorax, diaphragmatic injury, or mass lesions. Inadequate muscular effort and air movement suggest a neuromuscular disorder or drug effect as the cause of the cyanosis. No monitoring equipment in the pediatric ICU can substitute for a physical examination in detecting findings of this type.

The cardiac examination may suggest the cause and extent of cyanosis. Rate, location, and characteristics of precordial impulses, intensity of pulses, and blood pressure in the upper and lower extremities should be noted. Although tachycardia is common in patients with cyanosis of any cause, the development of bradycardia is a prognostic sign suggestive of profound cyanosis. A shift of the maximal impulse may occur as a result of ventricular hypoplasia or hypertrophy related to valvular or septal abnormalities or as a result of cardiac malposition (dextrocardia). The presence of a murmur may also indicate congenital heart disease, but it is important to remember that right-to-left shunts by themselves do not produce murmurs, since the flow required would be incompatible with life. This fact is important in certain disease states such as profound respiratory failure in the neonatal period when an enormous ductal flow producing a massive right-to-left shunt is inaudible. The specifics of cyanotic spells are covered below.

Examination of the abdomen may be diagnostic. A scaphoid contour indicates that abdominal contents have possibly been displaced into the thorax because of diaphragmatic herniation. Bowel sounds heard on auscultation of the chest add further support to this diagnosis. Hepatomegaly is suggestive of congestive heart failure as the cause of the cyanosis.

Although not commonly remembered, examination of the musculoskeletal system may be vital in the evaluation of a patient with cyanosis. Fractured bones, particularly long bones, can produce fat emboli which clearly can occur in children. Thromboembolism is generally more frequent in adults than in children, but pulmonary emboli also occur in children and have resulted in patients with cyanosis in our pediatric ICU.

CNS causes of cyanosis are well known but are not always considered. Isolated head trauma can produce both CNS-induced pulmonary edema and intrapulmonary shunting from alterations in neural control of matching pulmonary ventilation and flow.

Cyanotic Spells

Patients with cyanotic congenital heart defects, particularly with tetralogy of Fallot, may develop an alarming complication known by various names including "cyanotic spells," "paroxysmal hyperpnea," "tet spells," "hypoxic spells," "anoxic spells," "blue spells," or "syncopal episodes." These episodes are characterized by paroxysmal hyperpnea and increased cyanosis. Patients often proceed to exhibit limpness, generalized stiffness, and rolling back of the eyes. Systemic acidosis accompanies these attacks. Occasionally, convulsions, cerebral vascular accidents, and/or death may also occur. In the early stages, a patient may spontaneously assume the squatting (or knee-chest) position in order to alleviate the symptoms.

Patients range in age from 1 month to 12 years, with the peak incidence occurring in patients between 1 and 3 months of age. Although the paroxysms may occur at any time, the majority occur in the morning, usually upon awakening. The duration of an episode ranges from minutes to several hours, with most lasting 15–60 minutes. Several factors precipitating the attacks have been identified. Most commonly, these are crying, defecation, and feeding. There seems to be no correlation between the resting P_aO_2 and the incidence of the attacks.

Several causes have been suggested for the episodes, including spasm of the pulmonary infundibulum, acute rises in pulmonary vascular resistance (PVR), and sudden decrease in systemic vascular resistance (SVR). Regardless, the result is an increased ratio of PVR to SVR, with a decrease in pulmonary blood flow relative to systemic flow. In a normal person, hyperpnea is associated with a reduced P_aCO_2, an elevated P_aO_2, and an increased output from both the left and the right ventricle. In patients with decreased pulmonary blood flow, including those with tetralogy of Fallot, the response is altered. Although the cardiac output increases and systemic venous return also rises, the pulmonary flow can decrease. This results in a greater oxygen demand, an increase in P_aCO_2, a decrease in P_aO_2, and acidosis. Medical responses to cyanotic spells are covered in the section of this chapter dealing with therapy.

Laboratory Tests

Laboratory tests should complete the evaluation of cyanotic patients. Elevated hemoglobin (Hb) and/or Hct suggests the possibility of polycythemia. In infants and children, polycythemia may be secondary to hypoxia of cardiac, pulmonary, or other etiology. An elevated or depressed white cell count, with or without an increase in immature forms, implicates infections. A sample of blood drawn from a patient with suspected methemoglobin can be placed on filter paper and exposed to air. The blood will appear to be chocolate-brown after a few minutes.

Serum or blood glucose and calcium levels should be determined. Hypoglycemia is defined as blood glucose of ≤40 mg/100 ml in infants older than 4 days. However, between birth and 3 days of age, levels of <20 mg/100 ml on two determinations in premature infants and of 30 mg/100 ml in term infants are considered to be indicative of hypoglycemia. Calcium levels are normally in the range of 10 mg/100 ml; the ionized calcium is approximately 5 mg/100 ml. At levels of <3−4 mg ionized calcium, the patient may display symptoms of hypocalcemia, including cyanosis.

Arterial blood gas determinations provide important clues to the etiology of cyanosis. The P_aCO_2 is usually decreased in cyanosis of cardiac origin because of hypoxia-triggered tachypnea in the presence of normal gas exchange. Pulmonary disease associated with cyanosis indicates respiratory failure, which results in a normal or elevated P_aCO_2 despite the associated tachypnea. Most often, cyanosis is associated with hypoxic conditions and low P_aO_2. Commonly, in hypoxia due to hypoventilation or pulmonary disease, inspiration of 100% oxygen elevates the P_aO_2 significantly (>100−150 mm Hg). In the case of congenital cardiac defects, the response to 100% inspired O_2 may be minimal because of the effects of right-to-left shunts. Cyanosis may also be present in the face of a normal P_aO_2. This apparent paradox occurs in patients with polycythemia because of the desaturated blood normally present in the venous circulation as well as in smoke inhalation with carboxyhemoglobin elevation.

X-rays of the chest may provide extremely valuable information. Both anteroposterior and lateral X-rays should be obtained. Symmetry of the lung fields should be noted. Classic signs of pneumothorax, pulmonary parenchymal disease, lobar emphysema, or hyaline membrane disease may be apparent. A bowel gas pattern in the chest and a "gasless" abdomen point to diaphragmatic hernia. An elevated diaphragm is seen with eventration. Evaluation of pulmonary bloody flow should be conducted to determine whether it is elevated or decreased. This can be extremely helpful in differentiating certain cardiac lesions. The cardiac silhouette may prove helpful in the diagnosis of congenital heart disease in a cyanotic patient. A normal-sized heart with a cocked-up apex (couer-en-sabot or boot shape) caused by right ventricular dominance is the pathognomonic sign of tetralogy of Fallot. Commonly, the mediastinal shadow is narrow, the pulmonary vascular markings are decreased, and a right aortic arch is present in 25% of cases.

An ECG should be obtained on all cyanotic patients. Most patients with cyanosis of noncardiac etiology are expected to have a normal ECG. However, a child with upper airway obstruction or chronic hypoxia from other causes may develop cor pulmonale which would manifest as right-axis deviation and right ventricular strain and hypertrophy. A prolonged Q-T interval is observed in hypocalcemia. A decrease in body temperature below

30°C induces lengthening of all time intervals—R-R, P-R, QRS, and Q-T; and "J deflections" may be obvious in the midprecordial leads.

The use of the echocardiogram has been increasingly useful in patients with cyanosis. It has, of course, been instrumental in the diagnosis of anatomic cause of heart disease. It has also been used, with increasing sophistication, to localize and to quantitate shunts.

There are, of course, an unlimited number of tests that can be performed on cyanotic patients. In this era of concern about medical costs, we must be conscious of the fact that the history and physical examination must determine which laboratory tests are indicated, instead of the other way around.

Therapeutic Considerations
Cardiac

Successful management of congestive heart failure requires prompt identification of the underlying cause. In the interim, the patient should be resting in a semisitting position. Supplemental oxygen should be administered, and ventilatory support should be instituted as dictated by the clinical evaluation. Total fluid intake is usually restricted to maintenance and replacement of urinary output. Most patients with congestive heart failure also require pharmacologic treatment. Digoxin administration may improve myocardial performance and may yield a higher cardiac output. Guidelines and dosage schedules used in the authors' institution are presented in Table 8.3. Careful and regular monitoring of the ECG, monitoring of serum levels of digoxin and electrolytes, and monitoring of renal function are all required to prevent digoxin toxicity. Diuretic agents may be necessary in cases of severe congestive heart failure, to accelerate water excretion. However, serum levels of sodium, potassium, chloride, and bicarbonate must be monitored closely in order to prevent electrolyte disturbances caused by these agents.

Additional therapeutic measures may be necessary if initial therapy of congestive heart failure proves insufficient. Intravenous sympathomimetics, e.g., dopamine or isoproterenol, can improve cardiac output. Sedation with morphine (0.05 mg/kg) or diazepam (0.1 mg/kg) may decrease metabolic demands but must raise concerns about respiratory depression. In addition to the sedative effect, morphine produces systemic vasodilatation and increases cardiac output. In this setting, many pediatric intensivists are using vasodilators, with good results. If the congestive failure is still inadequately controlled with medical therapy, corrective or palliative surgery of the underlying cardiac defect, which may have been scheduled for a later date, will need to be performed.

Cyanotic Spells

Treatment of cyanotic spells is aimed at improving the arterial P_aO_2 and acidosis by decreasing obstruction to right ventricular outflow, improving

TABLE 8.3.
Digoxin Therapy[a]

Preparation	Route of Administration	Effect		Total Excretion	Oral Absorption	Digitalizing Dose	Daily Maintenance Dose
		Maximum Onset	Duration				
Digoxin (lanoxin) Available in Tablets (mg): 0.125 0.25 0.5 Elixir (mg/ml): 0.05 Ampules (mg/ ml): 0.1 0.25	i.v. i.m. p.o.	5–30 min 15–60 min 1–2 hr	2–5 hr 2–5 hr 4–8 hr	24 hr	48–72 hr	40–90%	p.o. (µg/kg) Preterm: 20–30 Full term: 25–35 1–24 months: 35–60 2–5 yr: 30–40 5–10 yr: 20–35 10 yr–adult: 10–15 i.m. or i.v. (µg/kg) Preterm: 15–25 Full term: 20–30 1–24 months: 30–50 2–5 yr: 25–35 5–10 yr: 15–30 10 yr–adult: 8–12	p.o. (µg/kg) Preterm: 20–30% of oral loading dose Full term to adult: 25–35% of oral loading dose Maintenance dose is given q 12 hr i.v. (µg/kg) Preterm: 20–30% of i.v. loading dose Full term to adult: 25–35% of i.v. loading dose

Parenteral digitalizing doses are 80% of oral digitalizing doses; $\frac{1}{2}$ TDD[b] is given stat, then $\frac{1}{4}$ TDD is given q 6–8 hr × 2.

[a] Adapted with permission from Cole CH (ed): *The Harriet Lane Handbook*, ed 10. Chicago, Year Book Medical, 1984, p 132.
[b] TDD, total digitalizing dose.

pulmonary blood flow, and reducing the PVR/SVR ratio. Supplemental oxygen is administered by face mask or oxygen hood. The patient is placed in a knee-chest position, which is physiologically similar to squatting. Squatting has been shown to increase effective pulmonary blood flow and to redistribute systemic flow to the upper body by increasing the SVR. During this maneuver, the arterial oxygen saturation remains unchanged, but the venous saturation increases, implying improved capillary and tissue oxygenation.

Hydration with intravenous fluids should be instituted. Acidosis is corrected by administration of $NaHCO_3$ after a sample for blood gas and pH has been obtained. Initially, the patient may be given $NaHCO_3$ at a dose of 2 mEq/kg (0.5 mEq/ml) over 5 minutes. Subsequent doses may be administered as needed according to the following formula:

$$NaHCO_3 \text{ dose (mEq)} = 0.3 \times \text{body weight (kg)} \times \text{base deficit}$$

Half the dose is given over 30 minutes, and the remainder is given over 4 hours.

Morphine administration (0.1–0.2 mg/kg subcutaneously or intravenously) is often quite effective in relieving a spell. The probable mechanism of action is a reduction of infundibular spasm and improved pulmonary blood flow. β-Adrenergic antagonists given intravenously may also reverse a spasm. Propranolol (0.2 mg/kg intravenously) has been shown to terminate a spell, probably by relaxing the right ventricular outlet. In addition, chronic oral therapy with propranolol (1–2 mg/kg 4 times daily) has been shown to decrease the frequency of the paroxysms. However, the use of propranolol in the newborn is discouraged because it may cause severe cardiac depression.

Pulmonary

Cyanosis may be a result of pulmonary parenchymal disease, such as adult respiratory distress syndrome, hyaline membrane disease, pneumonia, or aspiration. Its presence requires the administration of supplemental oxygen and may necessitate ventilatory support. Such support may take the form of continuous positive airway pressure or mechanical ventilation. These therapeutic measures are discussed at greater length in association with the individual diseases.

Metabolic

Metabolic abnormalities that produce cyanosis should be treated promptly while a concurrent search for cause is begun. Hypothermia can be reversed by the use of warming lights, warm coverings, and adjustment of the ambient temperature. Patients with symptomatic hypoglycemia should receive intravenous glucose. The usual dose of 25% dextrose (50% dextrose diluted 1:1 in sterile water) is 1–2 ml/kg. We avoid direct administration of 50% glucose in order to minimize adverse effects of hyperosmolality.

Therapy for methemoglobinemia (MetHb) starts with general supportive care and removal of any possible toxin. The latter may entail removal of

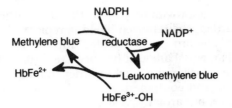

FIGURE 8.3. Conversion of methemoglobin ($HbFe^{3+}$-OH) to hemoglobin ($HbFe^{2+}$).

contaminated clothes, washing of the skin, and emptying of gastric contents with induced emesis or lavage. Because normal mechanisms convert MetHb to Hb over 15–20 hours, no other treatment for toxin-induced MetHb is needed in the absence of hypoxic symptoms. However, if signs of hypoxia are present or the level of MetHb is >30%, drug therapy should be considered. Pharmacologic treatment is aimed at converting the ferric iron (Fe^{3+}) in heme to the ferrous state. The preferred agent is methylene blue (tetramethylthionine chloride), which forms a nicotinamide adenine dinucleotide phosphate (NADPH)-dependent oxidation-reduction system for heme. This is accomplished through activation of NADPH-MetHb reductase, with methylene as a cofactor (Fig. 8.3).

The usual dosage of methylene blue is 1–2 mg/kg (in a 1% solution) administered intravenously over 5 minutes. Most MetHb should be converted within 30–60 minutes. If needed, the dose may be repeated after 1 hour (maximum dose, 7 mg/kg). Side effects are seen with higher doses and include precordial pain, dyspnea, restlessness, tremors, and apprehension. Dysuria and urinary frequency may also be present. High concentrations of methylene blue can occasionally cause mild hemolysis and may actually produce MetHb by reversing the reaction. Failure of methylene blue treatment may require blood transfusion or exchange transfusion therapy. Treatment failure suggests the possibility of glucose 6-phosphate dehydrogenase deficiency or sulfhemoglobinemia, for which no specific therapy exists. Therapy with transfusions, exchange transfusions, or hyperbaric oxygen may alleviate the acute symptoms. This intervention can be followed by treatment with ascorbic acid, which reduces MetHb slowly. Carboxyhemoglobin is generally associated with smoke inhalation, and its evaluation and treatment are covered in Chapter 24.

Treatment of polycythemia and/or hyperviscosity is an attempt to achieve an isovolemic reduction in the erythrocyte count. This is accomplished by performing a partial or "reduction" exchange transfusion. Catheters are placed for the withdrawal and infusion of blood. In the neonate, an umbilical venous or arterial catheter may be used. The total amount of blood to be exchanged is calculated as follows:

$$\text{Exchange volume} = \text{Weight (kg)} \times 85 \text{ ml/kg} \times \frac{\text{observed Hct} - \text{desired Hct}}{\text{observed Hct}}$$

The desired Hct is approximately 55%. Blood is withdrawn in 5–10-ml aliquots and discarded; the removed blood is replaced by an equal volume of plasma solution. The process is repeated until the calculated volume has been removed and an equal amount has been reinfused. The patient's temperature should be closely monitored in order to maintain normothermia. Resuscitation drugs and equipment should be readily accessible if severe hypotension, seizure, or cardiac arrest occurs.

SUMMARY

The traditional cardiology approaches to heart disease are a useful starting point for the intensivist caring for a child with pulmonary edema, myocardial ischemia, or cyanosis in the pediatric ICU. The approaches must be enlarged, however, by a knowledge of the myriad of unusual entities that can cause these conditions in the pediatric ICU patient without congenital heart disease. A knowledge of these entities is absolutely necessary if the intensivist is to be helpful in responding to the care of the children with these unusual but often fascinating conditions.

CHAPTER 9

Unusual Causes of Pulmonary Edema

PHYSIOLOGY OF PULMONARY EDEMA

Although the 1970s and 1980s saw the development of progressively more complex models of water and solute movement across the lung, the traditional principles of Starling are still a good place to begin the discussion of the physical factors determining fluid accumulation in pulmonary edema:

$$\dot{Q} = K_f(P_c - P_t) - \delta(\pi_c - \pi_t)$$

where $\dot{Q}$ equals net rate of flow across a unit surface area of capillary, K_f equals capillary filtration coefficient, P_c equals hydrostatic pressure in capillary, P_t equals hydrostatic pressure in interstitium, π_c equals oncotic pressure in plasma, π_t equals oncotic pressure in interstitium, and δ equals reflection coefficient, which is a measure of the ability of the pulmonary capillary to prevent protein from the plasma from crossing the capillary wall such that if δ equals 0, there is no restriction, while if δ equals 1, restriction is absolute.

In normal patients, the capillary hydrostatic pressure in the pulmonary capillary (P_c) is gravity dependent and, when measured with a pulmonary artery catheter, ranges from 8 to 12 torr. The hydrostatic pressure in the interstitium (P_t) is estimated as -10 torr. In the plasma (π_c) the colloid oncotic pressure is normally 25 torr, whereas in the interstitial fluid (π_t), it is $10-15$ torr. As a result, this balance of forces in the steady state means that there is a continuous filtration of a relatively small amount of fluid out of the vascular space. Because of the relatively low rate of formation of this fluid and the relatively impermeable nature of the alveolar epithelium, this fluid does not enter the alveolar space but is picked up in the interstitial space by the lymphatics.

SEQUENCE OF FORMATION OF PULMONARY EDEMA

A simple analysis of a Starling's equation approach to pulmonary edema would suggest that there are only two kinds of pulmonary edema: (a) cardiogenic-hydrostatic edema, which develops in the face of heart failure and increased pressure in the pulmonary capillaries, and (b) noncardiac edema,

103

caused by increased permeability of the pulmonary capillaries. In traditional hydrostatic edema, the time course of fluid accumulation described previously is generally slow and is related to the increased hydrostatic pressure in the capillaries. The fluid itself is traditionally thought of as low in protein. On the other hand, when there is capillary injury and increased permeability, the onset of edema can be very rapid, even in the face of normal hydrostatic pressure. Naturally, the increased capillary permeability allows the leakage of large-molecular-weight compounds, and protein concentration is increased in the edema fluid compared with that in cardiogenic-hydrostatic edema.

These two mechanism approaches to pulmonary edema are useful but are not complete physiologically, as research in the field has proven. A more comprehensive approach is shown in Table 9.1.

INCREASED PULMONARY CAPILLARY PRESSURE

Increased pulmonary capillary pressure is largely produced by cardiac disease and, from an etiologic viewpoint, is understandable as a series of diseases that impair left atrial or left ventricular filling, left atrial or left ventricular emptying, and left ventricular muscle function. A short list of these causes is included in Table 9.1. It is also important to recognize noncardiac causes of increased capillary wedge pressure. These include occlusive lesions of the pulmonary veins from fibrosis of multiple etiologies and mediastinal masses, which obstruct pulmonary venous return.

Altered Permeability

The more important causes of altered permeability of the lung that produce pulmonary edema are those associated with infections such as common pneumonia. These conditions result in a protein exudate in the interstitial and alveolar spaces of the lung. Similar injury results from toxic inhalants such as phosgene, ozone, oxides of nitrogen, and prolonged high-level oxygen exposure.

Specific subsets of this capillary leak pulmonary edema, such as near-drowning, aspiration, and adult respiratory distress syndrome, are discussed in some detail in the specific chapters dealing with the disease entities producing those conditions. Oxygen toxicity and aspirin-induced pulmonary edema, two of the more important remaining entities, are discussed at the end of this section.

Decreased Oncotic Pressure

Capillary oncotic pressure is dependent on plasma protein levels and may be important clinically, even in the face of normal capillary hydrostatic pressures. Patients with protein-losing enteropathies, hepatic failure, starvation, and other forms of malnutrition, producing decreased plasma levels of protein and decreased plasma capillary oncotic pressure, are all at risk for developing pulmonary edema.

TABLE 9.1.
Causes of Pulmonary Edema Based on Mechanisms[a]

Increased pulmonary capillary pressure
Systemic hypertension, aortic coarctation
Left ventricular outflow obstruction
Myocardial failure secondary to ischemia, myocarditis, high output, shunt, valvular regurgitation or obstruction, toxic antimetabolites (anthracycline)
Cortriatriatum, obstruction to/or high resistance in pulmonary veins
Noncardiogenic pulmonary venous disease, such as is secondary to mediastinal tumors

Altered permeability
Infectious bacterial and viral pneumonia
Inhaled toxic agents, such as phosgene, ozone, oxides of nitrogen, and prolonged high concentration oxygen administration
Circulating toxins, such as alloxan, snake venom, and α-naphthylthiourea
Vasoactive substances, such as histamine, kinins, and arachidonic acid metabolites, such as leukotrienes
Diffuse capillary leak syndrome, such as endotoxemia
Immunologic reactions, drug reactions, including salicylate pulmonary edema, allergic alveolitis, leukocyte sensitivity states, and blood transfusion reactions
Smoke inhalation and associated thermal injury
Disseminated intravascular coagulation
Near-drowning
Aspiration, including acid pneumonitis
Radiation pneumonia
Adult respiratory distress syndrome
Uremia

Decreased oncotic pressure
Hypoalbuminemia secondary to renal or hepatic disease, protein-losing enteropathy, or malnutrition

Lymphatic insufficiency
Congenital or acquired

Increased negative intrathoracic pressure
High negative pressure—Croup or epiglottitis, re-expansion pulmonary edema

Mixed or unknown mechanisms
Neurogenic pulmonary edema
Heroin (narcotic) pulmonary edema
High-attitude pulmonary edema
Pulmonary embolism
Eclampsia
Hypoglycemia
Pancreatitis

[a]Modified from Robin ED, Cross CE, Zelis R: Pulmonary edema. *N Engl J Med* 288:239, 292 (2 parts), 1973.

Lymphatic Insufficiency

The vital role of lymphatic drainage in maintaining fluid balance in the lung makes it immediately apparent that abnormalities in lymphatic drainage dramatically raise the likelihood of pulmonary edema. In patients, pulmonary lymphangitis or obstruction may produce a similar picture, and this has been of potential importance in a number of conditions, including lung transplantation.

Increased Negative Interstitial Pressure

Increased negative interstitial pressure is a particularly interesting theoretical possibility used to explain the development of pulmonary edema in children with croup and epiglottitis. Another variety of this physiology with clinical applications is re-expansion pulmonary edema. In this condition, rapid re-expansion of a lung collapsed with pneumothorax can result in pulmonary edema.

IMPORTANT CAUSES OF HEART FAILURE AND/OR PULMONARY EDEMA IN THE PEDIATRIC INTENSIVE CARE UNIT

Anthracycline Cardiotoxicity

The anthracycline antimetabolites doxorubicin (adriamycin) and daunomycin are commonly used antitumor agents, and both can cause bone marrow suppression and cardiotoxicity. Early signs of anthracycline cardiotoxicity are generally electrocardiographic changes, which can be transient. On the other hand, cardiomyopathy is a serious, dose-dependent, life-threatening complication.

The clinical features of anthracycline-induced cardiomyopathy are nonspecific and do not differ from those of other cardiomyopathies. The appearance of heart failure manifested by dyspnea, pulmonary edema, and peripheral edema with tachycardia and cardiomegaly are classic. This is particularly true in a patient who has received doxorubicin at more than 500 mg/m^2. Symptoms may arise any time up to 8 months after the last dose of doxorubicin.

Cumulative dose is important because clinically apparent cardiomyopathy occurs in < 1% of patients who receive a cumulative dose that is > 500 mg/m^2. However, there is a dose-dependent relationship such that of those receiving a total dose of 500–600 mg/m^2, 11% develop clinically apparent cardiomyopathy. If the total dose is > 600 mg/m^2, this incidence exceeds 30%.

If patients with anthracycline toxicity develop pulmonary edema, a mortality rate of at least 50–60% can be expected; awaiting development of clinical symptoms is impractical. Diagnostic evaluation with echocardiography, nuclear imaging, and, possibly, cardiac catheterization may quantify the severity of involvement early in the course and avoid further administration and toxicity.

Use of monitoring to prevent anthracycline toxicity is preferable to therapy of heart failure and pulmonary edema. Once present, however, fluid and salt restriction, diuretics, and judicious use of digitalis may be all that is required after anthracycline therapy is discontinued. When admission to the pediatric intensive care unit (ICU) is required, intensive inotropic support with dopamine or dobutamine and forced diuresis can be used. Both acute and chronic afterload reduction can be particularly beneficial. Because anthracycline cardiomyopathy may be reversible in children, intensive cardiac support including intubation and mechanical ventilation may be warranted to treat an acute episode of pulmonary edema.

Oxygen Toxicity

Although the systemic effects of oxygen toxicity can include a wide variety of physiologic alterations ranging from paresthesias and seizures to retrolental fibroplasia, in the pediatric ICU setting the most important toxic effects of oxygen involve the lung. In this section, we review generalized lung toxicity to oxygen and oxygen-induced pulmonary edema.

In normal humans, exposure to 100% oxygen at 1 atm generates symptoms after approximately 12 hours. A pattern of lung response to oxygen exposure is shown in Figure 9.1.

The mechanism by which oxygen produces its toxicity has been under intense investigation. Most authorities support the contention that oxygen toxicity involves oxygen-free radicals, which may be in the form of the superoxide ion (O_2^-), the hydroxyl radical ($\cdot OH$), or the free singlet ($'O_2$). It

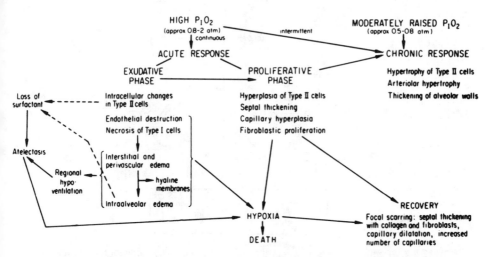

FIGURE 9.1. The lung's response to increased oxygen exposure. Note that the response to diffuse injury is limited and not specific to the injurious agent. P_IO_2, partial pressure of inspired oxygen. (From Winter PM, Miller JD: Oxygen toxicity. In Shoemaker WC, Thompson WL, Holbrook PR (eds): *Textbook of Critical Care Medicine*. Philadelphia, WB Saunders, 1984, p 218.)

has been recognized for some time that oxygen radicals could be the cause of pulmonary damage.

Immune Responses, Hypersensitivity, and Pulmonary Edema

Many allergic reactions involve the lung and include a series of cellular and biochemical events such as vasodilation, increased vasopermeability, and edema formation. It is clear that when immunoglobulin E (IgE) antibody and an antigen interact on the surface of a mast cell, many vasoactive substances are released. As can be seen in Figure 9.2, it is now believed that this mast cell activation results in primary mediator release as well as release of prostaglandin D_2 (PGD$_2$); it also results in the activation of other cell types. It is also now believed that mast cell activation results in secondary release of leukotriene and other oxidative arachidonic acid metabolites from pulmonary interstitial mononuclear cells.

It is now possible to consider at least that some of the pulmonary edema produced by allergic reactions involve IgE-mediated release of substances that activate leukotriene synthesis and release LTD$_4$ from pulmonary interstital cells. This results in increased pulmonary capillary fluid conductance and pulmonary edema.

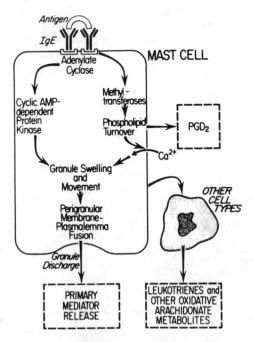

FIGURE 9.2. Pathway of mast cell activation-secretion to primary mediator release and arachidonic acid metabolism. Note the ultimate formation of leukotrienes. *Cyclic AMP*, cyclic adenosine monophosphate. (Reprinted by permission from Lewis RA, Austen KF: Mediation of local homeostasis and inflammation by leukotrienes and other mast cell-dependent compounds. *Nature* 293:103, 1981, ©1981, Macmillan Magazines Ltd.)

Salicylate-Induced Pulmonary Edema

Salicylate pulmonary edema is associated with high salicylate levels (>40 mg/dl), is noncardiac in origin, and is due to increased permeability to fluid and protein in the pulmonary vascular bed. Whereas general supportive measures for pulmonary edema, ranging from oxygen and diuretics to intubation and mechanical ventilation, may be needed, lowering of salicylate levels is a key ingredient in treatment.

Croup, Epiglottitis, and Pulmonary Re-expansion

There are three possible physiologic mechanisms for these events: (a) a catechol-mediated shift of blood volume for the systemic to the pulmonary circuit; (b) hypoxia-induced capillary leakage; and (c) an increase in negative pleural pressure, resulting in an increase in the alveolar capillary transmural pressure gradient. Together, these changes would increase the blood volume in the pulmonary capillaries, increase the pore size in the pulmonary capillaries, and increase the hydrostatic driving pressure of fluid into the lungs (Fig. 9.3).

Heroin- and Narcotic-Induced Pulmonary Edema

The edema fluid in heroin overdose is virtually identical with serum proteins. In fact, although heroin overdose can cause renal failure, myocardial infarction, brain infarction, and rhabdomyolysis, the lungs are the most frequent organ affected. There are several mechanisms postulated for the production, but most involve the cerebral edema documented in these pa-

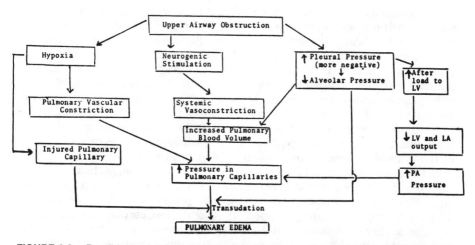

FIGURE 9.3.   Possible mechanisms in etiology of pulmonary edema associated with upper airway obstruction. *LA,* left atrium; *LV,* left ventricle; and *PA,* pulmonary artery. (Reproduced by permission of Travis KW, Todres ID, Shannon DC: Pulmonary edema associated with croup and epiglottitis. *Pediatrics* 59:695, 1977.)

tients and the lack of elevated wedge pressure in this syndrome. Most data suggest that the cause is not primary myocardial failure.

The consensus is that narcotic-depressed respiration caused by central nervous system (CNS) hypoxia produces a variety of neurogenic pulmonary hypoxia from CNS hypoxia. Additionally, CNS depression can cause loss of airway control and aspiration. Both of these may be implicated in the syndrome.

Neurogenic Pulmonary Edema

The relationship between neurologic injury and hemodynamic instability was recognized even before the description of the classic Cushing reflex, and pulmonary edema has been observed following head trauma in both adults and children.

The mechanism of neurogenic pulmonary edema may be conceptualized as a process in which trauma, hypoxia, or increased intracranial pressure initiates a hypothalamic reflex, which results in massive sympathetic discharge. This sympathetic discharge then causes a marked but transient increase in both systemic and pulmonary vascular pressures. The result is a shift of blood from systemic to low-resistance pulmonary circulation. The further increase in pulmonary capillary pressure leads to capillary wall damage and increased permeability, which persists and causes ongoing pulmonary edema. As the vascular pressures return to normal values, heart failure is averted. Unfortunately, the pulmonary edema persists and can be life threatening in itself.

TREATMENT

Physiologically, there are many different approaches to treatment of the patient with pulmonary edema. For instance chronic pulmonary edema in patients with heart disease treated with digitalis and diuretics may be compensated and may not require admission to the hospital, let alone to the pediatric ICU. One of the principles of management, however, is that patients with unexplained or unusual causes of respiratory distress thought to be pulmonary edema require admission to the pediatric ICU earlier than do patients with more usual forms of cardiac failure. The reason is the rapidity with which altered permeability pulmonary edema can develop. Early observation of these patients and assessment of the rate of change in the pulmonary edema are critical to their treatment plan.

In seriously ill or rapidly changing patients, particularly those who will need or already need respiratory support with positive end-expiratory pressure (PEEP) or continuous positive airway pressure (CPAP), the authors frequently employ a balloon-tipped thermodilution cardiac output catheter. The ability to measure left atrial "wedge" pressure for both diagnosis and therapy and the ability to measure intrapulmonary shunt, systemic vascular resistance, and other hemodynamic variables are often invaluable. The authors are not aware that various catheter techniques used to measure lung water in patients with pulmonary edema have proven to be useful in the treatment of infants and children with pulmonary edema.

All therapy for patients with pulmonary edema includes supplemental oxygen. The use of oxygen masks that have reservoir bags allows high levels of supplemental oxygen to be delivered. It does not generally allow the use of PEEP or CPAP, both of which require intubation in young children out of the neonatal period in distress who will not tolerate the face mask. Indications for intubation include progressive hypoxemia despite supplemental oxygen, an increasing P_aCO_2, or a respiratory rate and pattern indicating the likelihood of impending respiratory fatigue.

The intubation of patients in cardiorespiratory distress requires a knowledge of the use of rapid-sequence intubation techniques. Once the patient is intubated, the authors most frequently employ a trial of PEEP, which they have found to be successful in older children who will breathe spontaneously and cooperate with medical direction. Infants and small children often require controlled ventilation and have a higher incidence of need for paralysis in order to avoid inefficient ventilatory patterns. The mechanism by which PEEP works to improve hypoxemia and decrease right-to-left shunting is not by pushing fluid out of the alveoli, as was originally postulated. PEEP clearly increases functional residual capacity, expands fluid-filled alveoli, and improves compliance. The net effect is to improve arterial oxygen tension.

Specific measures beyond this clearly depend on the cause of the pulmonary edema. Cardiac failure may require digitalis, catecholamine, diuretics, and even afterload-reducing agents, depending on the specific nature of the cardiac failure. Morphine, which is commonly used in adults, is not generally used in small children as frequently because of concern about respiratory depression, although other supportive measures, such as head elevation, can be quite useful. The use of agents such as steroids directed at capillary permeability injury has not generally proved useful in any specific pulmonary edema syndrome and, because they may impair responses to infection, are not widely used at present. For similar reasons, the indiscriminate use of wide spectrum antibiotics is rarely indicated because of the possibility of subsequent nosocomial infections.

A point of therapy that should be emphasized is the high likelihood for development of pulmonary edema in patients during the recovery period as the patient is weaned from PEEP or CPAP. The increased venous return, which develops as PEEP or CPAP is decreased, often requires a decrease of fluid administration, diuresis, or both. Similar concerns should be expressed in critically ill patients with pulmonary edema, hypoxia, and hypercarbia who receive high levels of PEEP and CPAP. The harmful CNS effects of hypoxia or hypercarbia, when combined with the potential for elevated airway pressure to decrease blood pressure and increase intracranial pressure, must be considered when neurologic symptoms develop that are not explainable by the degree of hypoxia or hypercarbia.

CHAPTER 10

Dysrhythmias and Their Management

In the setting of pediatric critical care medicine, the rapid recognition of abnormal heart rates and rhythms is essential. In critically ill children, disorders of cardiac rate and rhythm frequently complicate noncardiac disease processes as well as primarily cause life-threatening conditions. Cardiac dysrhythmias may frequently go unrecognized until the child acutely decompensates and presents with either syncope due to central nervous system hypoperfusion or with the signs and symptoms of cardiac failure. In addition, the fact that cardiac output tends to rely more heavily on alterations in heart rate than on stroke volume in the fetus, neonate, and young child than it does in adults indicates that the pathological consequences of alteration in heart rate and rhythm in children differ from those in adults.

SPECIFIC DYSRHYTHMIAS

Bradydysrhythmias

Asystole

Asystole is the total absence of ventricular electrical activity. Total absence of ventricular electrical activity may result from either sinoatrial node arrest or complete sinoatrial ventricular conduction blockade. During complete atrioventricular (AV) blockade, asystole occurs when a subsidiary escape rhythm either from the AV node or from the ventricular site fails to occur. Because both the AV and the sinus nodes are under vagal influence, sinoatrial arrest and AV block may occur simultaneously. Fortunately, in most cases of sinoatrial generator arrest, an escape rhythm arises from the AV node or from the ventricles. This escape rhythm may or may not provide adequate hemodynamic function and generally indicates a need for therapy. Obviously, total asystole is fatal, and its therapy is the same as that outlined for cardiac arrest. Asystole occurs in the setting of severe myocardial damage and is the final stage after multiple severe systemic injury. Hypoxia, ischemia, direct myocardial injury, and severe electrolyte abnormalities are the major underlying causes of asystole.

Sinus Bradycardia

Sinus bradydysrhythmias may occur from either abnormally slow generator potential from the sinus node, the total absence of sinoatrial generator potential, or the conduction failure of this potential. Bradydysrhythmias may occur either with or without escape rhythms from subsidiary sites. The term "bradycardia" refers to the ventricular rate, and bradydysrhythmias other than sinus bradycardia are due to failure of subsidiary sites to serve as adequate pacemakers. In these rhythms the frequency of QRS complexes is abnormally slow either for the patient's age or for the clinical setting. For example, in an 18-month-old patient after cardiac surgery a sinus rate of 75 beats/min is abnormally slow, whereas in a sleeping child of the same age, this heart rate would be normal. A guide to the normal lower limit of heart rate in awake children is the following: over the age of 5, it is 60; up to the age of 5, it is 80; in the first year of life, it is 100; and in the first week of life, it is 95. During sleep, these limits are lower—below 50 for age 5 and above and below 60 for infants. When sinus bradycardia is severe, subsidiary pacemakers may arise. These escape rhythms may be nodal, originating from the AV node, and are frequently differentiated into high, medium, or low by the morphology and timing of the P wave with respect to the QRS complex. Frequently, these P waves show an abnormal axis, and they are often inverted. Most commonly, a junctional escape rhythm shows P waves positive in lead I and negative AVF, and if, in addition, the P wave occurs before the QRS complex, it is low atrial or high nodal in origin. P waves occurring either within or after QRS complex indicate that these are, in nature, truly junctional escape rhythms. Of course, idioventricular rhythms may also occur, and their QRS complexes may be morphologically identical to a premature ventricular contraction (PVC); however, they may also occur with a regular QRS pattern.

Sick Sinus Syndrome

Sick sinus syndrome may be caused by either a congenital abnormality or a direct injury to the sinus node and results in decreased sinus impulse formation or the inability of the generator potential to exit the sinus node (so-called "sinus exit block"). In children, these most frequently occur after surgery, especially after the Mustard procedure for correction of transposition of the great arteries. Sick sinus syndrome may also result from cardiomyopathies, ischemia, or myocarditis.

The electrocardiographic manifestations of sick sinus syndrome are varied and may include periods of sinus arrest and profound, unresponsive sinus bradyrhythms from subsidiary pacemakers. These escape rhythms may be quite varied and may be nodal or ventricular in origin, giving rise to tachydysrhythmias and, hence, the name bradycardia-tachycardia syndrome. Occasionally, atrial fibrillation occurs. Patients with sick sinus syndrome may present with either Stokes-Adams attacks or profound bradycardia and hypoperfusion. The diagnosis of sick sinus syndrome requires recognition of characteristics and electrocardiographic abnormalities such as sinus bradycardia and sinus arrest or the concurrence of bradycardia and tachycardia in the appropriate clinical setting. Absolute diagnosis generally requires intracardiac electrocardiographic measurement of sinoatrial conduction and sinoatrial recovery times after pacing. Patients with sick sinus syndrome who become symptomatic almost always require permanent intracardiac pacemaking.

Bradycardia frequently occurs in the clinical situation of increased vagal tone. In the intensive care unit (ICU), this is frequently associated with pharyngeal stimulation, such as occurs with nasogastric or endotracheal tube suctioning, elevated intracranial pressure, elevated blood pressure, abdominal distention, and increased intraocular pressure. Metabolic derangements, such as hypoglycemia, hypothermia, hypoxia, acidosis, and hypercalcemia, are also causes of acute bradycardia. Drug toxicity from digitalis or propranolol, for example, may also be a contributing factor. In addition to these general conditions, direct myocardial trauma, which may occur in multiple trauma but more commonly occurs after surgery, is also a leading cause of bradycardias. As escape rhythms frequently occur during bradycardias, it should be remembered that the clinical setting defined above is also the clinical setting in which escape rhythms are seen.

Conduction Abnormalities

Bradycardias also arise from conduction abnormalities between the normally generated sinoatrial action potential and the ventricles. This AV conduction delay or block results in an inordinately slow ventricular rate and decreased cardiac output or hemodynamically unstable escape rhythms. Conduction interference occurs in a broad spectrum including first-, second- and third-degree AV block. Recognition of AV conduction delay and complete AV nodal block are important because they may herald the catastrophic deterioration of cardiac rhythm with total loss of ventricular contraction. Identification of these may serve as a clue to underlying causes of syncopal episodes. This conduction blockade may occur at any level and may be within the atrium, the AV node itself, the bundle of His, or any of the bundle branches.

First-degree AV block occurs when all sinus impulses are conducted, with delay as indicated by a prolonged P-R interval. Developmental standards for the normal duration of the P-R interval exist and need to be referred to for exact diagnosis; however, conduction times of >0.20 seconds in children should raise suspicion.

Second-degree AV block is associated with failure of conduction of occasional, but not all, atrial beats to the ventricles and is divided into Mobitz type I and Mobitz type II block. Mobitz type I (Wenchebach phenomenon) describes a situation in which the P-R interval becomes progressively longer until eventually the atrial impulse is not conducted and a dropped beat occurs. This may occur over two, three, four, or even five beats before nonconduction happens. Mobitz type I heart block is invariably associated with conduction delay within the AV node. Mobitz type II block is recognized by the irregular and intermittent sudden dropping of beats expected to follow

P waves. These are not preceded by progressive P-R prolongation. Mobitz type II block is the more ominous abnormality of AV conduction because it frequently progresses to complete AV block. It is generally thought to occur via conduction blockade in the bundle of His or the bundle branches.

Complete AV block, either congenital or acquired, is the most common bradydysrhythmia in children. Complete AV block (third degree) means that there is total lack of conduction between the atria and the ventricles, and its diagnosis depends on the recognition of an abnormally slow QRS rate for a particular age and an irregular P-R interval. In children, the AV node is the most common site of conduction blockade, and for this reason, escape rhythms when they do occur originate from the bundle of His. One would, therefore, expect the QRS pattern to mimic that of normal sinus beats. Clearly, if there is concurrent damage to the conducting tissue of the bundle of His, which may occur during surgery, the QRS pattern either may be consistent with bundle branch blockade or may resemble a ventricular extrasystole. The remaining criterion for complete AV blockade is complete AV dissociation. For this reason, a nonconducted P wave should also be identifiable. As the AV node is generally refractory to 300–400 msec, P waves that occur within 400 msec of the preceding QRS complex are not normally conducted. However, P waves that occur 500–600 msec after the preceding QRS complex and that are not conducted are clearly abnormal. As a guide, the Q-T interval is approximately 400 msec in duration; thus P waves that occur during the T wave and that are not conducted are not an indication of AV blockade; however, P waves that occur after the end of the T wave and that are not conducted may be an indication of AV conduction blockade. Two final points need to be made: Total nodal dissociation can occur in the presence of any atrial rhythm, and generally, the ventricular rhythm is slow and regular.

Treatment of Bradydysrhythmias

Hemodynamic compromise manifested by hypotension and hypoperfusion are the indications for therapy of the bradydysrhythmias. In addition, certain dysrhythmias, such as Mobitz type II block, are so highly associated with catastrophic deterioration that therapy may also be indicated. Vagolytic medications such as atropine frequently increase heart rate and are the first line of therapy. Thus this treatment is useful in overriding lower escape rhythms of either junctional or ventricular origin. If atropine is unsuccessful in increasing heart rate, intravenous isoproterenol is often efficacious. Frequently, severely sinus node dysfunction, such as occurs in sick sinus syndrome, is refractory to such therapy. If sinus bradycardia persists and is associated with hemodynamic compromise, cardiac pacing may be indicated. Of course, it is also important to treat the underlying conditions, such as acidosis, electrolyte abnormalities, hypoxia, and ischemia.

The treatment of bradycardias associated with conduction delay and blockade also follows the same approximate schema. Although atropine is frequently used initially, it is often unsuccessful. Isoproterenol or even epinephrine may be required for conduction delay and may provide sufficient time for either transvenous or transthoracic pacemaking to be instituted. In the face of hemodynamic compromise associated with conduction delay, the possibility of providing temporary or permanent electrical cardiac pacemaking should be strongly considered. Obviously, cardiac pacemaking must be at the ventricular level in AV conduction defects. Ventricular pacemaking can be provided through a number of techniques. Whenever the threat of AV conduction delay occurs or sinoatrial node dysfunction can be expected, such as after surgery on the atrium or ventricular septum, ventricular pacing wires should be placed on the ventricle for several days after surgery. In the absence of ventricular pacing wires, there now exist balloon-tipped, flow-directed pacing catheters that may be passed with electrocardiographic and pressure monitoring in the absence of fluoroscopic guidance, and they can provide ventricular pacemaking. Transthoracic pacing can also be performed during acute circulatory failure and cardiac arrest from complete AV block. A newer approach to ventricular pacing is transesophageal pacing; however, this approach is inappropriate in the presence of AV conduction delay. The duration of pacemaking after the acute onset of AV conduction delay is a matter of concern. Frequently, normal conduction may be expected to return in 1–2 weeks. After 2 weeks, however, if AV conduction has not returned to normal, permanent cardiac pacemaking will probably be required.

Atrial Dysrhythmias
Atrial Extrasystoles

Atrial extrasystoles frequently occur in healthy individuals and children admitted to the pediatric ICU. Atrial extrasystole is readily recognized by the early occurrence of a P wave followed by a QRS complex (Table 10.1). The premature QRS complex may have the identical morphology to the preceding QRS complexes, or it may be aberrantly conducted and thus be dissimilar from preceding QRS complexes. Due to the extremely rapid rate of repolarization of the conducting tissue in the infant's myocardium, aberrant conduction does not occur in children under 18 months of age. Although simple premature atrial beats are frequently considered benign, they should still be sought, as they have the ability to generate serious cardiac dysrhythmias. Theoretically, the most serious atrial dysrhythmias always occur in response to an atrial extrasystole initiating multiple re-entry pathways leading to supraventricular tachydysrhythmias or atrial

TABLE 10.1. ─────────────────────────────────
Electrocardiographic Forms of Premature Atrial Contractions

Early P wave, normal QRS
Early P wave blocked in AV node
Early P wave, blocked in bundle banches, wide QRS with high likelihood of
  right bundle branch block

TABLE 10.2.
Comparison of Premature Atrial Contraction (PAC) and Premature Ventricular Contraction (PVC)

PAC—Resets sinus node, no compensatory pause
PVC—Does not reset sinus node, compensatory pause
PAC—Most have normal QRS, some have no QRS (blocked), some have right bundle branch block pattern
PVC—Wide and bizarre in any shape

---

fibrillation. Differentiation of atrial extrasystoles from ventricular extrasystoles may be difficult, especially in children (Table 10.2). The knowledge that aberrancy does not occur in children younger than 18 months of age should be borne in mind. In addition, the right bundle branch block pattern occurs more frequently in aberrantly conducted premature atrial contractions (PACs), and therefore, the recognition of the rsr' pattern in V_1 makes the extrasystole more likely an aberrantly conducted PAC than a PVC. Perhaps the most useful differentiating point is the occurrence of a compensatory pause, indicating ventricular ectopic beats. Finally, PVCs generally demonstrate a different initial vector from the preceding sinus beats, whereas PACs do not.

Supraventricular Tachydysrhythmia

Supraventricular Tachycardia

The most frequently observed pathologic dysrhythmia in pediatric practice is paroxysmal supraventricular tachycardia (SVT) or paroxysmal atrial tachycardia. This is defined as a rapid heart rate originating from an abnormal mechanism proximal to the bifurcation of the bundle of His, which, additionally, is morphologically dissimilar to atrial flutter. Morphologically, the electrocardiogram demonstrates regular R-R intervals and narrow QRS complexes (Fig. 10.1A). However, abnormal P wave morphology and a deranged P-R relationship with prolonged P-R intervals and absent or difficult to define P waves usually occur (Fig. 10.1B). In infants and neonates SVT may be at rates of 200–300 beats/min, whereas in older children, heart rates of 150–250 are more common. Characteristically, the onset of SVT is paroxysmal with a rapid sudden onset and offset. The majority of children with SVT demonstrate a normal P-R interval and a normal QRS complex. One exception to this is in the Lown-Ganong-Levine syndrome with a short P-R interval and a normal QRS complex. Between the ages of 3 and 16 years, the P-R interval is >100 msec, and in adults it is >120 msec, whereas in children under 3 years of age it is >80 msec. In the majority of patients with SVT, both atria and ventricles are beating abnormally rapidly.

SVT with aberrant AV conduction is extremely uncommon in children. For this reason, QRS morphology is generally normal and virtually invariably so in children under 18 months of age. When the QRS is abnormally wide, it is usually of a similar morphology to that seen during normal sinus

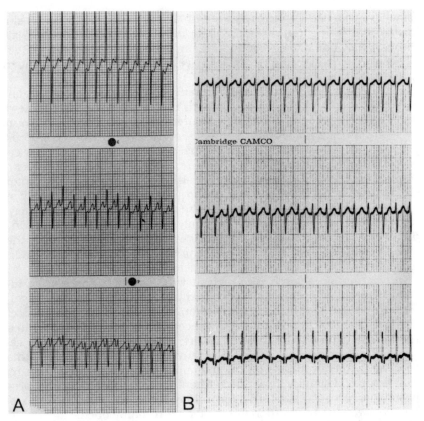

FIGURE 10.1. Two examples of neonatal SVT. Note narrow, regular QRS complexes, regular P-R intervals, and a heart rate of 300 beats/min. The regular P waves which are evident in *A* are not as clearly defined in *B*.

rhythm. When aberrancy does occur, it may be extremely difficult to differentiate SVT from ventricular tachycardia; however, a right bundle branch block pattern is more commonly seen with SVT, and a left bundle branch block pattern is more frequently seen with ventricular tachycardia.

SVT is caused by a so-called "re-entry phenomenon." This occurs when the atria are excited through the aberrant retrograde entry of the electrical impulse along a conducting pathway back into the atria, causing a circular movement of depolarization. This can occur through the AV node or, commonly, through accessory conducting tissue pathways such as the bundle of Kent or the bundle of James. The ability of atrial tissue to repolarize rapidly, especially in children, is the underlying reason why this aberrant circular movement can be effective. The Wolff-Parkinson-White syndrome was the first pattern of re-entry phenomena described in which the bundle of Kent leads to recurrent paroxysmal SVT. These patients characteristically have widened QRS complexes with a short P-R interval and a slurred upstroke (δ wave), indicating the aberrant pathway of early depolarization through the anomalously conducting bundle of Kent. Frequently, SVT can be seen to be triggered by a PVC that is conducted through this aberrant tissue and thus initiates the SVT.

In general, children with SVT present with congestive cardiac failure. SVT may occur in utero and result in the birth of a hydropic newborn infant. The diagnosis of fetal SVT in utero can be made by ultrasound or by fetal electrocardiographic studies. Frequently, in older children who present with failure, SVT may be confused with any of several other causes of low output, including cardiac failure, fever, sepsis, septic shock, and volume contraction. Chest pain may also be the presenting symptom in children with SVT, and screaming and irritability may be the only symptoms in infants. In older age groups, the onset of rapid heart rate may lead to the diagnosis of SVT. Most commonly, the onset of SVT occurs in children before 6 months of age and is slightly more common in boys than in girls. Although it may reflect underlying Wolff-Parkinson-White syndrome, frequently there are no predisposing factors.

In treating all children who present with SVT it is appropriate to consider using maneuvers that increase vagal tone. This increased vagal tone may interrupt electrical depolarization caused by the irregular circus movement and is frequently rapidly successful in converting SVT to sinus rhythm. In older children and in adults, these maneuvers include carotid sinus massage and the Valsalva maneuver. In younger children, this can be done by merely applying firm abdominal pressure, which often results in a bearing down response in children. Although use of ocular pressure is occasionally successful, this technique carries with it a high risk of retinal detachment and is therefore no longer recommended.

Another modality for treating SVT is eliciting the diving reflex. This complex neurologic reflex is elicited by providing an iced water (0°C) stimulus to the head and/or face of the child. This gives rise to both an increase in vagal tone and a withdrawal of sympathetic tone and, frequently, rapidly aborts SVT. This technique is particularly efficacious in infants and small children; however, it has also been successfully applied to older children. One important caveat is essential in performing all of these physiologic maneuvers; i.e., one should be prepared to treat rapidly profound bradycardias and even asystole that may result from vagotonic methods of aborting supraventricular dysrhythmias.

Two other techniques for increasing neurally mediated suppression of SVT deserve mention. Edrophonium bromide (Tensilon) can be given intravenously. This short-acting cholinesterase inhibitor increases concentrations of endogenous acetylcholine and thus vagal tone. Another means of suppressing SVT is the use of α-adrenergic sympathomimetic agents that result in an elevation in systemic vascular resistance and reflex vagal stimulation of the myocardium. Both methoxamine and phenylephrine have been reported to be useful for this purpose. In children who have already maximally compensated for decreased cardiac output secondary to SVT, a further increase in peripheral vascular resistance may lead to catastrophic myocardial decompensation. For this reason, this technique must be applied with caution, especially in older children.

In the past, digitalization was the standard first-line therapy for conversion of SVT in infants and older children. Rapid digitalization intravenously, if necessary over 4–6 hours, frequently converts supraventricular tachydysrhythmias. Continuation of digitalis in children who have been converted from SVT to sinus rhythm seems to be warranted; although the incidence of attacks may not be decreased, the rapidity of conversion of future attacks seems to be enhanced. Recent concerns about the use of digoxin in patients with Wolff-Parkinson-White syndrome have cast doubt on the wisdom of using digoxin as the first line of therapy in undiagnosed patients presenting with SVT. As digoxin may enhance AV conduction, it could cause early conduction of atrial beats to a nonrefractory ventricle, which could result in ventricular tachycardia (VT) or ventricular fibrillation. For this reason, the use of digoxin for initially converting SVT, atrial fibrillation, and atrial flutter in children may be contraindicated.

Propranolol, a β-adrenergic blocking agent, has proven useful in converting supraventricular tachydysrhythmias. β-Adrenergic blockade prolongs AV conduction time by increasing the refractory period of the conducting pathways. It is, therefore, useful for converting as well as preventing future episodes of SVT. Propranolol can be given intravenously, when indicated, and repeated hourly as long as the blood pressure and heart rate tolerate it. Propranolol is particularly effective in treating SVT resulting from Wolff-Parkinson-White syndrome. In severe cases of refractory SVT, other agents that block intraventricular conduction, such as quinidine and procainamide, may be useful in converting the tachydysrhythmia. Verapamil, a calcium channel blocker, has been reported to be useful therapy for converting SVT in infants and children. It is a useful alternative to propranolol as a first-line treatment to Wolff-Parkinson-White syndrome. Due to the myocardial depressant and peripheral vasodilator actions of verapamil, hypotension may be a complication. These two effects explain why it must be used with great care in combination with β-adrenergic blockade.

In the child who presents with hypoperfusion or becomes acutely hypoperfused, hypotensive, or acidotic or in whom pharmacologic therapy has been ineffective, further therapy is urgently required. Such is generally the situation in neonates with SVT and congestive heart failure. Synchronized direct current cardioversion with a dose of 0.5–2 J/kg is usually effective in cardioversion. Repeated attempts are indicated, and the dose may be increased to 5 J/kg.

Atrial Fibrillation and Flutter

Two remaining supraventricular tachydysrhythmias are atrial fibrillation and atrial flutter. They often occur in the pediatric ICU setting and need to be differentiated from more serious supraventricular tachydys-rhythmias. Atrial fibrillation results from rapid chaotic depolarization of multiple atrial foci and is accompanied by a variable response from the ventricles. Electrocardiographically, a rapid, irregular, ventricular response with irregular R-R intervals and absent P waves is seen (Fig. 10.2). Occasionally, distorted complexes indicating aberrant conduction are pres-

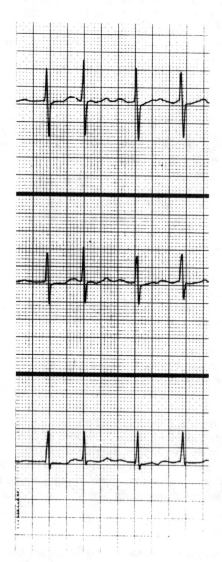

FIGURE 10.2. Atrial fibrillation. Note the absence of P waves and the irregular P-R interval with normal QRS morphology (V_{4-6}).

ent. Atrial fibrillation may result from rheumatic heart disease, mitral valve disease, hyperthyroidism, pericarditis, atrial septal defects, Ebstein's anomaly, and cardiomyopathies. The loss of atrial filling during atrial fibrillation is usually better tolerated in children than in adults.

Atrial flutter appears less frequently in children than in adults and is characterized by a rapid, uniform, sawtooth flutter wave that occurs between 250 and 500 times/min. Flutter waves are atrial depolarizations that last for up to 180 msec (Fig 10.3B). It should be noted that they may not be present in all electrocardiographic leads. Leads II, III, aVF, and V_1 are the leads that most frequently show flutter waves. AV conduction is almost always partially blocked, resulting in an irregular ventricular response (Fig. 10.3A). QRS morphology is the same as that for normal sinus beats, though aberrant conduction may also occur. A large percentage of these patients with atrial flutter have had an operation to correct a congenital heart defect. This was most commonly a Mustard or Senning procedure, atrial septal defect repair, Blalock-Hanlon septectomy, or a Fontan procedure. Other causes of atrial flutter are various types of congenital heart disease, cardiomyopathies, rheumatic disease, mitral valve prolapse, and pericarditis; occasionally, atrial flutter occurs in an anatomically normal heart. When atrial flutter occurs in a child younger than 1 year of age, it is likely to be associated with the Wolff-Parkinson-White syndrome.

Treatment. As in other dysrhythmias, the underlying hemodynamic status and diagnosis dictate the therapy. In patients who are hemodynamically stable, atrial flutter and fibrillation may best be converted with intravenous digitalization. However, if the underlying diagnosis includes the Wolff-Parkinson-White syndrome, digitalization is best avoided, and intravenous propranolol may be useful in showing the ventricular response. Procainamide and quinidine have also been useful in treating refractory flutter and fibrillation.

In the acutely ill child or one in whom the above pharmacologic maneuvers have been unsuccessful, the safest method of converting atrial flutter is overdrive atrial pacing. This can be performed via an indwelling intracardiac catheter or an esophageal pacing electrode. Atrial pacing should be at a rate approximately 20–30 beats greater than the intrinsic atrial rhythm and continued for at least 60 seconds. The pacing voltage should be 3 or 4 times greater than the atrial capture threshold. It should then be rapidly terminated. The underlying cause for atrial flutter and fibrillation could be sinus node disease, in which case rapid conversion could lead to an inordinately slow bradycardia and, potentially, to asystole. For this reason, means of atrial pacing and increasing atrial rate should be available.

The most efficacious way of converting atrial fibrillation and flutter is by synchronized direct current cardioversion. Again, standby pacing should be available, and appropriate anesthesia should be provided. If cardioversion is followed by rapid relapse, intravenous digitalization as well as the addition of procainamide may be indicated. An alternative to this tactic is the use of propranolol, which, through slowing AV conduction, may maintain the conversion to sinus rhythm.

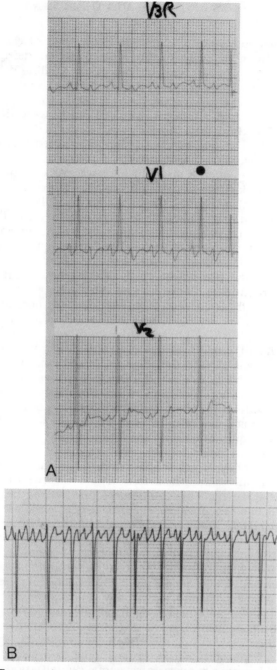

FIGURE 10.3. Two examples of atrial flutter. *A* shows flutter with a regular 2:1 AV conduction block and regular P-R intervals with a rate of 104 (leads I–III). This example of flutter is more subtle than that for another patient *(B)* (lead V₁), which shows the characteristic sawtooth pattern with variable R-R intervals.

Ventricular Dysrhythmias

Ventricular tachydysrhythmias can present dramatically and pose a serious threat to life. For this reason, the rapid recognition of predisposing factors and effective therapy is vitally important. A PVC is characterized by a wide, abnormal, slurred QRS complex, usually followed by a T wave with an inverted axis without a preceding P wave (Fig. 10.4). Differentiation from aberrantly conducted PAC is difficult. The best way to differentiate these two phenomena is to note the presence of a compensatory pause between QRS complexes, which indicates a ventricular ectopic beat. In addition, PVCs generally demonstrate a different initial vector from the preceding sinus beats, whereas PACs do not (Table 10.2).

PVCs can be described morphologically as uniform or multiform (unifocal or multifocal). The term multiform merely refers to the morphology of the QRS being different. It does not necessarily indicate multiple ectopic ventricular foci. In addition to aberrantly conducted atrial contractions, fusion of an ectopic ventricular beat also occurs. The electrocardiographic appearance results from the fusion of an ectopic beat with a supraventricular beat, and thus its morphology lies between that of a sinus beat and a PVC (Fig. 10.5). The significance of a fusion beat is the same as that of any other PVC. The significance of individual PVCs or couplets and triplets (ventricular tachycardia) of PVCs is that they indicate damaged areas of myocardium that result from ischemia, drugs, or direct trauma, which gives rise to an area of myocardial irritability. These damaged foci constantly pose the risk of deterioration to a sustained or ventricular fibrillation with hemodynamic collapse (Figs. 10.6 and 10.7).

VT can arise from an electrolyte or metabolic imbalance, cardiac tumor, cardiac damage after surgery, myocarditis, or a cardiomyopathy, or it may

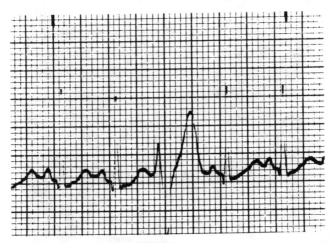

FIGURE 10.4. A single ventricular extrasystole. Note wide QRS with opposite vector from sinus QRS, abnormal T wave morphology, and fully compensatory pause.

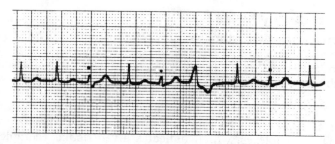

FIGURE 10.5. This rhythm strip shows an example of fusion beats which have been marked with a *solid dot* (·). There is also a ventricular ectopic beat. A fusion beat represents a combination of a ventricular ectopic beat with a supraventricular beat and is intermediate in form between the two. Their significance is the same as for ventricular ectopic beats.

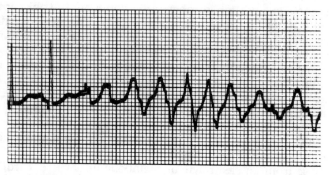

FIGURE 10.6. Sinus rhythm degenerating into VT.

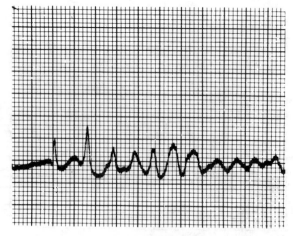

FIGURE 10.7. Bradycardia with a ventricular ectopic (R-on-T) initiating course ventricular fibrillation. Note disorganized, rapid chaotic electrical activity.

be idiopathic. It can also occur in the prolonged Q-T syndromes (Jervell, Lange-Nielsen, or Romano-Ward). Hemodynamic compromise follows VT and leads to syncope or sudden death. Ventricular fibrillation is manifest by chaotic, irregular ventricular depolarization and is characterized by the absence of regular recognizable QRS complexes. The therapy for ventricular fibrillation is the same as that for cardiac arrest.

It is frequently difficult to differentiate SVT from VT. Rates of >150 beats/min, wide QRS complexes, and inadequate circulation occur in both. Pre-existing AV dissociation, however, suggests VT, as does the presence of pre-existing fusion beats. Frequently, a trial of therapy is required to differentiate SVT and VT. Vagomimetic maneuvers rarely affect VT and frequently slow or abort SVTs.

Therapy for Ventricular Dysrhythmias

Treatment of rhythms that predispose to VT and ventricular fibrillation is indicated when there is either hemodynamic compromise or a rhythm that may rapidly deteriorate. The rhythms that may deteriorate are those with PVCs in couplets or triplets, multiform ventricular premature beats, PVCs occurring on or near the T wave (Fig. 10.7), and >6 PVCs/min. Although ventricular bigeminy is a stable dysrhythmia, the presence of hemodynamic compromise caused by the inadequate ventricular contractions during the ectopic beat may require therapy directed at preventing the PVCs (Table 10.3).

The acute therapy of PVCs is intravenous lidocaine. If this is unsuccessful in altering the pattern of PVCs, it may be repeated, and a continuous intravenous lidocaine infusion with serum levels to guide therapy is indicated. Intravenous procainamide is the next therapeutic step and may be continued either orally or intravenously. Disopyramide, a new quinidine-like drug, is an oral agent that prevents and suppresses PVCs and may eventually be available for intravenous use in the United States. Oral quinidine is also effective in the long-term suppression of PVCs.

The treatment of VT is again guided by the hemodynamic status of the patient. If cardiac output is maintained, the first drug of choice is intravenous lidocaine repeated twice and followed by a continuous infusion. If VT persists, intravenous procainamide or phenytoin is frequently successful. Recently, bretylium tosylate, an adrenergic nerve-blocking drug given intravenously, has proven very effective in terminating ventricular fibrillation and VT in children and should be considered in children with resis-

---

TABLE 10.3.
When to Treat a PVC

High frequency (>6/min)
Three or more in a row (VT)
Multifocal (different QRS forms)
Vulnerable period (PVC on T wave)

TABLE 10.4.
Classification of Antidysrhythmics

Class I—Sodium channel blockers
A. Quinidine
   Procainamide
   Disopyramide
B. Lidocaine
   Phenytoin
   Mixetelene
   Tocainide

Class II—β Blockers
Propranolol
Timolol

Class III—Prolonged repolarization
Bretylium
Amiodarone
Sotalol

Class IV—Calcium channel blockers
Verapamil
Nifedipine
Diltiazem

tant VT. Although it works within several minutes in ventricular fibrillation, it may take up to 2 hours to be effective in VT. Intravenous disopyramide has also proven efficacious for therapy of VT or ventricular fibrillation.

If pharmacologic treatment has been unsuccessful and hemodynamic compromise is present, electrocardioversion is the therapy of choice. Again, anesthetic and airway management aspects of the child should be assured prior to defibrillation. Doses of 1–4 J/kg are necessary and may be repeated until sinus rhythm occurs. For ventricular fibrillation or VT refractory to defibrillation, overdrive ventricular pacing may suppress an ectopic focus, and paired ventricular pacing may also be efficacious therapy.

THERAPEUTICS

To understand the mechanisms by which antidysrhythmic drugs are effective, it would be worthwhile to review the physiology of cardiac depolarization. This is not possible in this handbook. Therefore, please see Chapter 14 in the *Textbook of Pediatric Intensive Care*. For simple presentation we have included Table 10.4 on classification of drugs and Table 10.5 on drug dosages.

TABLE 10.5.
Drug Therapy for Dysrhythmias[a]

Drug	Dose	Route	Drug Level	Side Effects
Therapy for SVT				
Digoxin	See digitalizing schedule	p.o., i.m., i.v.	1–3 ng/ml	Dysrhythmias, conduction delay, diarrhea, nausea, vomiting
Edrophonium	0.04 mg/kg × 3	i.v.	—	Profound bradydysrhythmias
Methoxamine	5–15 μg/kg/min titrate to BP	i.v. infusion	—	Hypertension
Phenylephrine	0.5–5 μg/kg/min titrate to BP	i.v. infusion	—	Hypertension
Verapamil	0.05–0.15 mg/kg over 15 min × 2	i.v. bolus, p.o.	100–300 ng/ml	Hypotension
Therapy for ventricular dysrhythmias				
Bretylium	5 mg/kg bolus	i.v. bolus	—	Hypotension
Lidocaine	1–3 mg/kg, repeat if necessary 30–50 μg/kg/hr	i.v. bolus, infusion	1–6 μg/ml	Convulsions
Phenytoin	1–2 mg/kg	i.v. bolus, p.o.	10–20 μg/ml	Heart block
Therapy effective for SVT and ventricular dysrhythmias				
Disopyramide	2–5 mg/kg	p.o.	—	Hypotension, asystole, bronchospasm
Propranolol	0.01–0.1 mg/kg slowly	i.v. bolus	20–150 ng/ml	Nausea, vomiting, sudden death
Procainamide	3–10 mg/kg	i.v. bolus, infusion, p.o.	3–12 μg/ml	
Quinidine	15–60 mg/kg/day ÷ 4	p.o.	2–8 μg/ml	PVCs, AV block, hypotension
Therapy for bradydysrhythmias				
Atropine	0.01 mg/kg not <0.1 mg	i.m., i.v. bolus	—	Flushing, tachycardia, fever, pupillary dilatation
Isoproterenol	0.1–1.0 μg/kg/min titrated	i.v. infusion	—	PVCs, tachycardia

[a]BP, blood pressure.

CHAPTER 11

Shock

Shock is a clinical syndrome consisting of acute disruption of circulatory function and general insufficiency of tissue perfusion, which ultimately results in deranged homeostatic mechanisms. In general, all shock states eventually involve decreased delivery or impaired utilization of essential cellular substrates that cause disruption and eventual loss of normal cellular metabolism and function. Because circulatory function depends on blood volume, vascular tone, and cardiac function, all shock states result from abnormalities in one or more of these factors. It is worth emphasizing that hypotension is not the sine qua non of shock. Indeed, shock can occur with a normal blood pressure and a normal or even increased cardiac output.

CLASSIFICATION OF SHOCK STATES

Shock has been classified in many ways. We classify shock etiologically into (a) hypovolemic (lack of blood volume), (b) distributive (altered vascular tone, either primary or secondary to neurologic or neurohormonal alterations), and (c) cardiogenic (cardiac pump failure). In addition, septic shock, which has characteristics of all of these types of shock, is important enough and has enough unique characteristics to require separate classification (Table 11.1). Because the diversity of shock states makes classification difficult, several types cannot be neatly classified. Some of these are shown in the miscellaneous section of Table 11.1.

In addition to the above classification, it is helpful to consider three stages in shock: compensated, uncompensated, and irreversible. In the early compensated stage, homeostatic mechanisms are functioning to maintain essential organ perfusion. Blood pressure, urine output, and cardiac function may all seem to be normal. In the decompensated stage, this circulatory compensation fails due to ischemia, the elaboration of toxic materials, and, often, the initial compensatory mechanisms. Eventually, cellular function deteriorates and widespread abnormalities occur in all organ systems. When this process has caused such significant, irreparable functional loss in essential organs that death is inevitable despite temporary support, the terminal, or irreversible, stage of shock is reached. By this

TABLE 11.1. ————————————————————————————
Classification of Shock

Hypovolemic
Dehydration
  Gastroenteritis
  Deprivation
  Heat stroke
Burns
Hemorrhage

Distributive
Anaphylaxis
Neurogenic
Drug toxicity
Septic

Cardiogenic
Congenital heart disease
Ischemic heart disease
  Anoxia
  Kawasaki disease
Traumatic
Infectious cardiomyopathies
Drug toxicity
Tamponade

Septic shock

Miscellaneous
Heat stroke
Pulmonary embolus
  Blood
  Air
  Fat
Pancreatitis
Drug overdose
  Barbiturates
  β-Antagonists

stage, no matter what the initial classification of a given shock state may have been, there are gross abnormalities in volume status, vascular tone, and cardiac function.

Hypovolemic Shock

Hypovolemic shock results from decreased intravascular volume and, therefore, decreased venous return and myocardial preload. This intravascular fluid depletion may be due to hemorrhage, water and electrolyte losses, or plasma losses (Table 11.2), all of which may be either external or inter-

TABLE 11.2. ——————————————————————————
Causes of Hypovolemic Shock

Water and electrolyte loss
Diarrhea
Vomiting
Diabetes insipidus
Renal losses
Heat stroke
Intestinal obstruction
Burns

Hemorrhage
Trauma
Surgery
Gastrointestinal bleeding

Plasma losses
Burns
Nephrotic syndrome
Sepsis
Intestinal obstruction
Peritonitis

———————————————————————————————————————

nal (third-space losses). The major cause of world infant mortality is shock resulting from dehydration caused by the diarrhea and vomiting that accompany infectious gastroenteritis. It is estimated that between 5 and 18 million children die annually throughout the world from this condition. Although gastroenteritis affects many children in this country, it is effectively treated by volume resuscitation and electrolyte replacement. In the United States, trauma is the leading cause of death in children older than 1 year of age, and hypovolemic shock is a major contributor to the mortality caused by trauma.

Hemorrhagic shock resulting from trauma may occur because of external or internal blood loss. A ruptured viscus, usually the spleen or the liver, can lead to profound hypovolemic shock in a very short time and mandates immediate surgery. Soft-tissue trauma and long-bone fractures can also lead to massive blood loss and edema formation, thus causing shock that may be less obvious than frank external hemorrhage. Among the most obvious sites of external blood loss are vascular lacerations and scalp lacerations that may bleed profusely and rapidly compromise the circulation.

Gastrointestinal hemorrhage, another leading cause of hemorrhagic shock in children, can occur as part of a systemic illness or gastrointestinal infection, or it can result directly from a gastrointestinal tract primary lesion. Gastrointestinal hemorrhage occurs in patients with generalized coagulopathies such as those that occur in leukemias, in idiopathic thrombocytopenic purpura, after chemotherapy, or with disseminated intravascular coagulation from many causes, including septic shock. Severe gastrointestinal hemorrhage can accompany salmonellosis and shigellosis, further complicating the volume depletion that occurs in these diseases. Specific gastrointestinal lesions that may lead to hemorrhagic shock are different with different age groups. In infancy, the most likely diagnosable cause of hemorrhagic shock from the gastrointestinal tract is associated with coagulopathies, notably hemorrhagic disease of the newborn. However, it is worth noting that nearly 50% of the cases of gastrointestinal hemorrhage in the newborn remain undiagnosed. In children older than 1 year of age, upper gastrointestinal bleeding from ulceration, esophageal varices, or the Mallory-Weiss syndrome can lead to rapid, life-threatening exsanguination and requires emergent attention. Lower gastrointestinal bleeding can occur suddenly and profusely in children with intestinal polyposis (i.e., Peutz-Jeghers syndrome), colitis, and intussusception and rarely, but dramatically, from a Meckel's diverticulum.

The patient with early compensated hypovolemic shock presents with cool extremities, decreased peripheral perfusion, tachycardia, and decreased urine output as described earlier. Hemodynamically, these patients have normal to reduced filling pressures, increased systemic vascular resistance, decreased systemic vascular resistance, and decreased cardiac output but generally normal blood pressure. Flow is diverted away from the skin and splanchnic circulation to preserve central nervous system (CNS), myocardial, and central perfusion. Release of antidiuretic hormone (vasopressin) and stimulation of the renin-angiotensin aldosterone system tend to restore intravascular volume. In addition, alterations in the forces that control fluid flux across the capillary endothelium (Starling forces) lead to "autotransfusion" in the microcirculation from the periphery. With ongoing uncorrected volume loss, uncompensated shock leads to tissue damage, inadequate central circulation, and the release of products of tissue ischemia, which may further aggravate the already-serious situation. Hypotension, mental dysfunction, anuria, and respiratory and cardiac failure occur. Eventually, tissue hypoperfusion is so profound and so widespread that permanent myocardial damage and widespread cell death occur and recovery is impossible.

Distributive Shock

Abnormalities in vasomotor tone can cause maldistribution of a normal circulatory volume, which, if severe enough, may lead to shock. Consequent peripheral pooling and vascular shunting lead to a state of "relative hypovolemia." In addition, loss of arterial tone leads to marked hypotension. Although distributive shock may clinically resemble hypovolemic shock, it generally arises from different causes. Distributive shock occurs classically but not exclusively during anaphylaxis, drug toxicity, neurologic injury, and septic shock (Table 11.3).

Shock is one facet of anaphylaxis. The immune response is generated in a previously sensitized host when an antigen reacts with fixed immuno-

TABLE 11.3.
Causes of Distributive Shock

Anaphylaxis
Antibiotics
Vaccines
Blood
Local anesthetics
Iodine control media
Insects
Foods

Neurologic injury
Head injury
Spinal shock

Septic shock
Early phase

Drugs
Barbiturates
Phenothiazines
Tranquilizers
Antihypertensives

globulin E antibody. This triggers a complex series of reactions within circulating mast cells, eosinophils, and perivascular connective tissue mast cells and leads directly to complement activation, causing a massive release of a wide variety of vasoactive mediators. Among these are histamine, leukotrienes C_4 and D_4 (slow-reacting substances of anaphylaxis), eosinophilic chemotactic factor, bradykinin, and various vasoactive prostenoid compounds. Hemodynamically, the initial responses are widespread vasodilation, intravascular pooling, and decreased venous return, followed by capillary microvascular injury and intravascular volume depletion via this capillary leak. Clearly, profound hypotension can be the most dramatic manifestation of anaphylaxis; however, upper airway obstruction, obstructive airway disease, pulmonary edema, cutaneous manifestations, and gastrointestinal disturbances also occur and can be life threatening. In patients with anaphylactic shock, volume restitution and restoration of vasomotor tone are essential in preventing the development of uncompensated shock.

Neurogenic shock is most familiar after high spinal cord transection but also occurs in brainstem and isolated intracranial injuries. Hypotension accompanying CNS injuries can obviously have grave consequences with regard to the adequacy of CNS perfusion. Spinal shock occurs with cord transections above T1 that cause total loss of sympathetic cardiovascular tone. This leads to profound hypotension with systolic pressures of <40 torr and accompanied by bradycardia. Not surprisingly, mentation is affected, and urine output is very low. In the setting of trauma, the concurrence of hemorrhagic shock can be disastrous. Hypotension and bradycardia should alert one to the possibility of spinal cord transection in children after trauma.

Drug intoxication, which may be accidental in young children and self-inflicted in older children, can lead to profound peripheral vasodilation and distributive shock. This topic is further discussed in Chapter 22.

Cardiogenic Shock

Cardiogenic shock does not occur frequently in children, but it does account for a large number of admissions to pediatric intensive care units (ICUs). Cardiogenic shock can result from congenital heart disease, a wide spectrum of infectious and noninfectious acquired cardiomyopathies, trauma, ischemia, or surgical intervention. Hypoplastic left heart syndrome is a major cause of neonatal death and is the most common cause of cardiogenic shock in the first week of life. Recent advances in the surgical treatment of this condition make early recognition and effective therapeutic support more important than they were in the past. In the pediatric ICU, the major cause of cardiogenic shock is surgical repair of congenital heart disease. Myocardial impairment after inflammatory processes (myocarditis), ischemic infarction (as can occur in infants with anomalous left coronary artery, isoproterenol-treated asthmatics, or Kawasaki disease), primary cardiomyopathy (either obstructive or degenerative), secondary cardiomyopathy (infectious, toxic, and radiation), and high-output cardiac failure also contribute to the number of children seen with cardiogenic shock in the pediatric ICU. Other causes of myocardial impairment in children that may lead to shock include hypoglycemia, metabolic abnormalities, hypothermia, asphyxial episodes, various drug intoxications, and, of course, late sepsis. In addition to direct myocardial impairment, cardiogenic shock may result from cardiac dysrhythmias such as supraventricular tachycardia typically seen in neonates and ventricular arrhythmias.

Septic Shock

The exact incidence of septic shock in children is difficult to document. Estimates of the mortality in the United States (adults and children) from Gram-negative septic shock approach 100,000 deaths annually. In addition, viral, fungal, Rickettsial, and Gram-positive septic shock have significant mortalities. Clearly, septic shock is a serious and common disease. Septic shock arises in a variety of clinical settings. Most familiarly, in pediatrics it occurs in immunocompromised children such as neonates and those with leukemia and congenital immunodeficiencies; it also occurs after chemotherapy. Children with congenital urinary tract abnormalities and congenital heart disease are also at increased risk. Children with extensive burns or multiple traumas and critically ill children in ICUs frequently develop septic shock. In addition, reticuloendothelial depression follows hemorrhagic shock and can predispose children to developing septic shock.

Septic shock also occurs de novo in otherwise healthy children and can be rapidly fatal. Meningococcemia, pneumococcemia, and infection with *Haemophilus influenzae* are frequently complicated by septic shock, and these organisms have a particular predilection for children.

The pathogens responsible for initiating septic shock in children vary with age (Table 11.4). Although septic shock is generally caused by bacterial pathogens, it should be remembered that viral (dengue, herpes, varicella, influenza), Rickettsial (Rocky Mountain spotted fever and typhus), chlamydial, protozoal (malaria), and fungal *(Candida)* pathogens may be accompanied by septic shock. Although in the past it was believed that the type of pathogen determined the pattern of hemodynamic response, this now seems less likely. A wide variety of pathogens appear to be able to trigger the mechanisms responsible for septic shock and to initiate common metabolic and hemodynamic consequences. Although the pattern of response does not rely on the exact pathogen, much previous work has made Gram-negative shock and endotoxin shock synonymous with septic shock. Vast numbers of animal studies with endotoxin have contributed to our understanding of septic shock. Although all of the response to pathogenic invasion are not the result of the elaboration of endotoxins, these have been best categorized.

Septic shock, regardless of the organisms involved, undergoes distinct physiologic stages. The early compensated stage of septic shock in humans

TABLE 11.4.
Common Pathogens Causing Septic Shock

Neonates
Group B β-hemolytic streptococci
Enterobacteriaceae
Listeria monocytogenes
Staphylococcus aureus

Infants
H. influenzae
Streptococcus pneumoniae
S. aureus

Children
S. pneumoniae
Neisseria meningitidis
S. aureus
Enterobacteriaceae

Immunocompromised
Enterobacteriaceae
S. aureus
Pseudomonadaceae
Candida albicans

is characterized by decreased vascular resistance (distributive shock), increased cardiac output, tachycardia, warm extremities, and adequate urine output. At this stage, coexisting hypovolemia may result in a decreased output, but overt myocardial depression is not characteristic of the early, hyperdynamic shock secondary to sepsis. Later, the uncompensated phase occurs, with intravascular volume depletion and myocardial depression becoming more apparent. The child is now cold, listless, anuric, and in respiratory distress and has a high vascular resistance and decreasing cardiac output. This clinical picture progresses with the addition of ischemic injury to that caused by endotoxins, and irreversible shock is reached when myocardial damage is profound.

Miscellaneous
Heat Stroke

Children who develop high fevers, are overbundled, and may have a congenital failure of the heat-dissipating mechanism (Riley-Day syndrome) are clearly at risk. In addition, heat stroke is obviously more common in hot weather. Limitation of liberal water intake, as may occur in infants, or intentional deprivation is also an aggravating feature. In children who present with acidosis, hemodynamic dysfunction, and fever of > 42°C, heat stroke is a major, life-threatening consideration.

Pulmonary Embolism

Acute massive pulmonary thromboembolism can occur in children after surgery, especially pelvic surgery; instrumentation of the heart vessels; cardiac catheterization; hemodialysis; hyperalimentation; ventriculojugular catheterization; pulmonary artery catheterization; trauma, especially to the pelvis; and hypercoagulopathies such as polycythemia. It may also occur secondary to other illnesses, such as dehydration and heat stroke, and although it is not embolic, sickle cell disease can lead to massive pulmonary artery thrombosis, which has characteristics in common with massive pulmonary embolism.

Fat embolism occurs in a wide variety of clinical settings that give rise to bone trauma. Although traumatic fracture is the most common of these, it may also follow orthopedic surgery and even occur in sickle cell disease. Although fat embolism after long-bone fracture is said to be rare in children, it still requires consideration. The picture of acute massive fat embolism is that of shock secondary to low output due to sudden right ventricular failure. As in pulmonary thromboembolism, fat globules in the pulmonary arteries lead to pulmonary vasoconstriction and pulmonary capillary endothelial damage with resulting shock. CNS and clotting abnormalities also occur.

Entry of air into central vessels may be rapidly fatal or may give rise to a shock state. Air emboli can occur when large vessels are lacerated after trauma, during spinal surgery or neurosurgery, and iatrogenically by accidental air entry during intravenous therapy. "Air block" of the right ventricular outflow tract, main pulmonary artery, or distal alveolar arterioles results in decreased right ventricular output and decreased systemic perfusion. There is also reflex pulmonary vasoconstriction which increases right ventricular afterload. In addition, systemic emboli may occur, giving rise to CNS signs and myocardial ischemia. Profound hypotension and cyanosis with hyperpnea indicate a grave shock state.

Acute Pancreatitis

Acute hemorrhagic pancreatitis can readily give rise to hypotension, hemoconcentration, anuria, hypocalcemia, fever, and acidosis, which may require therapy aimed at correcting the shock state. Although cholelithiasis and alcoholism are the leading causes of this condition in adults, in children it is most commonly associated with drug therapy (thiazides, prednisone, azathioprine), congenital biliary disease, or mumps or occurs idiopathically.

Drug Overdose

A shock-like picture is frequently seen after inadvertent and intentional drug overdoses. This is covered in Chapter 22.

DIAGNOSIS OF SHOCK STATE

The early diagnosis of shock requires a high index of suspicion and a knowledge of which conditions predispose children to shock. Clearly, the age of the child will provide some diagnostic clues, and previous medical conditions such as congenital heart disease, immunodeficiencies, suspected ingestions, and a history of trauma will all raise the suspicion that the child may be suffering from a shock state. In children, shock can also occur after surgery, especially cardiac surgery. Clearly, children who are febrile, have an identifiable source of an infection, or are hypovolemic from any cause are at great risk of developing shock. It may be very difficult to determine which children have crossed from being dehydrated and febrile to having fully developed shock.

With regard to the physical examination, it is possible to identify signs reflecting the underlying physiologic process. Decreased tissue perfusion can be identified by changes in body surface temperature, capillary refill, and impaired function of several organ systems. Body surface temperature is a time-honored, simple, and effective method of assessing adequate tissue perfusion. Cold extremities or increased peripheral core temperature gradients (>2°C) indicate intact homeostatic mechanisms that have decreased nonessential cutaneous perfusion in the face of contracted intravascular volume. This system is very efficient and therefore serves as an early indicator of decreased intravascular volume. Decreased capillary refill is also a sensitive indicator of tissue perfusion. The exact technique for determining capillary refill must be determined by each physician because there are no recognized standards. The rate of refill after firm compression of soft tissues and nail beds for 5 seconds is related to the site of determination due to the intricacy of the capillary bed, the temperature, and the amount of circulation through the microvasculature. In general, refill over the face is faster than that over the chest, which is faster than that over the hands and feet. Normally, a blanched area disappears extremely rapidly, in less than 3 seconds. Capillary refill that takes longer than 5 seconds is clearly abnormal. Although this is a very nonspecific indicator of tissue hypoperfusion, it is also a very sensitive one. In addition, stasis due to pheripheral vasoconstriction may lead to peripheral cyanosis. Although peripheral hypoperfusion is the physiologic response to intravascular volume contraction, it does not, in itself, indicate shock; however, it clearly heralds it. In addition, the physical findings of dehydration may also be present and can indicate the severity of hypovolemia (Table 11.5). Vital organ hypoperfusion can be assumed to occur if oliguria from renal hypoperfusion coexists or if altered mentation occurs, indicating CNS hypoperfusion.

The physical findings of acidosis are primarily respiratory. Decreased CNS pH is a potent stimulus to the chemoreceptors located in the medulla. Chemoreceptor stimulation causes increased minute ventilation by increasing both tidal volume and respirator rate. Therefore, tachypnea, hyperpnea, and hyperventilation are frequently seen as early findings in shock states. Respiratory alkalosis is frequently an early accompaniment of all stages of all types of shock, but with severe shock, decreased respirations may add respiratory acidosis to metabolic acidosis.

Further assessment of the severity and cause of shock states is greatly assisted by several laboratory investigations. Routine laboratory tests such as serum electrolytes, blood cell counts, platelet counts, and hematocrits (for the reasons discussed earlier) are obviously necessary to delineate the extent of metabolic disturbance. Serum calcium should be determined in

TABLE 11.5.
Dehydration in Children: Clinical Signs[a]

Clinical Signs	Mild	Moderate	Severe
Activity	Normal	Lethargic	Lethargic to coma
Color	Pale	Gray	Mottled
Urine output	Decreased (<2–3 ml/kg/hr)	Oliguric (<1 ml/kg/hr)	Anuria
Fontanel	Flat	Depressed	Sunken (retreated)
Mucous membrane	Dry	Very dry	Cracked
Skin turgor	Slight decrease	Marked decrease	Tenting
Pulse	Normal to increased	Increased	Grossly tachycardic
Blood pressure	Normal	Normal	Decreased
Weight loss	5%	10%	15%

[a]Hypernatremic dehydration may occur with only moderate changes in clinical signs.

all shock states because hypocalcemia occurs frequently and can further compromise respiratory muscle, myocardial, and metabolic function. Measurements of serum protein, albumin, and colloid oncotic pressure serve as guides to volume replacement and the severity of the capillary endothelial defect.

Probably the most frequently performed and most valuable laboratory investigation is the arterial blood gas analysis. Clearly, arterial oxygen content and carbon dioxide tension aid in the evaluation of the adequacy of ventilatory function which is frequently impaired in shock. In addition, determination of pH and base deficit serves as one of the most readily available methods of quantifying tissue hypoperfusion.

Shock can be divided into four classes according to the amount of blood loss and the severity of symptoms. Table 11.6 shows these classes as defined by the Advanced Trauma Life Support Standards of the American College of Surgeons. This classification can be used to guide therapy, assess severity, and standardize various shock states as well as to provide a useful basis for information transfer between caretakers of children in shock.

TABLE 11.6.
Advanced Trauma Life Support Classification of Shock

Class I
15% or less acute blood volume loss
Blood pressure normal
Pulse increased 10–20%
No change in capillary refill

Class II
20–25% loss of blood volume
Tachycardia > 150 beats/min
Tachypnea 35–40 breaths/min
Capillary refill prolonged
Systolic blood pressure decreased
Pulse pressure decreased
Orthostatic hypotension > 10–15 torr
Urine output > 1 ml/kg/hr

Class III
30–35% blood volume loss
All of the above signs
Urine output < 1 ml/kg/hr
Lethargic, clammy, and vomiting

Class IV
40–50% blood volume loss
Nonpalpable pulses
Obtunded

MONITORING OF SHOCK

It cannot be emphasized too strongly that the most effective and sensitive physiologic monitoring available is the repeated and careful examination of the child's physical status by a competent and experienced observer. Observations for alteration in peripheral perfusion, color, presence of cyanosis, characteristics of the pulse, blood pressure, respiratory pattern, and level of consciousness are absolutely essential in the continuous, ongoing monitoring of children with shock. Careful nursing observation of vital signs and the activity of the child and clear, concise display of these data form the central core of information from which the child's therapy is determined. In addition, the minimum monitoring of a child with shock or at risk for shock includes continuous electrocardiographic monitoring and temperature and blood pressure measurements. In younger infants, blood glucose should be determined frequently (Dextrostix). In all but the most mild cases, blood pressure determination will probably necessitate invasive intra-arterial cannulation. In addition, these indwelling arterial cannulas can be used for continuous monitoring of blood gases that, as mentioned earlier, provide the key laboratory measurements in monitoring patients with shock. Relying on sphygmomanometry in children with shock has many pitfalls and is remarkably unreliable. The unstable and potentially catastrophic compromise in circulation requires beat-to-beat continuous blood pressure measurement and display. In addition to electrocardiographic and blood pressure monitoring, close attention to intake and output and urine production is essential. Urine output in children is normally 2–3 ml/kg/hr, and urine outputs of <1 ml/kg/hr are indicative of renal hypoperfusion in shock states. It is usual for oliguria to occur early in shock states and injury before the alterations in blood pressure or the development of the significant tachycardia. Alterations in urine-specific gravity should be noted. (Naturally, intake should be carefully recorded, and the patient's weight should also be monitored.)

In patients with severe shock and certainly in children with myocardial compromise, consideration must be given to invasive venous and pulmonary arterial pressure monitoring. In the past decade, there has been increasing use of this form of monitoring in critically ill children. It now has a firmly established role to play in providing quick, accurate assessment not only of cardiac performance as determined by cardiac output but also of both right and left filling pressures and alterations in pulmonary vascular resistance.

TREATMENT OF SHOCK

General Principles

Base deficits of >10 mEq/liter in septic or cardiogenic shock are generally associated with a poor outcome; profound metabolic acidosis due to hypovolemia and renal bicarbonate loss, however, is generally better tolerated. A base deficit of >6 mEq/liter should probably be corrected in acute shock states. This is now a debatable point, but we find it helpful.

Bicarbonate supplementation can be given by repeated slow boluses of 1–2 mEq of sodium bicarbonate per kg; in infants, a solution of 0.5 mEq/ml is used to avoid acute change in osmolarity which may lead to intraventricular hemorrhage. Frequently, 10–20 mEq/kg may be required to correct profound acidosis. The formula, 0.3 (body weight) × (base deficit) = mEq of NaHCO₃, required to half-correct acidosis, may serve as a rough guide. If bolus therapy is not effective or the metabolic acidosis persists or grows more severe, a continuous intravenous sodium bicarbonate infusion may be required.

If sodium bicarbonate supplementation is ineffective, peritoneal dialysis may be necessary to remove excess acid, lactate, phosphate, and hydrogen ion, as well as to correct hypernatremia and to allow further bicarbonate administration. In sever metabolic acidosis with hemodynamic collapse, which may occur in aspirin overdose and with inborn errors of metabolism of sepsis, peritoneal dialysis may be lifesaving not only by removing excess acid by also by alleviating the underlying cause of shock. Adequate peritoneal perfusion is necessary for effective peritoneal dialysis, so initial blood pressure resuscitation is mandatory.

Cardiovascular Support

Stroke Volume

Preload Augmentation

Rapid intravascular volume expansion guided by the clinical examination and urine output is frequently adequate to restore blood pressure and peripheral perfusion in children with shock. In the case of otherwise normal cardiorespiratory function, volume overload resulting in pulmonary edema is rare. Volume replacement of 10–20 ml/kg over 10 minutes can generally be safely given. Replacement of losses due to excess urine output, stool output, or hemorrhage can be guided by body weight changes and careful monitoring of intake and output. When volume resuscitation of > 50–70 ml/kg in the first 4–6 hours is required, more invasive monitoring should be considered. Severe third-space losses due to capillary leak can occur.

Another method of increasing venous return and augmenting preload is by application of military antishock trousers, which are manufactured in pediatric sizes. Application of these in the field or hospital for children suffering from severe hypotension may prove lifesaving and provide a means of maintaining blood pressure until more definitive therapy is provided.

The use of colloid versus crystalloid replacement for shock is an ongoing debate in pediatrics. For simple dehydration, the estimated fluid and electrolyte deficits should be replaced. For sepsis and trauma, the underlying arguments of vascular leak, intravascular oncotic pressure maintenance, pulmonary edema (adult respiratory distress syndrome), and cost versus risks are ongoing. At present, a judicious mixture of crystalloid, blood products to maintain hemoglobin and clotting factors, and colloid (albumin and hetastarch) to maintain colloid oncotic pressure seems appropriate and most reasonable. Recent evidence suggests that hypertonic fluid replacement may have a role to play. Table 11.7 provides guidelines for fluid therapy in dehydration.

Cardiac Contractility Augmentation

The use of pressor agents to increase myocardial function in children is well described. Although for years digitalis glycosides have been advocated, their use in children with potential electrolyte abnormalities, myocardial impairment, irritable myocardium, acid-base disturbances, and question-able renal function carries a high risk. For this reason, more specific ino-tropic agents with a rapid onset of action, ability to be titrated, and short half-lives are preferable. The use of dopamine, dobutamine, isoproterenol, and other catecholamine pressor agents is well described in both infants and older children (Table 11.8). Although there is some question on the value of dopamine in neonates because of their functionally immature au-tonomic nervous system, it is frequently of value in increasing hemody-namic performance. All of these agents augment myocardial contractility.

Specific Catecholamines

The complexity of the cardiovascular derangement in shock states makes it difficult to predict the response to individual hemodynamically active therapeutic agents. This has two implications. First, the response to any agent may not be the textbook response. For example, dobutamine in a volume-depleted patient may cause significant vasodilation (systemic and

TABLE 11.7.
Fluid Therapy Guidelines

	H_2O (ml/kg)	Na	K (mEq/kg)	Cl	HCO_3
To Correct 10% Dehydration					
Isotonic	150	7–10	7–10	4–8	8–15
Hypotonic (Na < 130 mEq/liter)	75	10–15	10–15	5–10	10–20
Hypertonic (Na > 150 mEq/liter)	125	2–5	2–5	2–4	4–10

	Maintenance 900/m²/day or by		
Calories	weight:		
		1–10 kg	100 cal/kg
		11–20 kg	1000 + 50 cal/kg
		>20 kg	1000 + 20 cal/kg
Water	100 ml/100 cal/day		
Electrolytes[a]	Na = 3–5 mEq/kg/day		
	K = 2–3 mEq/kg/day		
	Ca⁺ = 2–5 mEq/kg/day		

[a]Balance anion as chloride, bicarbonate, or phosphate guided by laboratory tests.

TABLE 11.8.
Specific Agents

Agent	Site of Action	Dose (μg/kg/min)	Effect[a]
Dopamine	Dopamine receptor	1–3	Renal vasodilator Inotrope
	$\alpha > \beta$	5–20	Peripheral vasoconstriction Increased PVR Dysrhythmias
Dobutamine	β_1	1–20	Inotrope Vasodilation (β_2) Lowers PVR Weak α-activity Tachycardia and extra-systolic
Isoproterenol	β_1 and β_2	0.05–2.0	Inotrope Vasodilation Lowers PVR $M\dot{V}O_2 \uparrow$ Dysrhythmias
Epinephrine	$\beta > \alpha$	0.05–1.0	Inotrope Tachycardia Decreased renal flow $M\dot{V}O_2 \uparrow$ Dysrhythmias
Norepinephrine	$\alpha > \beta$	0.05–1.0	Profound constrictor Inotrope $M\dot{V}O_2 \uparrow$, SVR $\uparrow \uparrow$
Sodium nitro-prusside	Vasodilator—Arterial greater than venous	0.5–10	Rapid onset, short duration Increases ICP $\dot{V}/\dot{Q}$ mismatch
Nitroglycerin	Vasodilator—Venous greater than arterial	1–20	Cyanide toxicity Decreases PVR Increases intracranial pressure

[a]PVR, pulmonary vascular resistance; SVR, systemic vascular resistance; ICP, intracranial pressure; and $\dot{V}/\dot{Q}$, ventilation/perfusion.

pulmonary) and increased intrapulmonary shunting and, therefore, actually decrease cardiac output and oxygen delivery despite enhancing contractility. Second, as the response may vary, invasive hemodynamic monitoring and measurement of cardiac output are indicated in children ill enough to require advanced hemodynamic support. This needs to be remembered during the coming discussion of the cardiovascular support drugs. Table 11.8 summarizes key points concerning these agents.

Isoproterenol was the first synthetic catecholamine and has found extensive application in a wide host of clinical settings. Isoproterenol is almost a pure β-adrenergic agonist and is thus a positive inotropic and chronotropic agent. In addition, both peripheral vasodilation, as manifested by a fall in diastolic blood pressure, and pulmonary vasodilation occur. Also, renal, splanchnic, muscle, and cutaneous flows are increased. The latter may unfortunately lead to perfusion of nonessential vascular beds and a relative "steal" phenomenon. In addition, the fall in diastolic pressure may have adverse effects on myocardial perfusion, as this maximally occurs during diastole. This, in combination with markedly increased myocardial oxygen consumption ($M\dot{V}O_2$) due to its positive inotropic and chronotropic effects, may lead to aggravated myocardial ischemia. Isoproterenol is also a potent pulmonary vasodilator. As such, it is a very useful agent in children with right heart failure after elevated pulmonary vascular resistance. Isoproterenol blunts hypoxic pulmonary vasoconstrictor activity and may thus increase intrapulmonary shunting. For this reason, oxygen delivery should be monitored in the critical situation with significant lung disease when isoproterenol is administered. Finally, isoproterenol has β-adrenergic metabolic effects causing hyperglycemia, albeit less than those seen with epinephrine, and increased release of free fatty acids.

Dopamine remains the most commonly used therapeutic agent in shock states. This is true in spite of or perhaps because of its less than pure effects. Dopamine stimulates α-adrenergic, β-adrenergic and dopaminergic sympathetic receptors and thus has a variety of effects. In low doses (1–3 $\mu g/kg/min$), it acts primarily by causing renal and splanchnic vasodilation, thus serving as a diuretic and protecting renal profusion. In medium doses (3–10 $\mu/kg/min$), increasing inotropic effect is seen, with increased stroke volume and cardiac output. In larger doses (>15 $\mu/kg/min$), increasing α-adrenergic vasoconstrictor activity is seen, and decreased peripheral and renal perfusion and increased myocardial afterload may occur. The exact degree to which these mixed effects occur in an individual varies, and careful monitoring to assess the response to dopamine in each patient is required. Tachycardia and extrasystole may occur but is less of a problem with dopamine than with the previously mentioned agents. Pulmonary vascular resistance may be increased, and this should be remembered in treating newborns and patients at risk for pulmonary hypertension. In addition, due to the arguments given earlier concerning the neonatal myocardium, there is some debate concerning its efficacy in neonates.

Epinephrine stimulates both α-adrenergic and β-adrenergic receptors. The response to it mimics that of generalized autonomic stimulation. In general, increased cardiac output, blood pressure, and heart rate, a hypermetabolic state, CNS stimulation, and increased $M\dot{V}O_2$ occur. Both pulmonary and systemic vascular resistances are elevated, and renal ischemia is a potential complication. Tachydysrhythmias and ventricular dysrhythmias are serious threats. Epinephrine can certainly always be expected to enhance myocardial contractility and to lead a still heart to beating, but its myriad untoward activities cause its use to be reserved only for dire cases.

Norepinephrine has a long, if somewhat unglorified, clinical position. Although it is both an α-adrenergic and a β-adrenergic agonist, its potent peripheral vasoconstrictor effects overshadow the positive inotropic effects. Severe systemic, pulmonary, peripheral, renal, and splanchnic vasoconstriction occur with its use, and these acutely elevate the blood pressure. In addition, cardiac contractility is enhanced, but in the setting of massively increased myocardial afterload, cardiac output may not be increased, and the markedly enhanced $M\dot{V}O_2$ may cause profound myocardial ischemia. For these reasons, its use had largely been abandoned. Recently, however, clinicians have again begun to consider it as a potentially valuable therapeutic agent.

Afterload Reduction

Afterload reduction plays a role in improving myocardial performance in children with cardiogenic shock after surgery, myocarditis, or ischemic heart disease or in the later stages of septic shock with myocardial failure. In the late stage of septic shock, high systemic vascular resistance, poor peripheral perfusion, and decreased cardiac output may respond to afterload reduction. Afterload-reducing agents may also benefit children who require epinephrine or norepinephrine as an inotropic agent to decrease the α-adrenergic effects of increased systemic vascular resistance. This combination of afterload reduction with increased inotropy may provide the optimal support for a profoundly impaired myocardium. Both nitroprusside and nitroglycerin lower systemic vascular resistance in children and are useful afterload-reducing agents. It has been suggested that nitroglycerin is a more potent venodilator and pulmonary vasodilator than is nitroprusside, whereas nitroprusside has more potent peripheral arterial vasodilating effects.

Steroids

There is no specific evidence in the literature concerning the use of steroids in children with shock. However, there seems to be supportive evidence in the adult literature that prednisone at a dose of 30 mg/kg, given early and repeated once or twice in septic shock, improves the outcome. When adrenal function may be impaired, such as in the Waterhouse-Friderichsen syndrome after meningococcal or *H. influenzae* infection, glucocorticoid replacement is essential, and mineralocorticoid replacement should be considered.

Naloxone

Naloxone has been shown to reverse hypotension and improve survival in many experimental studies. Unfortunately, in humans the results are mixed at best. Although the discovery of the role of endophins in shock states provides interesting insights and potentially valuable therapeutic implications, these have not as yet been realized.

Supportive Therapy

Coagulation abnormalities probably occur to some extent in all forms of septic shock and may complicate hypoperfusion states of any etiology. Monitoring of prothrombin time, partial thromboplastin time, and platelet count and observation for excessive bleeding are essential. Therapy specifically designed to replace absent clotting factors seems to provide the most advantageous therapy currently available. Use of vitamin K, fresh frozen plasma, and platelet transfusions should correct most coagulopathies.

Gastrointestinal disturbances after hypoperfusion and stress include bleeding and ileus. Ileus may result from electrolyte abnormalities and may result in abdominal distention with respiratory compromise. Gastrointestinal blood loss from either acute gastritis or peptic ulceration should be prevented by using antacids and/or an H_2-receptor blocker such as cimetidine.

Renal support is essential to avoid prolonged renal shutdown in hypoperfusion states. Volume augmentation and diuretics such as mannitol, furosemide, and ethacrynic acid have been advocated for early use to encourage renal blood flow and to maintain tubular function. Low-dose dopamine (3–5 μ/kg/min) also improves renal blood flow and may be beneficial in preventing acute renal failure in shock states.

Respiratory Support for the Child in Shock

The child with acute circulatory failure may have ineffective oxygen delivery not only on a hemodynamic basis but also on a decreased respiratory muscle function basis, causing hypoventilation and hypoxemia. This may be due to decreased respiratory muscle perfusion, acidosis, hypoxia, and electrolyte abnormalities. A second cause of respiratory failure in shock is the development of intrapulmonary shunting due to noncardiac pulmonary edema (adult respiratory distress syndrome), which may further aggravate ventilation/perfusion abnormalities. For these reasons, increased inspired oxygen is essential in all children with shock. Furthermore, in order to ensure the airway provides optimal relief from respiratory muscle fatigue and facilitates provision of positive airway pressure, early intubation of the trachea should be considered in all children with shock.

SUMMARY

An aggressive multimodality approach to the treatment of shock consists of consideration of all of these therapies, often simultaneously. Ensuring a patent airway and adequate oxygenation is, as always, the first step. Preload augmentation with intravascular fluid therapy should rapidly follow and is the most important therapy in nearly every instance. It should be considered at every stage of shock therapy and for every type of shock. Therapy directed at the underlying cause, whether it be instituting antibiotics, converting a cardiac dysrhythmia, or stopping hemorrhage, should occur concurrently. Frequently, oxygenation, ventilation, and fluid therapy

TABLE 11.9.

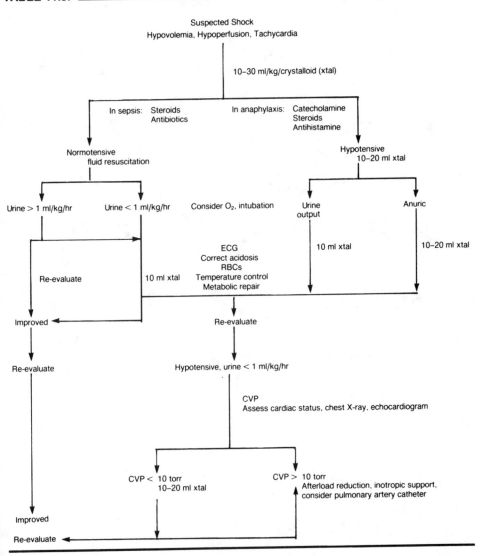

are all that is required and, even in severe circumstance, will often delay further deterioration to allow more aggressive therapy. The administration of pharmacologic agents, including agents from steroids to pressor agents, aimed at correcting metabolic abnormalities and restoring cardiovascular function is the final step in completing the multimodality therapy of shock states. Table 11.9 provides an abbreviated algorithm for shock therapy.

CHAPTER 12

Evaluation of the Comatose Child

Although this chapter will focus on the physical examination, evaluation, and practical approach to the comatose patient, it is important for the reader to remember the general aspects of intensive care. Careful attention to the "ABCs" of patient care—focusing on airway, breathing, and circulation—apply just as much to the comatose patient as to the more general intensive care unit (ICU) patient. The reader is referred to the introductory chapters of this book to review these subjects.

EMERGENT NEUROLOGIC ASSESSMENT

The Glasgow coma scale is particularly useful for emergent neurologic assessment of the comatose child. The information required for the scale is always available in the emergent setting, and no reliance is placed on historical information. The components of the score are shown in Table 12.1

Scores of <9 are suggestive of very severe injury, and these patients should have airway support. Such patients have considerable mortality and are potential candidates for intracranial pressure monitoring and other invasive hemodynamic monitoring. Children with higher scores generally recover. Thus for purposes of quick prognostic estimates, this score is very helpful. The goal is to identify high-risk patients for more invasive therapies—not to decide patients from whom to withhold therapy.

The Glasgow coma scale has two advantages over a more thorough neurologic examination: simplicity and direction. Its simplicity permits very frequent re-examination and recording of the scores. It is easy to see that the scale is directed at measuring arousability, the specific deficit with which the child presents. The Glasgow coma score is a useful "vital sign" to record on the emergency room and intensive care flow sheets. This sequential examination may be performed by personnel who are less sophisticated in neurologic assessment and who can provide backup monitoring for the physician or nurse who should perform more thorough, sequential examinations as described later in this chapter.

In addition to assessment of the depth of coma of the child, further assessment of the child's neurologic status must be accomplished in the

151

TABLE 12.1.
Glasgow Coma Scale

Eye opening	Points
No response	1
Response to pain	2
Response to voice	3
Spontaneously	4
Verbal response	
No response	1
Incomprehensible sounds	2
Inappropriate words	3
Disoriented conversation	4
Oriented and appropriate	5
Motor response	
No response	1
Decerebrate posturing	2
Decorticate posturing	3
Flexion withdrawal	4
Localizes pain	5
Obeys commands	6
Maximum score	15

emergency period. Children can be divided into three categories: (a) traumatic injuries involving the head and other systems, (b) traumatic injuries restricted to the head, and (c) medical brain injuries. The priorities of assessment are slightly different.

Systemic Trauma Involving the Head

Children with mixed systemic and central nervous system (CNS) traumatic injuries are evaluated by a trauma team that includes a general (pediatric or otherwise) surgeon. The essential question to answer is whether an abdominal or thoracic injury offers an acute threat to the patient's life. Hypotension in such patients is due to systemic trauma, not head injury, and efforts must be made to control shock. If the child has a life-threatening major abdominal or thoracic injury requiring operative intervention, this intervention has priority over most head injuries, but during such therapy, the clinician must anticipate the possibility of cerebral herniation and must be prepared to treat it appropriately. If it is possible without threat to life for the child to have a neurosurgical assessment prior to going to the operating room, this should be accomplished. For instance, if the military antishock trouser suit permits the blood pressure to stabilize, even in the suspected presence of abdominal trauma, some patients can be quickly evaluated via a computed axial tomography (CAT) scan before going to the operating room. However, neurosurgical evaluation is usually less important than care of the general surgical emergencies. If the pupils are unequal or a subdural or epidural hematoma is strongly suspected, evaluation should proceed in the operating room while the abdominal or thoracic emergency is treated.

Traumatic Injuries Restricted to the Head

The child with isolated head trauma must also be evaluated by the general surgeon, whose job is to ensure that systemic trauma is not missed by the remainder of the trauma team. Generally, systemic trauma is not going to pre-empt neurosurgical intervention or evaluation in such patients, but careful evaluation and attention to hemodynamic stability must be maintained throughout the evaluation. If the child is severely comatose or is going to the operating room for a neurosurgical procedure, then peritoneal lavage or minilaparotomy may be indicated in certain patients. The liver-spleen radionuclide scan is of value for assessing the abdomen and may be accomplished in the ICU after emergent neurologic assessment has been accomplished. Chest films usually rule out acutely life-threatening chest trauma. In short, the child with an "isolated head injury" should be considered a child with mixed injuries in whom the systemic injury is so mild as to be of less concern in the emergency treatment phase. In this category of patient, the head injury is more likely to harm the patient than are the systemic injuries, and neurosurgical intervention takes priority.

Medical Brain Injury

Finally, comatose children with no history of trauma also require expeditious evaluation of their CNS. When airway, ventilation, and circulation are established, the question becomes: "Does this patient require emergency neurosurgery?" The absence of a trauma history does not rule out either trauma or neurosurgical intervention; spontaneous intracerebral hemorrhage may present with sudden coma, and brain tumors become manifest in similar fashion, which may include sudden coma. The most important tool for the clinician is the physical examination. The emergency neurologic examination includes assessment of motor function (e.g., spontaneous, responsive to pain or voice, obedient), verbal function, the pupils (equality and reactivity), and eye opening. Unfortunately, in comatose patients there is generally little verbal or eye response, and motor response is often described as "withdrawal from pain." If the pupils are acutely unequal or unreactive, this is highly suggestive of a progressive mass lesion and requires emergency treatment of impending herniation. Although surgical intervention is likely, it is still useful to obtain CAT scans of such patients prior to operative intervention (if possible). Thus, in a comatose child the CAT scan is an early priority in management.

PHYSICAL EXAMINATION

It is useful to point out the need for two different types of neurologic assessment. The first type, as discussed in the previous section, is emergent assessment of the severity of neurologic injury and sequential monitoring of the patient. This requires a relatively simple method of examination, such as the Glasgow coma scale. The second type is a more thorough neurologic examination aimed at lesion localization and differential diagnosis of the child's illness. This latter type of examination is not practical to accomplish in the CAT scan room every 5 minutes, nor is the Glasgow coma scale an adequate neurologic assessment of the patient who, having been stabilized, can be subjected to more thorough examination.

Neurologic Examination

Any examination presumes a history has been taken and the examiner has specific questions that remain unanswered. The examination should provide answers for these questions. For the intensivist dealing directly with a poorly responsive child, initial historical information need not be detailed and is often limited by the absence of an informed historian. The physician must immediately concern himself or herself with four questions:

1. What is the stability of the patient?
2. What is the pathologic process?
3. What therapies should be initiated immediately?
4. What further diagnostic tests are needed?

The goal of the physical examination is to develop the best possible answers to the first two questions. With this information, answers to the third and fourth questions follow from the acuity and nature of the illness.

The neurologic examination begins with the assessment of vital signs (Table 12.2) and physical examination of the other systems of the body (Table 12.3). Neurologic assessment is likely to be invalid in older children if, for instance, the blood pressure is <50 mm Hg. Either hyperventilation

---

TABLE 12.2.
Vital Signs and Differential Diagnosis of Coma[a]

System	Sign	Disorder
Temperature	Fever	Infection (especially meningitis, encephalitis), diabetic acidosis, or thyrotoxicosis
Heart rate	Increased	Hypovolemic shock, diabetic acidosis, adrenal insufficiency, congestive heart failure
Blood pressure	Increased	Hypertensive encephalopathy, as in acute glomerulonephritis
	Decreased	Hypovolemia, adrenal insufficiency
Respiratory rate	Increased	Pneumonia, congestive heart failure, metabolic acidosis (especially diabetes)
	Irregular	Pickwickian syndrome (obstructive sleep apnea, CO_2 narcosis)

[a]Adapted with permission from Lockman LA: Coma. In Swaiman K (ed): *The Practice of Pediatric Neurology.* St. Louis, CV Mosby, 1982, p 150.

TABLE 12.3.
Physical Examination and Diagnosis of Coma[a]

System	Sign	Disorder
Skin	Dry	Dehydration, myxedema, adrenal insufficiency
	Wet	Syncope
	Pigment	Addison's disease
	Nevi	Tuberous sclerosis with seizures
	Petechiae	Bacteremia, subacute bacterial endocarditis, idiopathic thrombocytopenic purpura
	Cyanosis	Hypoxia, congenital heart disease with cerebral embolism
	Erythema	Carbon monoxide, atropine, or mercury intoxication
	Butterfly rash	Lupus erythematosus, tuberous sclerosis
	Desquamation	Vitamin A intoxication, scarlatina
	Nail changes	Splinter hemorrhage—Endocarditis Mycotic infection and hypoparathyroidism Periungual fibroma (tuberous sclerosis)
Breath odor	Fruity	Diabetic ketoacidosis
	Feculent	Hepatic encephalopathy
	Garlic	Selenium toxicity, paraldehyde intoxication, arsenic poisoning
	Almonds	Cyanide poisoning
Scalp	Contusions	Trauma
	Vasodilation	Sagittal sinus thrombosis
Eyes	Chemosis	Cavernous sinus thrombosis
	Periorbital ecchymosis	Blow out orbital fracture
	Subhyaloid hemorrhage	Subarachnoid hemorrhage
	Vasospasm	Hypertensive encephalopathy
Ears	Hemorrhage	Basilar skull fracture
	Otitis media	Brain abscess, lateral sinus thrombosis
Nose	Cerebrospinal fluid rhinorrhea	Basilar skull fracture
Mouth	Scarred tongue	Seizure disorder
	Pigmentation	Addison's disease
	Lead lines	Plumbism (lead intoxication)
Neck	Rigid	Meningitis, pneumonia, subarachnoid hemorrhage, encephalitis

TABLE 12.3.—*continued*

System	Sign	Disorder
Thyroid	Enlarged	Myxedema, thyrotoxicosis
Heart	Murmur	Subacute endocarditis, brain abscess
Abdomen	Hepatomegaly	Leukemia, hepatic failure, heart failure
Extremities	Fracture	Trauma, fat embolism
	Ecchymosis	Trauma, hemorrhagic diathesis

[a]Adapted with permission from Lockman LA: Coma. In Swaiman K (ed): *The Practice of Pediatric Neurology.* St Louis, CV Mosby, 1982, p 150.

or hypoventilation may alter the neurologic examination, to say nothing of the possibility of reflecting a central disorder of ventilation. Motor response will be altered by spinal cord transection, but the careless examiner might believe the patient to be comatose. Numerous neurologic disorders are typified by systemic findings.

The general appearance of the child should be noted. Asymmetries of posture may denote focal motor abnormalities. The shape of the head may indicate important disorders; frontal bossing, macrocephaly, microcephaly, split sutures, and tense fontanel are findings of significance. The head circumference should be measured and plotted on an appropriate growth curve; it is surprising how often this step is omitted in the intensive care setting. Finally, the skull can be assessed by percussion ("cracked pot sign," indicative of hydrocephalus), transillumination in infants (which may demonstrate hydrocephalus, subdural effusions, or subdural hematomas), and auscultation (to detect arteriovenous malformations). After these maneuvers, the neurologic examination can be started.

The level of consciousness should be assessed first. Is the child arousable or not? Sequential stimulation with loud voice, touch, and, finally, pain should be used. If the child is arousable, he or she is not comatose but rather is in either a normal or some intermediate state. If the child maintains alertness without further stimulation, he or she is awake or conscious. However, if the child becomes unresponsive again, then his or her level of consciousness falls into the intermediate category. For simplicity, the term that is used in this chapter for such a situation is stupor. In the emergent setting, stupor should be treated similarly to coma. The examiner can move to other issues if the patient is aroused easily and can maintain arousal without further sensory inputs. However, if the patient is stuporous or comatose, the examiner should quickly attempt to answer the above questions. The next thing to do is assess cerebral hemispheric function by determining the motor response to pain (Fig. 12.1).

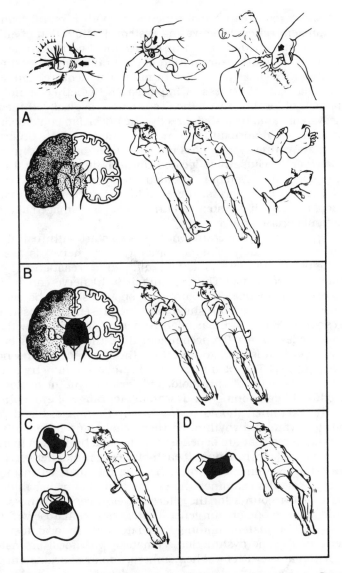

FIGURE 12.1.   Motor responses to noxious stimulation in comatose patients. *Panel A* demonstrates localization of pain as the patient reaches for the inciting stimulus. *Panel B* shows decorticate rigidity. *Panel C* demonstrates decerebrate rigidity. *panel D* shows a flaccid patient with no response to pain. (From Plum F, Posner JB: *The Diagnosis of Stupor and Coma,* ed 3. Philadelphia, FA Davis, 1982, p 66.)

Consciousness requires normal function of both cerebral hemispheres and the brainstem reticular activating system. Dysfunction of either both hemispheres or the reticular activating system must occur in order to count for stupor or coma. Thus, examination of the brainstem by testing cranial nerve activity is the next piece of information to acquire. The examiner now knows that consciousness is impaired and whether or not there is any component of focal hemispheric dysfunction. Logically, if the reticular activating system could be tested directly, the physician could define where the abnormality or abnormalities of neural function exist. Unfortunately, the reticular activating system does not lend itself to simple direct bedside testing. However, because it is located diffusely in the central pons and midbrain regions, this system is situated closely to cranial nerves III–VIII. By testing these cranial nerves, the examiner can then infer that the adjacent reticular activating system is either intact or damaged at a site near a nonfunctional cranial nerve.

The best approach to the cranial nerves is to start with rostrally located nerves and move caudally. The oculomotor (third nerve) is assessed by studying the pupils. Pupils should be examined for reaction to light, size, and symmetry of response. The trigeminal (fifth) nerve can be assessed with the corneal response. The corneal response should be elicited and compared as to sensitivity (threshold) and the presence or absence of consensual response. The vestibular (eighth) nerve is examined with the vestibulo-ocular reflex (VOR). To accomplish this, the doll's eyes or calorics test should be administered to ascertain the presence or absence of an intact VOR pathway. The examiner should compare symmetry of response both for the sensitivity of threshold and for the type of oculomotor response produced (e.g., conjugate, dysconjugate, range of eye motion).

Finally, the examiner should review briefly the pulse, blood pressure, and respiratory rate and rhythm, as these vital signs have central intergrating mechanisms that are dependent on normal brainstem (particularly pontine and medullary) function. If each of these cranial nerve reflexes are intact, then the examiner can infer that the reticular activating system also is intact. Now the examiner should integrate his or her findings into a statement that accounts for the altered level of consciousness. The patient should fall into one of four general categories: comatose without focal hemispheric or brainstem findings, comatose with focal (asymmetric) hemispheric neurologic dysfunction, comatose with focal brainstem dysfunction, or comatose with focal hemispheric and focal brainstem dysfunction.

Metabolic etiologies of coma strongly tend to produce symmetric hemispheric responses and spare brainstem reflex pathways. This is not to say that early unilateral disease, such as subdural or epidural hematomas, cannot present as symmetric hemispheric responses. Structural lesions most often produce hemispheric dysfunction that is focal and are often accompanied by brainstem dysfunction if there is a rostral-to-caudal compartment shift (a herniation syndrome).

Motor Response

Motor response is one of the three components of the Glasgow coma scale. As discussed previously, motor performance is the most reliable form of cognitive testing in the stuporous patient. Purposeful motor behavior requires that the patient be "aware of self and environment" and have intact motor pathways. The motor system originates in the pyramidal cells of the precentral gyrus. It forms a discrete corticospinal tract that passes through the anterior brainstem into the spinal cord, where it innervates the motor neurons.

A normal motor system is one that effects voluntary movements. The speed, strength, and symmetry with which the patient performs work with his or her motor system are all functions that can be quantitated in detail when the patient is awake. For the stuporous or comatose patients, these functions are best described qualitatively and more often require a noxious stimulus to elicit a response. Such stimuli include supraorbital pressure, vigorous rubbing of the sternum, or subungual pressure to the finger or toenails. Eye opening or any form of speech, including poorly defined grunts and groans, suggests wakefulness or some degree of reticular activating system function. Speech and/or purposeful withdrawal from painful stimuli is a sign of cortical function and, hence, cortical preservation. Decorticate postures (i.e., arm, wrist, and finger flexion with leg extension) are associated with cortical or hemispheric dysfunction. Decerebrate postures (i.e., arm and leg extension) correlated with high pontine and midbrain destructive lesions. Flaccidity and the absence of any motor response is indicative of severe low brainstem dysfunction (pontomedullary, junction, and caudal). When asymmetry is noted in the motor response, the limb in question should be stimulated several times to validate the finding. The correct motor execution of verbal commands is an excellent sign for the return of consciousness. The muscle tone of an extremity and the deep tendon reflexes should be evaluated when time permits. These will often confirm the finding of an asymmetric response to pain. Hypotonia occurs acutely with hemispheric, medullary, and spinal cord lesions. Hypertonia is usually a sign of pre-existent corticospinal tract injury. The major exception is acute injury to the midbrain or pons. When this occurs, the vestibulospinal motor system continues to exert a tonic influence on the spinal cord, but the more rostral corticospinal system is disrupted. Hypertonia, hyperreflexia, clonus, and the Babinski sign can be elicited acutely in this situation. Decerebrate rigidity can be thought of as an extreme manifestation of these unopposed vestibulospinal reflexes. Flaccidity strongly suggests spinal shock and should be associated immediately with cervical spine and medullary lesions; both are acutely life threatening.

Pupillary Response (Fig. 12.2)

Pupillary constriction is controlled by parasympathetic fibers in the third nerve. Dilation is mediated by the sympathetic system, which travels dif-

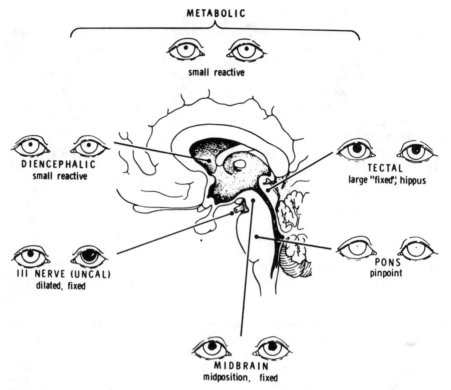

FIGURE 12.2. Pupils in comatose patients. (From Plum F, Posner JB: *The Diagnosis of Stupor and Coma,* ed 3. Philadelphia, FA Davis, 1982, p 46.)

fusely from the hypothalamus to the cervical spinal cord and then to the superior cervical ganglia. Bilateral lesions of the midbrain or pontine tegmentum will interrupt this pathway. Midposition unreactive pupils suggest disruption of both parasympathetic and sympathetic pathways by a midbrain lesion. Pinpoint pupils occur when the parasympathetic innervation is intact but a pontine lesion has disrupted the sympathetic nerves.

The pupillary response is very resistant to metabolic causes of coma, and the absence of pupillary reaction is strongly suggestive of structural disease. Unilateral dilation of a pupil is suggestive of uncal herniation and is caused by unilateral compression of the oculomotor nerve. Metabolic etiologies of coma may cause a variety of pupillary changes, but generally the pupils remain reactive. Atropine and scopolamine cause full dilation of the pupils, which will be unreactive. Glutethimide has variable effects on pupillary size but may cause them to be nonreactive to light. Narcotics generally cause pinpoint pupils that are, however, reactive. Cardiac arrest generally results in fixed, dilated pupils, which will become responsive soon after successful, expeditious resuscitation. If severe anoxia is suffered, reactivity may not be restored.

Corneal Response

The corneal response assesses the integrity of fifth nerve sensory and seventh nerve motor innervation. Afferent inputs are produced by touching the cornea with a cotton wisp and observing the stimulated eye for constriction of the orbicularis oculi or a blink response. The contralateral eye should produce a simultaneous (consensual) blink. If the consensual response is the only response that occurs, then sensation is intact on the stimulated side, and there is an ipsilateral facial nerve palsy. For some obtunded patients, light touch will not produce a response but gentle scleral pressure with cotton swab elicits obicularis oculi constriction.

A weak motor response can be noted by closely following the lower eyelid's medial lashes; they deviate toward the midline and then relax. This reflex is a good test for mid and low pontine dysfunction. In order to test other branches of the seventh nerve, a cotton swab can be used to irritate the nasal mucosa. This produces widespread facial muscular contraction with a grimace response.

Vestibulo-ocular Response (Fig. 12.3)

Doll's Eyes

The doll's eye reflex is also termed the oculocephalic response. There is some confusion among clinicians who are familiar with modern toy dolls. The reflex is elicited by sharply turning the patient's head from the midline to a lateral gaze position with open eyelids. Old-fashioned dolls often had mobile eyeballs that displayed inertia. Thus, a rapid turn of the head was unaccompanied by a similar movement of the eyes. The eyes of these dolls seemed to have the contraversive movement that the oculocephalic response generates in humans. Such a result in the patient is a "positive" oculocephalic reflex.

The reflex can be elicited in all four directions. The head is grasped firmly, the eyelids are held open, and the head is turned to one side quickly. A positive response is indicated if the eyes continue to gaze straight ahead, which reflects active deviation of the eyes in the opposite direction from the turn. This maneuver is repeated in the opposite lateral direction. Vertical movements can be elicited by sequential extension and flexion of the head and neck.

This reflex should never be tested in children with suspected cervical injuries! This includes children who have arrived in the emergency room or the intensive care setting following major head injury. The information that is obtained can be duplicated by testing the caloric response (see below), or its obtainment should wait until adequate assessment of the integrity of cervical spine occurs. The authors' practice is not to perform this

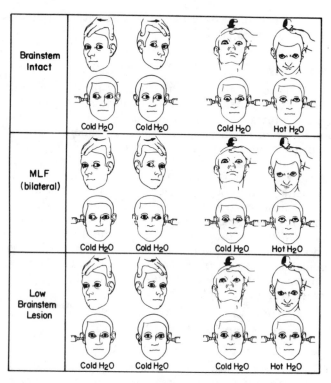

FIGURE 12.3. Vestibulo-ocular response in unconscious patients. In patients with intact brainstem function *(upper panel)*, a positive doll's eye response is elicited, and cold water stimulus causes tonic deviation toward the cold side. *Middle panel* illustrates the findings with involvement of the medial longitudinal fasciculus *(MLF)*. Severe brainstem disease results in abolition of the VOR *(lower panel)*. (Adapted with permission from Plum F, Posner JB: *The Diagnosis of Stupor and Coma,* ed 3. Philadelphia, FA Davis, 1982, p 55.)

reflex during the stabilization period of any child with neurologic disorder.

A normal awake patient may have a positive response if he or she voluntarily fixates vision on an object. In patients with diffuse hemispheral disease and supratentorial coma, the reflex is present and easily elicited. As cortical depression worsens, the reflex becomes more prominent. The presence of the reflex indicates the absence of cortical influence on the brainstem oculomotor centers. The presence of a brisk VOR suggests that the patient does not appreciate visual stimuli and, hence, is comatose. It also proves that brainstem vestibular and oculomotor centers are intact.

With lesions involving the brainstem, oculomotor, or vestibular centers, this reflex is impaired or lost completely. Thus, in the evaluation of a patient for brain death, the clinician seeks the presence of this reflex to indicate brainstem function.

Caloric Response

The caloric response tests the same pathways as the oculocephalic but can be accomplished even in patients with cervical injuries. It is necessary to check the tympanic membrane because the test should not be attempted if the membrane is not intact. To test lateral eye movements, the head is elevated 30° (accomplished by elevating the head of the bed, not requiring neck flexion), and ice water of up to 120 ml is introduced slowly over several minutes into the canal. A small catheter can be made by cutting the tubing of a scalp vein needle; this catheter is placed gently in the auditory canal, and fluid is slowly injected over 2 minutes. The absence of the reflex should not be diagnosed until the maximum volume has been used; lesser volumes can obviously be used if the response is apparent. Testing of the opposite ear should not be attempted for at least 5 minutes; this assures the clinician that the vestibulo-ocular system has stabilized since the previous test.

To test vertical eye movements, both auditory canals should be irrigated simultaneously. Cold water is used to produce a downward gaze, and warm water is used to produce an upward gaze.

In awake patients, nystagmus is produced by these maneuvers, with the slow component toward the cold stimulus and the fast component in the opposite direction. As supratentorial disease develops, including metabolic depression of cortical function, the fast component disappears, and tonic deviation of the eyes toward the cold stimulus develops. Such deviation may persist for several minutes. As metabolic depression continues to severe levels (such as barbiturate coma) or in the presence of brainstem damage, the caloric reflex is abolished.

The oculovestibular reflex is more persistent than the oculocephalic reflex and thus may be present despite absence of the oculocephalic reflex. The elicitation of the caloric response does not require movements of the neck, and in the presence of intact tympanic membranes, this test offers significant advantages over the oculocephalic reflex. As already stated, the oculocephalic reflex ought not to be attempted during the emergent management of comatose children. Where head and neck injury are likely, similar information can be obtained by performing caloric testing.

PRACTICAL APPROACH TO THE COMATOSE CHILD

Causes of coma may be classified in numerous ways, and from a diagnostic standpoint, the classic approach is based on the concept that consciousness is produced by normal function of the brainstem reticular activating system and both cerebral hemispheres. Hence, altered level of consciousness represents bilateral hemispheric dysfunction and/or brainstem reticular activating system dysfunction. By careful consideration of the history, and primarily the physical examination, it is possible to classify comatose patients into one of four pathophysiologic categories:

1. Supratentorial mass lesions
2. Subtentorial mass lesions or destructive lesions

3. Metabolic disorders
4. Psychogenic coma

Specific disease entities within each of these categories have an appropriate and expeditious diagnostic approach, and it is useful to try to classify these patients in order to decide how to approach the work-up of the coma. However, for the physician greeting such a patient in the emergency room or ICU, it is often easier to know what to do than it is to know what the cause might be. For this situation, an alternative classification is preferable:

1. Metabolic coma that is immediately treatable
2. Rapidly progressive supratentorial or subtentorial masses or destructive lesions
3. Nonprogressive (stable) coma

At first glance, this classification may seem less insightful, but its purpose is different. The purpose of this system is not the complete evaluation of the differential diagnosis of the comatose child. The primary goal of the system is to ensure that the clinician prevents early death or permanent sequelae to the patient during the diagnostic process.

Immediately Treatable Metabolic Coma

The term *immediately treatable* metabolic coma eliminates immediate consideration of the many esoteric causes of metabolic coma. In fact, the classification is made even simpler by restricting considerations to metabolic disorders that are also immediately damaging. The primary entity is hypoglycemia, which not only is easily treated but may rapidly cause irreversible CNS damage if not treated. For this reason, the child should be treated with glucose, 2 ml of 25% dextrose per kg. When the intravenous line is established, it is desirable to obtain a blood sample prior to injecting the glucose solution, in order that the diagnosis will not be obscured. However, administration of the sugar should not be delayed until laboratory test results are obtained, nor should such administration await the results of dipstick glucose determinations. The risk of this therapy is nil, and the risks of nontreatment are immense. Dipstick methods are often incorrectly performed or interpreted. In summary, all comatose patients (without other obvious cause) should receive glucose as soon as the intravenous line is established.

In adult patients, thiamine is often administered at this stage, and naloxone hydrochloride or scopolamine are also considered in patients because of possible narcotic or cholinergic overdose. Thiamine deficiency is exceedingly unusual in children. For adult patients, thiamine at a dose of 50 to 100 mg is administered intravenously shortly after glucose is given. If the patient is stable, however, the use of narcotic antagonists is not extremely urgent because the airway, breathing, and circulation are being maintained. Instead of administering such drugs, and waiting for the results, the authors' pragmatic approach is to classify narcotic overdose as "nonprogressive (stable) coma" and consider rapidly progressive intracranial lesion first. Thus, the authors' classification scheme is a therapeutic classification, not a diagnostic approach. Management of metabolic coma at this stage consists of glucose administration, and then consideration must proceed to other intracranial lesions. If the child has fever or meningismus, and meningitis is considered a possibility, then lumbar puncture should be accomplished when the child is stabilized. Antibiotics should be instituted promptly, and if the child is too unstable for lumbar puncture, antibiotics should be administered prior to lumbar puncture.

Rapidly Progressive Intracranial Lesions

Supratentorial lesions cause coma by depressing function of large parts of the cerebral cortex, and thus relatively small focal supratentorial lesions are unlikely to cause coma. Subtentorial lesions may depress consciousness by exerting pressure upon or causing dysfunction or destruction of the brainstem, including the reticular activating system. Unlike supratentorial lesions, a small lesion in the brainstem is capable of depressing consciousness. In either case, onset of coma can rapidly develop with any major intracranial lesion. The differential diagnosis of supratentorial lesions and subtentorial lesions is different, but the ramifications for the emergent management and approach are similar.

As a general rule, metabolic causes of coma lead to a symmetrical neurologic examination. Conversely, the finding of focal abnormalities is strongly suggestive of intracranial mass lesion pathology. However, this rule is often broken, and supratentorial mass lesions may present as fairly symmetrical on examination. Thus, although focal findings support the possibility of intracranial pathology, their absence should not reassure the physician into believing that the coma is based on metabolic cause.

Any patient in whom brainstem abnormalities can be demonstrated should be considered to have a mass lesion until the clinician can rule out such a possibility. Such abnormalities include cranial nerve palsies, abnormal oculovestibular reflexes (calorics), and abnormal oculocephalic reflexes. Whether such abnormalities arise from a supratentorial or a subtentorial source may be suggested by the progression of the patient's illness. Clear rostral-to-caudal deterioration is highly suggestive of a supratentorial mass. For example, if the physician has the opportunity to talk to the obtunded patient, later to intubate him or her, and finally to see one pupil dilate, it is likely that a supratentorial mass lesion is present. The emergency room or intensive care physician rarely has the opportunity to see the full course of rostral-caudal deterioration. However, on a pragmatic level, patients with brainstem abnormalities should be presumed to have serious intracranial pathology with the potential for further deterioration. This situation requires immediate and further delineation, and the most expedient way is via the CAT scan. Great care must be taken, however, to ensure airway and circulation control in such patients.

Once the clinician has decided that the patient is stable enough to undergo a CAT scan and has appropriately prepared the patient (by intubation, appropriate intravenous access, etc.), then the CAT scan should be procured on an emergent basis. The physician should be in attendance at the scan and should monitor the patient intensively during the scan. Specifically, respiration and pulse should be monitored continually, and blood pressure should be checked every 5–10 minutes. If possible, a brief neurologic examination should be accomplished at the time of blood pressure measurement. The study should be reviewed immediately with the attending radiologist and neurosurgeon or neurologist. Further management may be aimed at the demonstrated lesions. If the CAT scan is unremarkable, then supratentorial and subtentorial lesions have been effectively eliminated as acute causes of coma, and consideration is given to nonprogressive (stable) coma.

Nonprogressive (Stable) Coma

It is correct to infer that nonprogressive (stable) coma refers to all causes of coma except for hypoglycemia, cerebrospinal fluid infections (Table 12.4), and intracranial mass lesions. Obviously, this collection of diagnoses is termed stable only in the context of good intensive care; it is assumed that ventilation and circulatory support can be provided to all comatose children in the intensive care environment. Patients with coma from etiologies falling into this category certainly suffer mortality and morbidity in the absence of compulsive intensive care. By the time the clinician arrives at this point, all emergent therapies have been started, and most treatable causes of coma have been identified. At this point, the physician can more carefully consider the history, conduct the physical examination, and plan his or her work-up of the patient.

Differential Diagnosis of Coma

By this point, the clinician has stabilized and examined the child, excluded rapidly progressive and destructive processes, and must reconsider

TABLE 12.4. _____
Infectious Causes of Coma[a]

Bacterial meningitis
Brain abscess with ventricular rupture
Epidural empyema
Subdural empyema
Fungal meningitis
Protozoan infections—Amebic, malarial, cysticercosis
Tuberculous meningitis
Viral encephalitis
Postinfectious encephalomyelitis
Acute hemorrhagic leukoencephalopathy
Severe systemic infection, sepsis

[a]Adapted with permission from Lockman LA: Coma. In Swaiman K (ed): *The Practice of Pediatric Neurology*. St Louis: CV Mosby, 1982, p 153.

the wide differential diagnosis of coma. It is useful to return to the traditional classification:

1. Supratentorial mass lesions
2. Subtentorial mass lesions or destructive lesions
3. Metabolic disorders
4. Psychogenic coma

Rapidly changing lesions have been excluded by several physical examinations and by CAT scans. In the course of obtaining this study, the diagnosis of supratentorial and subtentorial mass lesions may already be clear. If the CAT scan is negative, then the clinician is left with the likely diagnosis of coma due to metabolic etiologies, although early cerebral infarction has not been excluded. Psychogenic coma is a possibility with adult patients but is extremely rare in pediatrics and therefore will not be discussed further here.

At the onset, comatose patients can be divided into those who have a traumatic injury and those who do not. Patients with head trauma are then studied with a CAT scan, which reveals the extent of injuries or simply shows areas of swelling or ischemia. Patients without surgical lesions are presumably comatose from the concussive force of injury, which may have caused neuronal disruption, destruction, etc. These primary injuries may result in secondary neuronal damage, but there is little requirement for further differential diagnosis of coma itself. Table 12.5 lists various traumatic and physical causes of coma.

Children who have not suffered a traumatic event have either structural disease or metabolic disease. Structural disease is either supratentorial or subtentorial, and the mechanism of coma with supratentorial structural disease is increased intracranial pressure, resulting in global ischemia or cerebral herniation. Herniation may present as one of two syndromes termed "central" or "uncal" herniation. Central herniation is typified by a study rostral-caudal pattern of deterioration, with loss of consciousness first, fol-

---

TABLE 12.5.
Traumatic and Physical Causes of Coma[a]

Acute subdural hematoma
Chronic subdural hematoma
Concussion
Contusion
Decompression sickness (caisson disease)
Electrocution
Epidural hematoma—Middle cerebral artery laceration
Extreme hypothermia
Heatstroke
Sunstroke

---

[a]Adapted with permission from Lockman LA: Coma. In Swaiman K (ed): *The Practice of Pediatric Neurology.* St Louis, CV Mosby, 1982, p 153.

lowed by bilateral pupillary dilatation and stereotyped motor responses (Fig. 12.4). A change of posturing from decorticate to decerebrate suggests a midbrain lesion and further caudal progression of the shift in intracranial contents. Uncal herniation proceeds more suddenly, with near simultaneous onset of coma and a unilateral dilated pupil (Fig. 12.5). An ipsilateral third nerve paresis is often demonstrated with the VOR response, and a hemiparesis (contralateral to the lesion) is seen on motor examination. Both types of herniation eventually cause midbrain compression. Thus, uncal herniation syndromes eventually develop a symmetrical appearance

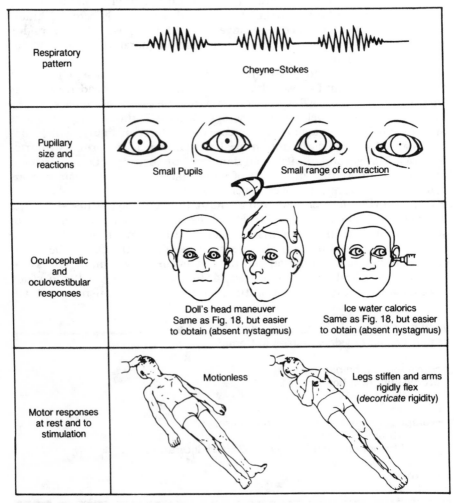

FIGURE 12.4.   Signs of central transtentorial herniation. (From Plum F, Posner JB: *The Diagnosis of Stupor and Coma*, ed 3. Philadelphia, FA Davis, 1982, p 104.)

and become indistinguishable from midbrain and pontine level central herniation syndromes (Fig. 12.6). Both forms of herniation, unless treated, are rapidly destructive to vital brainstem centers. The outcome is either fatality or severe neurologic debilitation. Successful reversal can occur when either syndrome is identified in its early stages. In fact, the main purpose of a CAT scan early in the management of comatose children is to rule out lesions that are causing or are likely to cause cerebral herniation. The therapy for herniation is dealt with earlier in this chapter.

Children with subtentorial disease have either a compression of brainstem structures (as might be seen from a posterior fossa hematoma or tumor) or a dysfunction (hemorrhage or ischemia) of those structures.

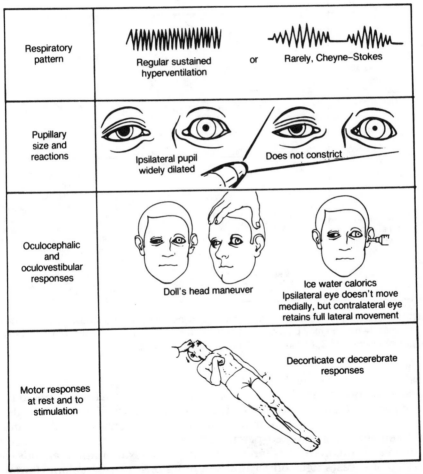

FIGURE 12.5. Signs of uncal herniation, demonstrating third-nerve involvement. (From Plum F, Posner JB: *The Diagnosis of Stupor and Coma*, ed 3. Philadelphia, FA Davis, 1982, p 110.)

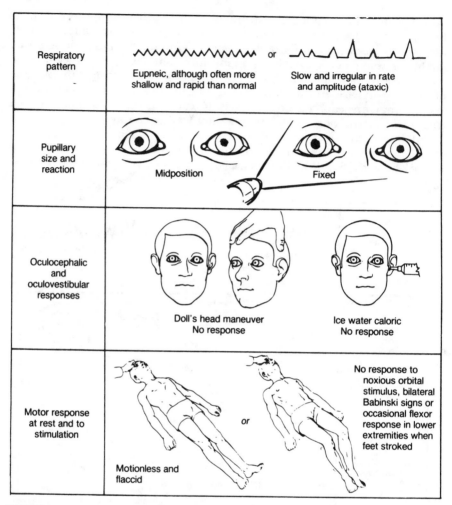

Respiratory pattern	Eupneic, although often more shallow and rapid than normal	or	Slow and irregular in rate and amplitude (ataxic)
Pupillary size and reaction	Midposition		Fixed
Oculocephalic and oculovestibular responses	Doll's head maneuver No response		Ice water caloric No response
Motor response at rest and to stimulation	Motionless and flaccid	or	No response to noxious orbital stimulus, bilateral Babinski signs or occasional flexor response in lower extremities when feet stroked

FIGURE 12.6.   Signs of late herniation, with lower pons-upper medulla involvement. Either central or uncal herniation may progress to this stage. (From Plum F, Posner JB: *The Diagnosis of Stupor and Coma,* ed 3. Philadelphia, FA Davis, 1982, p 108.)

Posttraumatic swelling may also cause destruction, compression, or ischemia of subtentorial structures. Lower cuts of the CAT scan should produce good visualization of these structures and allow relatively facile diagnosis of lesions in this area. In addition, evoked responses (visual, auditory, and somatosensory evoked potentials) can provide electrical evidence of function throughout this area. The physical examination already described also casts light on localization of lesions in this region. However, the precise differential diagnosis of subtentorial lesions is not as important as the mere recognition that such a lesion exists. A CAT scan should reveal whether such a lesion is ischemic, destructive, or hemorrhagic. Further substantiation of the etiology may require angiography.

A metabolic etiology of possibly endogenous or exogenous origin is suggested in comatose patients with no evidence of supratentorial or subtentorial lesion (Table 12.6). The clinician should be tipped in the direction of metabolic disorders if the neurologic examination (including physical findings, electrophysiologic studies, and CAT scans) cannot be reconciled. That is, if there are sporadic findings that do not reflect a lesion in a particular area, metabolic causes should be considered. For example, if a patient has no respiration but has reactive pupils, this is difficult to reconcile with a structural lesion. Any structural lesion that completely eliminates respiration should have compressed or destroyed medullary structures, and supramedullary structures would precede in such destruction; thus, fixed and dilated pupils would be expected. In fact, the pupillary reflex is usually intact in children with metabolic etiologies of coma, abnormal motor responses are common (and usually symmetrical, in contrast to structural supratentorial lesions), and loss of respiration is very common.

Endogenous causes of metabolic coma include: hyperammonemia, either neonatal or acquired; abnormal electrolytes, such as severe hyponatremia, hypoglycemia, and azotemia; and very severe acidosis, as might be seen in diabetic ketoacidosis. In addition, hypoxia should be considered as a met-

TABLE 12.6. ——————————————————————————
Metabolic Causes of Coma[a]

Hypoglycemia
Infection (see Tabel 12.5)
Acidosis
Alkalosis
Hepatic failure, portosystemic shunts
Hyperammonemia
Hypercalcemia and hypocalcemia
Hypercapnia (Pickwickian syndrome)
Hypermagnesemia, hypomagnesemia
Hypoxia
Hyperosmolar states
Hypertonic dehydration
Porphyria
Uremia
Vitamin deficiency/dependency states
   Nicotinic acid
   Pantothenic acid
   Pyridoxine
   Thiamine (Leigh's disease)
   Vitamin B$_{12}$

[a]Adapted with permission from Lockman LA: Coma. In Swaiman K (ed): *The Practice of Pediatric Neurology.* St Louis, CV Mosby, 1982, p 153.

abolic etiology for coma, although of course it is presumed that the clinician already has diagnosed and treated hypoxia appropriately.

Ingestions of substances and infections complete the spectrum of metabolic disorders. Various drugs and poisons are capable of causing coma, and these are generally diagnosed by laboratory screening. Specific findings in poisoning are covered in Chapter 22.

SUMMARY

This chapter has presented a pragmatic approach to the comatose patient. This approach includes appropriate management of the airway, breathing, and circulatory systems. Hypoglycemia is treated pre-emptively, antibiotics are begun if meningitis is probable, and the timing of CAT scanning is considered. Thereafter, the clinician has the opportunity to begin again, carefully considering the myriad causes of coma, knowing that major life-threatening causes of coma have already been treated. In this manner, the intensive care physician can combine emergent management with an intelligent diagnostic approach and be ready to organize or define further neurologic care.

CHAPTER 13

Status Epilepticus

Status epilepticus is a medical emergency that requires prompt recognition and immediate vigorous treatment. Death or permanent neurologic sequelae may occur if patients are untreated or poorly treated or if treatment is delayed. Because status epilepticus is a common neurologic emergency, the pediatric intensivist should be familiar with the underlying pathophysiology, required evaluation, and treatment of these patients.

Status epilepticus is the most severe condition of a seizure. An often-quoted definition* states that status epilepticus represents "epileptic seizures that are so frequently repeated or so prolonged as to create a fixed and lasting epileptic condition." Another definition† includes "convulsive status epilepticus, in which the patient does not recover to a normal alert state between repeated tonic-clonic attacks"; still another definition‡ states "status epilepticus may be defined as a single generalized convulsion that lasts longer than 30 minutes or recurrent tonic-clonic convulsions occurring so frequently that the patient remains obtunded between seizures." Clearly, there is no universally agreed upon definition of status epilepticus. Thus, any type of seizures, if it becomes frequent enough, may by definition constitute status epilepticus. Generalized tonic-clonic status, which represents the most common and dramatic form, has served as the focus for pathophysiologic and therapeutic studies. However, with a greater degree of clinical awareness and improved monitoring techniques, nonconvulsive status epilepticus, such as absence status (spike and wave stupor) and complex partial status, has been recognized. Epilepsia partialis continua represents continuous partial seizures without loss of consciousness.

---

*International League against Epilepsy: *Epilepsia* 5:305, 1964.

*Roger J, Lob H, Tassinari CA: Status epilepticus. In Vinken PJ, Bruyn GW (eds): *Handbook of Clinical Neurology.* Amsterdam, North-Holland, 1974, p 145.

†Delgado-Escueta AV, Wasterlain C, Treiman DM, Porter RJ: Management of status epilepticus. *N Engl J Med* 306:1337, 1982.

‡Morris HH: Current Treatment of status epilepticus. *J Fam Pract* 13:987, 1981.

ETIOLOGY

The true incidence of generalized tonic-clonic status epilepticus is unknown, but it has been estimated that 60,000–160,000 persons in the United States have at least one episode of convulsive status epilepticus in a given year. In children, estimates are that 5.8% of epileptic children admitted to the hospital have status epilepticus.

The etiology of status epilepticus differs widely among studies, reflecting a variety of factors that includes the age of the group studied and the referral base of the institution performing the analysis (Table 13.1). In general, the largest status group consists of patients with known epilepsy who are suffering from an acute exacerbation of seizures. In adult epileptic patients, a significant precipitating factor is related to secondary changes in medication (13–23%), including irregularities of ingestion, withdrawal, and changes in regimen. In contrast, 15–20% of patients with status epilepticus had anticonvulsant drug levels in the therapeutic range, and their etiology would be considered idiopathic. In other epileptic patients, status epilepticus may be related to a progressive underlying disease or systemic

TABLE 13.1.
Etiology of Status Epilepticus in Adults and Children

Diagnostic Category	Aicardi[a]	Rowan[b]	Zhang[c]	Aminoff[d]
Cerebrovascular diseases	—[e]	3	33	15
Infections	29	4	15	4
Traumatic	7	5	10	3
Brain tumors	—	2	5	4
Metabolic disorders	27	1	5	8
Birth injury or perinatal	14	7	3	2
Drug intoxication	—	—	2	10
Encephalopathy	10	—	5	—
Idiopathic	126	9	9	15
Anticonvulsant withdrawal	—	13	40	27
Total number of cases	239	42	100	98

[a]Pediatric series: Aicardi J, Chevrie JJ: Convulsive status epilepticus in infants and children: A study of 239 cases. *Epilepsia* 11:187, 1970.
[b]Rowan AJ, Scott DF: Major status epilepticus: A series of 42 patients. *Acta Neurol Scand* 46:573, 1970.
[c]Zhang Z, Feng Y: A clinical study of 100 status epilepticus cases. *Chin Med J* 95:113, 1982.
[d]Aminoff MJ, Simon RP: Status epilepticus: Causes, clinical features, and consequences in 98 patients. *Am J Med* 69:657, 1980.
[e]Dashes indicate not specifically noted in series described.

central nervous system (CNS) infection. In addition, because almost any CNS insult can precipitate status epilepticus, acute central nervous lesions in nonepileptic patients constitute a second large group. Thus, a variety of cerebrovascular diseases, infections, head trauma, neoplasms, anoxia, metabolic disorders, and toxins may all precipitate status epilepticus.

In children, approximately one-half of the status episodes were idiopathic, and one-half were caused by definable precipitants. In the latter group, slightly more than half were due to acute injury (meningitis, encephalitis, dehydration, etc.) and slightly less than half were in children with prior cerebral damage. Of the children with no demonstrable cause, more than half of the episodes of status were associated with fever. The highest incidence of the fever-associated episodes occurred in children between 6 months and 3 years of age.

PATHOPHYSIOLOGY

The morbidity and mortality from status epilepticus seem related to one or a combination of the following pathophysiologic processes:

1. Damage to the CNS caused by the acute insult precipitating status
2. Systemic stress from repeated generalized tonic-clonic convulsions
3. Injury from repetitive epileptic discharges within the CNS

The interaction of these three processes had complicated the understanding of status epilepticus. In order to help present the pathophysiology of status epilepticus in a clear fashion, Table 13.2 is included which lists the medical complications of status epilepticus by organ system. Table 13.3 lists many of the systemic complications that occur during prolonged seizures and summarizes much of the work discussed in this section.

Arterial and Cerebral Venous Blood Pressures

At the onset of seizure activity, both arterial and cerebral venous blood pressures rise dramatically, with arterial systolic pressures often over 200 mm Hg. The rise of arterial pressure appears to be due to a massive sympathetic discharge and can be blocked with phentolamine hydrochloride. Within an hour, the blood pressure returns to normal or subnormal levels, but the mean arterial pressure does not drop below the level normally considered adequate for cerebral perfusion (e.g., 60 mm Hg).

In summary, arterial blood pressure and cerebral blood flow increase during status epilepticus and are accompanied by large increases of cerebral venous and intracranial pressure. The acute vasodilation of the cerebral vessels may even result in microvascular rupture. Late in status epilepticus, while arterial blood and cerebral venous pressures return to normal or even hypotensive levels, cerebral blood flow continues to be higher than normal. Although the increase in cerebral blood flow is compensatory for the increased metabolic rate of the brain, in premature infants such an increase might, in itself, be harmful (vis-à-vis premature cerebral vasculature, germinal matrix rupture, and intraventricular hemorrhage).

TABLE 13.2.
Medical Complications of Status Epilepticus[a]

Interictal coma

Cumulative anoxia
Cerebral and systemic

Cardiovascular complications
Tachycardia, bradycardia
Cardiac arrest
Cardiac failure
Hypertension
Hypotension, shock

Respiratory system failure
Apnea
Cheyne-Stokes
Tachypnea
Neurogenic pulmonary edema
Aspiration
Pneumonia
Respiratory acidosis
Cyanosis

Renal failure
Oliguria, uremia
Acute tubular necrosis
Rhabdomyolysis
Lower nephron necrosis

Autonomic system disturbances
Hyperpyrexia
Excessive sweating, vomiting
Hypersecretion (salivary, tracheal)
Airway obstruction

Metabolic/biochemical abnormalities
Acidosis (metabolic, lactate)
Anoxemia
Hypernatremia
Hyponatremia
Hyperkalemia
Hypoglycemia
Hepatic Failure

Infections
Pulmonary
Bladder
Skin

[a]Adapted from Glaser GH: Medical complications of status epilepticus. *Adv Neurol* 34:396, 1983, reprinted with permission of Raven Press, New York.

TABLE 13.3. ─────────────────────────────
Systemic Complications of Status Epilepticus

Parameter	Early (<30 min)	Late (>30 min)	Complication
Blood pressure	Increase	Decrease	Hypotension
P_aO_2	Decrease	Decrease	Hypoxia
P_aCO_2	Increase	Variable	Increased intracranial pressure
Serum pH	Decrease	Decrease	Acidosis
Temperature	Increase 1°C	Increase 2°C	Fever
Autonomic activity	Increase	Increase	Arrhythmias
Lung fluids	Increase	Increase	Atelectasis
Serum potassium	Increase	Increase	Arrhythmias
Serum creatine phosphokinase	Normal	Increase	Renal failure
Cerebral blood flow	Increase 900%	Increase 200%	Cerebral bleed
Cerebral oxygen consumption	Increase 300%	Increase 300%	Ischemia

Blood Gases

Profound changes occur in arterial blood gas values during status epilepticus. The blood pH drops dramatically, and serum bicarbonate is reduced dramatically. The arterial PCO_2 is increased, exacerbating the acidosis. Finally, arterial oxygen tension drops, though arterial oxygen gradually improves.

These changes could exacerbate other events, and studies dealing with cortical oxygen metabolism are highly suggestive of inadequate oxygen delivery. The increase in carbon dioxide may contribute to cerebral vasodilation; the combination of increased metabolic activity due to seizures and the vasodilatory effects of CO_2 probably result in a maximally dilated, nonautoregulated cerebral vascular bed. This would be expected to cause significant cerebral edema, prolonged intracranial hypertension, and ultimately, if brain edema is severe, regional cerebral ischemia. Indeed, cerebral herniation has been observed in this animal model.

Glucose, Lactate, and Electrolyte Levels

Serum glucose often increases initially and drops to normal or hypoglycemic levels later.

Arterial lactate rises immediately when status epilepticus is induced, reaching very high levels within minutes; this eventually returns to normal. Measurement of arterial and cerebral venous lactate suggests net uptake of lactate by the brain, which supports the notion that lactate production results from tonic-clonic manifestations of status epilepticus.

Changes in lactate levels can be explained by the following mechanism:

Cerebral glucose consumption during early status epilepticus greatly exceeds cerebral oxygen consumption (stoichiometrically), gradually decreasing to equal oxygen consumption by 1 hour. Anaerobic glycolysis is required, and lactate is produced. When the glucose consumption rate drops to match oxygen consumption, lactate production decreases, a fact consistent with the finding that cerebral lactate levels stop increasing after the first hour of status epilepticus.

Severe Hyperpyrexia

Severe hyperpyrexia develops during prolonged seizures. Temperatures can reach as high as 43°C (109.3°F). After seizure activity ceases, the temperature drifts downward, eventually becoming subnormal. The increase of temperature during status is blunted, but not abolished, by paralysis; hyperpyrexia may reflect hypothalamic dysfunction as well as increased total oxygen consumption in the body.

Brain Metabolism

Clearly, status epilepticus may injure the brain. The mechanism, however, is unclear. It is speculated that the tremendous vasodilation from early seizures may injure the brain, uncouple cerebral blood flow from metabolism, and result in an "unautoregulated" cerebral vasculature. As a result, cerebral oxygen delivery is not adequate during repetitive seizures. This impairment of oxygen delivery might explain the mechanism for ischemic histologic changes documented in neuropathologic studies.

CLINICAL MANAGEMENT

Status epilepticus is a neurologic emergency that requires immediate effective treatment to avoid severe brain damage or death. Because the longer a generalized convulsive status epilepticus persists the worse the morbidity and mortality, it is critically important that the treatment sequence be preplanned. One such approach is given in Table 13.4.

In the section, "Pathophysiology," it is apparent that the goals in managing status epilepticus are:

1. To stabilize the patient
   - Ensure adequate cardiorespiratory function and brain oxygenation
   - Stabilize metabolic balance by prevention or correction of hypoglycemia, lactic acidosis, electrolyte imbalance, and dehydration
2. To treat the treatable
   - Stop electric and clinical seizure activity as soon as possible, preferably within 30 minutes
   - Prevent recurrence of seizures
   - Prevent or correct any other systemic complications
   - Evaluate and treat possible causes of status epilepticus

TABLE 13.4. ————————————————————————————————
Emergency Management of Status Epilepticus

Immediate actions
Airway protection, using endotracheal tube and 100% O_2
Breathing support, using muscle relaxants if needed
Circulation, verifying and providing blood pressure support
Establish intravenous line (securely) and draw laboratory samples for glucose, blood urea nitrogen, electrolytes, calcium, phosphate, complete blood count, toxicology screen, and anticonvulsant levels
Administer 2–4 ml of 25% dextrose in water per kilogram
Administer diazepam (0.3 mg/kg over 2 minutes, up to 10 mg) *or* lorazepam (0.05 mg/kg over 2 minutes, up to 10 mg)

Next 40 minutes
Administer phenytoin (18–20 mg/kg over 10 minutes up to 1000 mg); monitor blood pressure and electrocardiogram; administer no faster than 50 mg/min
If still seizing, administer phenobarbital (20 mg/kg by intravenous drip no faster than 30 mg/min); intubate patient if respiratory depression occurs

Next hour
If seizures persist, give paraldehyde (0.1 ml of 4% solution per kilogram per hour by intravenous continuous drip)
If still seizing, consider general anesthesia

Stabilizing the Patient

The overwhelming priorities in the management of a patient with status epilepticus are preservation of the airway, maintenance of ventilation, assurance of oxygenation, and support of the circulation. Patients with status epilepticus often have hypoxia and impaired ventilation. The patient should be positioned to avoid aspiration, suffocation, or physical injury. Adequate aeration should be ensured, and a plastic airway may be placed if it can be done easily. The forced use of such an airway or the use of tongue blades or metal objects may cause severe oral injury and should be avoided. In the presence of poor air exchange, the child should be intubated. The authors also recommend that a patient who does not cease seizure activity after appropriate anticonvulsants should be prophylactically intubated and ventilated. It is wrong to await the development of cyanosis, severe acidosis, or hemodynamic instability before proceeding to intubation.

In order to accomplish intubation, often it is necessary to use muscle relaxants. Moreover, these patients often vomit because they have been relatively healthy in the previous period and often have eaten. Thus, particular attention needs to be paid to avoidance of factors that result in aspiration. The muscle relaxation that is employed, if needed, should be a short-acting relaxant because the clinician will be unable to titrate the anticonvulsant therapy if a long-acting agent is used.

After intubation is accomplished, or it is deemed unnecessary, the child should be placed on 100% oxygen until arterial blood gases can be obtained and hyperoxygenation can be documented. There is experimental evidence that suggests that maintaining cerebral oxygenation might have a beneficial effect on the outcome of status epilepticus, and thus avoidance of hypoxia is to be strictly enforced.

Implementing Drug Therapy

To control status epilepticus quickly and to prevent recurrences, a therapeutic serum concentration of a long-acting anticonvulsant medication must be achieved. Clinical experience suggests that it is not the choice of drug but rather the timing, route, and vigor of therapy that are major determinants of the duration of status epilepticus and subsequent morbidity. This same experience suggests that vigorous intravenous therapy early in a seizure may abort status epilepticus and that early therapy is far more effective than later therapy. Knowledge of the pharmacology and pharmacokinetics is essential. The physician must be familiar with loading dose, the half-life of the drug, and potential toxicities. The ideal drug for treatment of status epilepticus should enter the brain rapidly, have an immediate onset of activity, not depress consciousness or respiratory function, and have a long therapeutic half-life. It should also be effective in treating somatic manifestations as well as electric activities. The three most commonly used classes of drugs for the treatment of status epilepticus include benzodiazepines, phenytoin, and phenobarbital. Others less widely used are paraldehyde, valproic acid, lidocaine, clonazepam, chlormethiazole, and general anesthesia.

Benzodiazepines

Diazepam (e.g., Valium) is most often used as the initial agent for managing status epilepticus, having gained its popularity because of rapid distribution in the brain (within 10 seconds) and its relatively low toxicity. Studies in the pediatric age group have shown 85–90% initial control rates, but it may be less effective in status epilepticus of organic causes. The drug is effective for virtually all types of status epilepticus, including grand mal, focal motor, absence, myoclonic, and secondarily generalized grand mal seizures. The major disadvantages of the drug are its tendency to depress respiration and consciousness and its short half-life in the CNS. Studies in adults have shown that a diazepam serum level of 0.5 μ/ml is needed to control interictal paroxysmal activity. In adults, a 10-mg injection over 1–2 minutes produces a serum level between 0.3 and 2.0 μ/ml. However, serum diazepam concentrations frequently decrease by more than 50% during the first 20 minutes because of rapid and extensive redistribution. This may account for the frequent recurrence of seizure activity 20–30 minutes after initial injection of the drug. *Cessation of a convulsion after a single dose of diazepam should not be considered sufficient*

*treatment, and diazepam must be used in conjunction with, or be fol-
lowed by, loading with a long-acting anticonvulsant.* In cases in which
mental status is of prime importance, the combination of diazepam and
phenytoin is recommended.

Diazepam is available for use in 2-ml ampules containing 10 mg of drug.
Because of its relative insolubility in intravenous solutions, the drug should
be drawn into a small-volume syringe, which is then attached directly to
the hub of the catheter and directly injected. A large vein is recommended
to prevent vascular irritation. The initial dose is 0.3–0.5mg/kg administered over a 2-minute period, up to a maximum of 10mg/single dose. The
dose may be repeated in 10 minutes if status persists. If control has not
been achieved after two to three doses, another anticonvulsant medication
should strongly be considered. It has been suggested that a slow intravenous infusion of benzodiazepam (50 mg in 250 ml of 5% dextrose in water
at a rate of 40 ml/hr) provides a serum level of 0.2–0.8μ/ml in adults and
provides control of interictal paroxysmal activity in patients not responding to the original bolus injections of this drug.

The side effects of this drug include sedation, respiratory arrest, hypotension, and (rarely) cardiac arrest. The risk of respiratory depression is
intensified in the presence of phenobarbital. When status epilepticus is
being treated, the risk of respiratory depression from use of diazepam should
not be considered a serious complication but should be anticipated and
easily treated with assisted ventilation. Other effects include drowsiness,
delirium, dysarthria, and paradoxical excitement.

A newer benzodiazepine, lorazepam (e.g., Ativan), has recently been advocated for treatment of status epilepticus because of its longer CNS action. Despite the fact that the peak effect occurs at 45–60 minutes and
lorazepam penetrates the blood-brain barrier slowly, most workers have
noted an onset of effective action in less than 3 minutes. Thus, although
slower in onset than diazepam, lorazepam produces acceptable effects for
acute management, and it prevents recurrence of seizures for period of 2–
72 hours, a significant advantage over the effect provided by diazepam.
Doses of 2–10 mg (total) in adults and doses of 0.05–0.23 mg/kg in children have been recommended. The drug is administered intravenously over
a 2-minute period, though faster administration does not seem to increase
complications. Drowsiness is the most common side effect, and even high
doses of lorazepam have not caused respiratory depression, bradycardia,
or sudden hypotension.

Phenytoin

Phenytoin (e.g., Dilantin) is extremely effective in controlling tonic-clonic
status epilepticus in adults and children and in neonates and young infants. Many have suggested its use as the initial agent of choice. The major
advantage of phenytoin, besides its effectiveness, is its relatively long half-
life (24 hours) and its lack of CNS depression. Phenytoin is highly fat soluble, enters the brain within minutes, and rapidly reaches brain levels
adequate to control seizures. Intravenous loading produces equal plasma

and brain tissue levels within 3 minutes, and within 20 minutes, the brain tissue levels exceed plasma levels. Despite this rapid equilibration, it has been suggested that phenytoin takes 20 minutes to exert its antiepileptic effect and, therefore is often used in combination with diazepam.

Phenytoin is highly insoluble in intravenous solutions. It is therefore recommended that a syringe containing prediluted drug (50 mg/ml) be directly attached to the hub of the intravenous catheter. An initial loading dose of 18–25 kg is infused intravenously at a rate not to exceed 50 mg/min. The current available preparation of phenytoin contains both propylene glycol and ethanol; the former is a cadiotoxic agent. Thus, the heart rate, blood pressure, and electrocardiogram should be monitored during phenytoin infusion. If bradycardia or hyptension occurs, the rate of infusion must be decreased. Extreme care should be exercised in the administration of phenytoin to patients with known cardiac disease, especially those with sinus bradycardia, atrial block, or congestive heart failure. Maintenance doses are begun 12–24 hours after the initial injection, with adjustments made on the basis of measured drug levels. If the child's seizures do not respond to loading-dose phenytoin infusion, other agents should be utilized because administration of more phenytoin merely results in toxic levels.

Phenobarbital

Phenobarbital is highly effective in the therapy for status epilepticus and was the initial agent of choice for many years. It was superseded by diazepam, and current literature generally supports the use of diazepam or phenytoin as initial agent. However, phenobarbital is safe and effective, and many still regard it as the agent of choice for status epilepticus, particularly in children.

Phenobarbital has several advantages: a long half-life, effectiveness against generalized and partial seizures, and a long history of usage. Phenobarbital is said to be slowly absorbed by brain parenchyma and to require 10–20 minutes for its antiepileptic effects. In contrast to other anticonvulsants, phenobarbital, which is packaged in 1-ml vials containing 130 mg, may be diluted with normal saline. A loading dose of 15–25 mg/kg, administered at a rate not to exceed 30 mg/min, is recommended. The initial dose is 5–10 mg/kg administered over 10 minutes. This may be repeated in 20 minutes and again in 40 minutes if seizures persist. In neonates, an intravenous dose of 15–20 mg/kg produces serum levels ranging from 16 to 23 mg/ml. In infants, the half-life of phenobarbital varies (59–129 hours) from infant to infant and daily within the same infant. Thus, in the seriously ill neonate, optimal control must be based on repeated serum determinations. The older infant and child distribute and metabolize phenobarbital in a more uniform manner than does the neonate or young infant, with a serum half-life of 72–96 hours.

High dose of phenobarbital cause marked sedation, respiratory depression, hypotension, and cardiovascular collapse. The depression of respiration is more profound in patients initially treated with diazepam, and ventilatory support is frequently required. Once status epilepticus is controlled, a maintenance dose of 5 mg/kg/day may be instituted 12–24 hours after the initial loading dose. Further adjustments are made on the basis of serum measurements.

Other Agents

Paraldehyde may be used to treat status epilepticus that is refractory to benzodiazepines, phenytoin, and phenobarbital therapy. Paraldehyde has been used intermittently for treatment of status epilepticus but has not been well studied. It may be administered rectally or intravenously. Intravenously, the drug should be administered in a dilute solution, usually a 4% solution (20 ml of paraldehyde in 500 ml of normal saline). The infusion may be administered as rapidly as necessary to control seizures, but the therapeutic dose is probably in the range of 0.1–0.2 ml/kg/hr. The drip rate is titrated downward after the seizures are controlled.

A fresh solution should be used because paraldehyde rapidly oxidizes to acetaldehyde and acetic acid on exposure to air and light. In addition, plastic may be dissolved by the concentrated drug. Thus, paraldehyde should be mixed in glass bottles, and the plastic tubing systems should be changed every 12 hours. Ideally, the drug should not be administered through plastic tubing. Paraldehyde may be administered rectally, but absorption is not reliable, and this route is not appropriate for status epilepticus. The drug should not be used in children with pulmonary edema, chronic lung disease, or liver disease. Paraldehyde has been reported to cause pulmonary hemorrhage, pulmonary edema, acidosis, hepatitis, nephrosis, and bleeding diatheses.

Several other anticonvulsants may be considered if patients do not respond to previous agents. *Valproic acid* is not available in parenteral form but has been used rectally for the treatment of status epilepticus. A major disadvantage is its relative slowness in absorption, compared with drugs that are administered intravenously. *Lidocaine* (50–100-mg bolus in adults) may be effective in some persons when other drugs have failed, but higher doses of this drug are epileptogenic, and its use is not advocated in children. *Clonazepam* and *chlormethiazole* have also been used in the treatment of status epilepticus with some success, but they have not gained widespread acceptance, particularly for use in children.

In view of the potential morbidity and mortality associated with generalized tonic-clonic status epilepticus, numerous authors have recommended the use of *general anesthesia* or *barbiturate coma* to minimize the metabolic sequelae of prolonged seizure activity or to suppress the process permanently. Few guidelines exist regarding the depth or duration of anesthesia or the advantages of inhalation anesthesia versus intravenous agents, and the use of anesthesia for this purpose is not universally accepted. With general anesthesia, with or without neuromuscular blockade, the motor manifestations of status are clearly masked. However, electrical activity may persist, and electroencephalographic monitoring is helpful during such therapy. In addition, convulsion-like activity indicated on the electroencephalogram may be provoked via general anesthesia with halothane, enflurane, or etomidate. The anesthetic must be periodically decreased to determine whether continued therapy is required. Despite the controversy about this modality of therapy, the experimental physiologic data concerning status epilepticus support aggressive therapy and suggest that the most severe, refractory patients be considered for general anesthesia or barbiturate coma to stop the seizures.

FURTHER EVALUATION

Although the control of seizures is of utmost importance, evaluation of their etiology should be initiated within the first few minutes after the patient is seen. Laboratory tests should include determination of serum electrolytes, glucose, calcium, hepatic enzymes, urea nitrogen, and when indicated, a toxicology screen and serum magnesium. A Dextrostix test performed at bedside can be an immediate clue to ruling out hypoglycemia. If the patient is known to have epilepsy, serum anticonvulsant levels should be measured. If meningitis is suspected, a lumbar puncture should be carried out when the child is stabilized. Evidence of increased intracranial pressure or a focal neurologic examination mandates consideration of computerized axial tomography scanning or other neurologic studies as soon as possible.

SUMMARY

Status epilepticus causes significant mortality and morbidity and must be regarded as a medical emergency. The longer the seizures are permitted to continue, the more difficult they become to control, and the worse the prognosis. What is surprising is that some physicians continue to tolerate periods of status epilepticus that are much longer than ought to be permitted. Delayed treatment disregards an enormous amount of pathologic evidence that status epilepticus, per se, is harmful to the CNS. Immediate, rational, and potentially aggressive therapy is essential to reduce the mortality and long-term morbidity of status epilepticus.

CHAPTER 14

Reye Syndrome

Reye syndrome is a disorder of unknown etiology in which a child recovering from a viral prodrome suddenly develops pernicious vomiting and eventually develops neurologic changes. The syndrome was first formally described by several groups in 1963 and is associated with significant mortality and morbidity even today. Understanding of the etiology and pathophysiology of the disease remains poor despite immense numbers of research reports, and the disorder remains an unsolved enigmatic puzzle, although its relationship with aspirin administration is, in part, clear.

EPIDEMIOLOGY

Reye and coworkers described this syndrome in 1963, providing pathologic details on 21 children who had presented with viral prodromes, developed repetitive vomiting, and had elevated serum transaminase levels, a 90% mortality rate and, on autopsy, fatty infiltration of their viscera. Hence, the disease has been named Reye syndrome or, on occasion, Reye-Johnson syndrome, although in the remainder of this chapter it will be referred to as Reye syndrome.

The following diagnostic criteria were developed for case definition (not clinical staging) by the Centers for Disease Control:

1. There must be acute noninflammatory encephalopathy with
   A. Microvesicular fatty metamorphosis of the liver confirmed by biopsy or autopsy or
   B. Serum glutamic oxaloacetic transaminase (SGOT), serum glutamic pyruvic transaminase (SGPT), or serum ammonia (NH_3) of more than 3 times normal.
2. If cerebrospinal fluid is obtained, it must have >9 leukocytes/mm^3.
3. There should be no other more reasonable explanation for the neurologic presentation or the hepatic abnormalities.

Usually there is acute onset of a change in mental status in the "biphasic" illness, in which the first phase is the viral prodromal syndrome. This is accompanied by pernicious vomiting. On physical examination, the child is obtunded, with generalized cerebral depression but not usually

185

including focal changes. The child is usually afebrile and anicteric, although hepatomegaly may be seen in about 40% of patients. Abnormalities related to hepatic failure may occur, including enzyme elevations, coagulation disorders, and alterations of carbohydrate, amino acid, and lipid metabolism. Other accompaniments of multisystem failure may occur, including myocardial failure, dehydration and shock, acute renal failure, peptic ulcers, pancreatitis, and sepsis. Patients who die have severe cerebral edema and fatty infiltration of the viscera, including the heart and kidneys. Patients may die without herniation from myocardial failure, gasatrointestinal bleeding, status epilepticus, renal failure, respiratory failure, or cardiovascular collapse, but the usual cause of death is herniation secondary to intracranial hypertension.

The differential diagnosis of the disorder is broad and, in infants, includes a variety of genetic metabolic disorders. A differential diagnosis list is given in Table 14.1.

Reye syndrome is largely a disease of children, and although it has been described increasingly in adults, most cases occur in children under 15 years of age. Table 14.2 shows the age distribution of children who fell victim to the disorder between 1966 and 1976 in Ohio. As can be seen, the original time period was associated with somewhat younger children, and as diagnosis of the disorder has improved because of patient and physician awareness, more older children are noted in the later series. For comparison, the mean age of children dying from Reye syndrome in Michigan was 5.5 years.

The temporal patterns of Reye syndrome outbreaks in this country have matched the patterns of influenza outbreaks, peaking in the winters. The varicella-related cases have also peaked in the winter, just as has varicella. Thus the age distribution of Reye syndrome might be related to the incidence of these viral diseases in those age groups, and for varicella-related disease, this has been demonstrated. The rarity of Reye syndrome in adults may therefore reflect the fact that most adults have been exposed to the infectious agents that cause Reye syndrome and have been prescreened" for susceptibility to the disease.

Neonatal Reye syndrome probably occurs but is rare. It has been described, but there are difficulties in the interpretation of liver histology

TABLE 14.1. _____
Differential Diagnosis of Reye Syndrome

Inflammatory encephalopathies
Toxic ingestion (especially aspirin)
Ornithine transcarbamoylase deficiency
Carnitine deficiency
Pyruvate dehydrogenase and pyruvate carboxylase deficiencies
Argininosuccinate deficiency
Fatty acid abnormalities
Urea cycle abnormalities

TABLE 14.2.
Age Distribution of Reye Syndrome Patients in Ohio, 1966–1976[a]

Age (yr)	1966–1973		1974–1976	
	No.	%	No.	%
0–2	18	27	11	10
3–4	16	24	13	12
5–6	12	18	22	21
7–8	8	12	15	14
9–10	5	5	14	13
11–12	3	4	14	13
13–14	3	4	14	13
15–16	2	3	4	14

[a]From Sullivan-Bolyai JZ, Corey L: Epidemiology of Reye syndrome. *Epidemiol Rev* 3:7, 1981.

and cerebral pathology in that age group. Furthermore, it has been increasingly appreciated that in neonatal and young infant "Reye syndrome" there is a higher incidence of congenital metabolic abnormalities (Table 14.3) than had been previously believed.

Of all the epidemiologic information available, the dramatic decrease in incidence of Reye syndrome since aspirin administration in children with viral illnesses has been curtailed is remarkable. Although this disease was once frequent, it is now a rare cause of intensive care admission in children.

PATHOPHYSIOLOGY

The etiology of Reye syndrome is unknown. Our understanding of the disease is hampered by the inability to produce adequate laboratory models in animals, although criteria by which to judge animal models have been proposed. In ferrets, a hyperammonemia syndrome can be produced with an arginine-deficient diet; in this model, various abnormalities associated with Reye syndrome can be produced with the combinations of aspirin, influenza virus, and elevated ammonia. Clearly, this mimics the human disease. Influenza virus alone can cause some of the findings of Reye syndrome in mice, and aspirin has been demonstrated to enhance varicella virus production in an in vitro cell culture.

Multiple viral illnesses have been predecessors of Reye syndrome, particularly influenza and varicella, but also adenoviruses, coxsackieviruses A and B, cytomegalovirus, dengue virus, echoviruses, Epstein-Barr virus, herpes simplex virus, mumps, parainfluenza virus, poliomyelitis virus, reovirus, respiratory syncytial virus, rotavirus, rubella, rubeola, vaccinia virus and, possibly, live viral vaccines. Viruses cannot be grown out of brain, liver, or any other specific organs on autopsy of these patients, however, and no one has identified viral particles on ultrastructural studies of children with Reye syndrome.

TABLE 14.3.
Selected Clinical, Laboratory, and Pathologic Findings in 50 Infants under Age 10 Months with Diagnosis of Reye Syndrome[a]

Data	No. of Infants
Clinical	
Sex	25/47 (females/total)
Vomiting	43/50
Seizures	43/44
Respiratory changes	20/22
Mortality	36/59
Severe CNS sequelae	9/59
Normal recovery	14/59
Recurrent attacks	4/59
Laboratory	
SGOT > twice normal	59/59
Prothrombin time < 75%	31/34
Glucose < 50 mg/dl	26/33
Pathologic	
Hepatic steatosis	52/52

[a]From Huttenlocher PR, Trauner DA: Reye's syndrome in infancy. *Pediatrics* 62:88, 1978.

One might also anticipate the possibility that toxins of some sort, such as salicylates, are involved. Indeed, a host of potential toxins have been proposed, as is shown in Table 14.4. Each of the items in the table has been associated in some manner with Reye syndrome, but few have actually remained consistent contenders as etiologic agents in the disease, with the exception of salicylates. This requires special discussion.

Salicylates have been associated with Reye syndrome in three case-controlled studies. In addition to case-matched control studies, salicylate lev-

TABLE 14.4.
Toxins and Medications Associated with Reye Syndrome-like Illness[a]

Salicylates	Isopropyl alcohol
Aflatoxins	Antiemetics
Endotoxins	Pteridine
Hypoglycin	Valproic acid
Insecticides and related chemicals	Warfarin

[a]From Sullivan-Bolyai JZ, Corey L: Epidemiology of Reye syndrome. *Epidemiol Rev* 3:13, 1981.

els have been demonstrated to be relatively high in many patients with Reye syndrome, and the histology of fatal salicylate intoxication is similar in some respects to that seen in Reye syndrome. Despite the limitations of the case control studies, the epidemiologic evidence convinced the Committee on Infectious Diseases of the American Academy of Pediatrics to issue a statement suggesting that salicylates be used with caution, if at all, in children with varicella or influenza. A pilot study was released in 1985 by the Institute of Medicine, the results of which suggest that aspirin is associated with an increased risk of acquiring the disease. Specifically, 96% of the 29 children who developed Reye syndrome had been given aspirin, but only 45% of 143 case controls had received the drug. Ultimately, this resulted in warning labels on salicylate-containing products in the United States and a dramatic decrease in the incidence of Reye syndrome. The pathophysiologic relationship between the syndrome and aspirin, however, is still unclear.

Finally, some children still appear to get Reye syndrome with no aspirin exposure. As a result, the precise nature of the interaction of viral infection, genetic predisposition, toxin exposure, and other factors is not known, and it makes sense that several factors are probably involved in the pathogenesis of the disease. It is pointed out that the disorder is associated with a mitochondrial disturbance of unknown etiology, that the histology of the disorder, including that demonstrated by ultrastructural data, is well described, and yet none of these avenues of research have explained the physiology of the disease.

CLINICAL PRESENTATION AND STAGING

The key symptoms of Reye syndrome are a viral prodrome followed by the unexpected and acute onset of repetitive vomiting. Most often the prodromal illness is chickenpox or influenza but may be viral gastroenteritis or some other viral illness. The child then has the onset of altered behavior, which may consist of lethargy, confusion, and combativeness or may rapidly progress to decerebrate posturing, flaccidity, and death. In infants, seizures may be the presenting evidence of central nervous system (CNS) disease. The children are not jaundiced and are usually afebrile, but they have hepatomegaly. In infants, hyperventilation, apnea, and shock are often seen.

The laboratory findings of Reye syndrome include elevated transaminase levels (SGOT and SGPT), usually elevated serum ammonia, prolonged prothrombin times, other evidences of hepatic failure, and an essentially normal lumbar puncture. These is no evidence of inflammation in the cerebrospinal fluid (<9 cells/mm^3), but if the patient has systemic hypoglycemia, the glucose may be lower than normal. Hypoglycemia is common in infants (Table 14.3), but the glucose is usually normal in children over the age of 4 years. The bilirubin is nearly always normal.

Liver biopsy demonstrates fatty infiltration in the absence of necrosis. It is certainly not mandatory to perform a liver biopsy in all children with suspected Reye syndrome because there are significant risks associated with the procedure performed in a critically ill child with a bleeding diathesis. However, biopsy may be helpful in certain cases, such as in the case of suspected recurrence of Reye syndrome either in the same child or in the same family or in instances in which a typical prodromal illness cannot be defined. Biopsy should be performed only after correction of the coagulopathy.

The National Institutes of Health sponsored a consensus conference that led to a consensus statement in 1981, which resulted in a short description of the syndrome as well as a recommended staging system. This system is shown here because it has largely replaced the earlier criteria which included the electroencephalogram.

1. Stage I—Lethargy, follows verbal commands, normal posture, purposeful response to pain, brisk pupillary light reflex, and normal oculocephalic reflex
2. Stage II—Combative or stuporous, inappropriate verbalizing, normal posture, purposeful or nonpurposeful response to pain, sluggish pupillary reflexes, and conjugate deviation on doll's eye maneuver
3. Stage III—Comatose, decorticate posture, decorticate response to pain, sluggish pupillary reaction, conjugate deviation on doll's eye maneuver
4. Stage IV—Comatose, decerebrate posture and decerebrate response to pain, sluggish pupillary reflexes, and inconsistent or absent oculocephalic reflex
5. Stage V—Comatose, flaccid, no response to pain, no pupillary response, no oculocephalic relex

CLINICAL MANAGEMENT

Children with stage I disease may not require intensive care admission, and if appropriate management can be provided at a nontertiary center, referral is not necessary. However, all children with stage II or worse Reye syndrome should be referred to a tertiary pediatric center with an intensive care unit (ICU) team that is experienced with the disease. The progression of the disease from stage II to stage V may be extremely rapid; hence, despite any controversy of therapy at stage II, the child should be transferred immediately.

Children who are in stage I require close neurologic evaluation (at least hourly), frequent glucose determinations (2–4 hours apart), and daily determinations of ammonia, transaminases, and electrolytes. Hypoglycemia is avoided by the provision of intravenous glucose (10–15%), coupled with close monitoring of the glucose level. Children with stage I Reye syndrome have an excellent prognosis with hospital observation and glucose and electrolyte intravenous therapy.

Children who are in stage II or worse require significantly more care and must be admitted to the ICU setting. There is some controversy about the therapy of children with stage II disease. Some advocate aggressive therapy including intracranial pressure monitoring and control for patients in "deep" stage II, as the progression of the disease can be quite rapid. Others emphasize the invasive and dangerous nature of the therapies that are employed in the management of these patients. The National Institutes of Health consensus panel was unwilling to endorse a regime for Sfagell patients or to commit themselves to a particular stage of the disease at which such intracranial pressure management should be considered. Our practice includes aggressive therapy (intubation, hemodynamic monitoring, intracranial pressure monitoring and control, and ammonia reduction therapies) of all patients with stage III disease or worse; additionally, children with stage II who are progressing toward stage III are treated aggressively. Occasionally, children with stage II disease do not progress, and these children do not require intubation or intracranial pressure monitoring.

General Care
Fluids and Electrolytes

Several types of electrolyte disturbances are seen in Reye syndrome, the most well known of which is hypoglycemia. Abnormalities of potassium, calcium, and phosphorus may also be seen, and in the presence of the syndrome of inappropriate antidiuretic hormone secretion (SIADH) or diabetes insipidus, water balance is disordered.

Hypoglycemia is to be avoided, and prevention of hypoglycemia is the main therapeutic intervention in stage I Reye syndrome, as is mentioned previously. A 10–15% dextrose solution is used to maintain the glucose between 200 and 300 mg/dl, and the glucose is monitored on a frequent basis. At more severe stages, hypoglycemia is less of a problem, and hyperglycemia may even occur, depending on other types of therapies (i.e., large numbers of drugs being infused through various lines which all contain glucose).

Largely as a complication of intracranial hypertension and CNS dysfunction, either diabetes insipidus or SIADH may be seen. Either disorder will complicate the management of intracranial hypertension, described in a later section, because the presence of antidiuretic hormone (ADH) will cause free water retention, exacerbating cerebral edema. Patients with diabetes insipidus should be treated only with intravenous (never by any other route) ADH, or one may inadvertently achieve a long-lasting ADH effect that causes the same problem. The serum sodium should be checked at least every 4 hours, and additional fluid restriction should be instituted if hyponatremia begins to develop.

Calcium and phosphate depletion may also be seen in these children and should be replenished. The safest approach to this management is frequent (every 4 hours) monitoring of these electrolytes and appropriate supplementation.

Respiratory Support

Stage I patients should not require sophisticated respiratory support, but the adequate oxygenation of such children should be assured. More severe stages of the disease require aggressive support because prevention of hypoxia and hypercapnia is a foundation of good neurointensive care.

All children with stage III Reye syndrome should be electively intubated by using appropriate sedation and muscle relaxation. Some children with stage II Reye syndrome may not require intubation, but practice of the authors includes intubation of any stage II patient who begins to deteriorate further. The presence of spontaneous hyperventilation does not preclude the need for intubation in these critically ill comatose children. Once intubated, the airway is assured, ventilation and oxygenation are better controlled, and rapid institution of means to control intracranial hypertension may be accomplished without the risk of respiratory arrest (i.e., thiopental).

We believe arterial lines should be placed in children with stage II or stage III Reye syndrome. This facilitates the obtainment of blood gases and serum electrolyte measurements and permits on-line continuous blood pressure monitoring. Although there are obvious risks to arterial line placement, close monitoring of the child with Reye syndrome is vitally important and is greatly facilitated with such a line.

Finally, it is worthwhile to point out the possible effects of positive end-expiratory pressure (PEEP) on intracranial pressure. Intrathoracic pressure may be transmitted to the intracranial vault and may further exacerbate intracranial hypertension. As a corollary statement, PEEP should be as minimal as is permissible by oxygen delivery. However, if hypoxia can only be appropriately treated with PEEP, this must take priority over concerns about the intracranial pressure resulting from PEEP.

Hemodynamic Monitoring and Support

One of the therapeutic goals in Reye syndrome is to prevent or minimize cerebral edema, and a primary modality of treatment is a combination of fluid restriction and diuresis. The goal of this therapy is to maintain an adequate fluid volume status (i.e., adequate left atrial pressure), thus preventing overload, and a slightly hyperosmolar (i.e., 300–310 mOsm/liter) state. Such management is treacherous, and hemodynamic monitoring and support are often required.

Arterial lines are the mainstay of hemodynamic monitoring in all children with stage II or worse Reye syndrome, permitting continuous knowledge of arterial blood pressure. If intracranial pressure monitoring is performed, an arterial line is mandatory to permit the calculation of cerebral perfusion pressure. Additionally, many therapies used for intracranial hypertension have adverse effects on blood pressure on a moment-to-moment basis, and continuous measurement of blood pressure is absolutely necessary.

Although it may be argued that a central venous catheter can provide some assessment of the filling pressure of the heart, in Reye syndrome a number of factors complicate the use of this simple monitoring device. The true "filling" of the left ventricle is the end-diastolic left ventricular volume, not the left ventricular pressure. Measurement of left atrial pressure permits an estimate of this volume if one presumes that there is a relatively constant ventricular compliance. The assumption that the left side of the heart is filled to the same degree as the right side has led pediatricians to use the central venous pressure (right atrial pressure) to assess the volume-filling status of the left ventricle. This is a tenuous relationship in a healthy patient; in the patient with Reye syndrome the situation is even less certain.

In short, the pulmonary arterial catheter provides a wealth of information, bearing on a number of physiologic parameters that are clearly abnormal in severe Reye syndrome, either because of the disorder itself or because of the therapies engineered to treat intracranial hypertension. In stage III or worse patients, we believe a pulmonary artery catheter should be used.

To assess preload, both the central venous and the pulmonary arterial wedge pressures are examined, not only in a steady state but also in response to a fluid challenge. This allows the clinician to gauge the compliance of the right and left atria and permits valid conclusions about ventricular preload. For instance, if the administration of 10 ml of fluid per kilogram over 20 minutes only changes the wedge pressure by 1 mm Hg, additional volume may be administered. The reason is that the left atrium is still very compliant, and the volume bolus has resulted in minimal pressure change. Once a volume bolus alters the wedge pressure significantly, however, pharmacologic agents are necessary.

The choice of pharmacologic agent depends on the specific goals that are suggested by the hemodynamic profile. If, for instance, the systemic vascular resistance is normal and the cardiac output is low, inotropic support such as dobutamine ($5-10\mu g/kg/min$) is needed. If the cardiac output is high and the systemic vascular resistance is low, the patient has peripheral cardiovascular collapse and needs an agent such as norepinephrine or epinephrine ($0.1-0.5\mu g/kg/min$) or high-dose dopamine ($>10\mu g/kg/min$) to increase vascular tone. If the heart rate is very low, isoproterenol may be used to raise it; this is done at the risk of arrhythmias and peripheral vasodilation. It should be clear to the reader that the specific choices of drip medications can be made rationally by obtaining hemodynamic measurements; this is our reason for recommending pulmonary artery catheterization in these patients.

Coagulopathy

Children with Reye syndrome should be given vitamin K (5 mg slowly intravenously for children and 0.25 mg/kg for infants). Children with clinical bleeding should be given fresh frozen plasma. Children with a bleeding diathesis demonstrated with laboratory tests should be given fresh frozen plasma (10 ml/kg) immediately before any invasive procedures, such as liver biopsy. The prothrombin time and partial thromboplastin time should be monitored every 12 hours for the first several days.

Temperature Control

It is important to control the temperature of these children because decreases in temperature may contribute to hemodynamic instability and increases will cause an increase of cerebral metabolic rate. Cooling and warming mattresses can be used with a feedback probe to achieve optimal control of temperature. Temperature should be measured with a rectal or esophageal probe or with the thermistor of a pulmonary artery catheter.

Intracranial Pressure Management

As stated earlier, it is our practice to insert intracranial pressure monitoring devices as part of aggressive therapy in stage III patients or even in rapidly deteriorating stage II patients.

Monitoring Techniques

There are numerous methods for monitoring intracranial pressure. The most commonly used devices are subarachnoid bolts and intraventricular drains. The former are probably safer, particularly in the presence of a coagulopathy, and are easily inserted in children but may be unstable in small infants. Intraventricular drains permit the drainage of cerebrospinal fluid to reduce intracranial pressure, but there are increased risks associated with the traversal of brain tissue. Furthermore, insertion may be difficult in the presence of severe cerebral edema compressing the lateral ventricles. The intraventricular drain is a more reliable monitor, and if a subarachnoid monitor is used, the clinician must constantly verify the proper function of the device to avoid the underestimation of the actual intracranial pressure.

Goals of Management

There are two major goals: (a) maintenance of adequate cerebral perfusion and (b) prevention of cerebral herniation.

Any perfusion pressure is calculated as the "upstream" pressure. The upstream pressure is the carotid arterial pressure, which is clinically assumed to be the same as the systemic blood pressure. In patients in the ICU with intracranial pressure monitoring, the intracranial pressure is universally used as the downstream pressure, and thus cerebral perfusion pressure (CPP) is calculated from mean arterial pressure (MAP) and intracranial pressure (ICP) as

$$CPP = MAP - ICP$$

Clinically, the goal is to maintain the cerebral perfusion pressure above the lower limit of autoregulation or approximately 50 mm Hg in children above the neonatal or young infancy period.

The other therapeutic goal of intracranial pressure monitoring and control is to prevent cerebral herniation; severe cerebral edema and swelling will eventually cause herniation and death. Herniation may occur after acute events such as endotracheal suctioning or painful stimuli; in these instances, routine herperventilation or administration of short-acting barbiturates may protect the patient from acute rises in intracranial pressure.

Fluid Restriction and Osmotherapy

Reduction of intracranial pressure can be accomplished by lowering the amount of intracranial blood volume, such as with hyperventilation. Additionally, cerebrospinal fluid may often be drained. The third constituent of the intracranial vault, the brain itself, swells severely in Reye syndrome, and fluid restriction and osmotherapy are primarily aimed at the reduction of brain swelling.

It is certain that cerebral edema can be worsened by the administration of excessive free water, such as would be contained in 5% dextrose in water. After the glucose is metabolized, the free water reduces serum osmolality, and cellular edema results. It is also certain that acute administration of mannitol or furosemide can reduce intracranial pressure, an action that has been presumed to be due to cerebral dehydration. However, certain aspects of this subject are less clear-cut. For instance, it is not at all certain whether intentional dehydration is helpful. Indeed, if fluid restriction and mannitol are combined aggressively and the patient becomes hyperosmolar, the clinician may be worse off in terms of options because neither further osmotherapy nor fluid administration can then be used. Thus if the osmolality has been permitted to approach 340 mOsm, it is impossible to administer mannitol for subsequent spikes in intracranial pressure. Conversely, if the child becomes hemodynamically unstable and requires fluid administration, all available intravenous solutions are much less osmolar than 340 mOsm! The prudent course, in the opinion of the authors, is to maintain a relatively normal osmolality (approximately 300 mOsm/liter) by using judicious amounts of mannitol to treat intracranial hypertension (0.25 g/kg up to every 4 hours). Alternately, small doses of nonosmotic diuretics can also be used. Intravenous solutions should not contain excessive water, and saline, half-normal saline, or Ringer's lactate are appropriate fluids. Finally, the circulating blood volume should not be excessive, but dehydration should not be accomplished to the point of hemodynamic instability.

Head Position

The cerebral blood volume is a function of cerebral blood flow into the cranial vault as well as impedance to outflow from the vault. It is important to maintain the child's head in the midline position, or compression of the jugular vein may caue an increase in intracranial pressure. Although this is a minor event in children or adults without neurologic disease, jugular obstruction may cause significant rises in intracranial pressure in patients with cerebral edema as is encountered with Reye syndrome. Whether elevation of the head of the bed 30–45° is useful is open to discussion. Nevertheless, it also is a routine position.

Hyperventilation

Although hyperventilation is quite effective in reducing cerebral blood flow and accordingly reducing the intracranial pressure, obviously the use of hyperventilation to lower intracranial pressure by producing cerebral vasoconstriction has some inherent clinical limitations. There is very little information available on this subject. Some centers use jugular bulb oxygen tensions to assess cerebral extraction. This allows aggressive use of hyperventilation; when the degree of hyperventilation actually compromises cerebral blood flow, the cerebral oxygen extraction rises. Hyperventilation becomes less effective over a prolonged period of time, presumably because the cerebrospinal fluid bicarbonate is reduced over a period of time. Hyperventilation to extreme degrees is probably not helpful in the long term, and the authors recommend maintaining the carbon dioxide tension between 25 and 35 mm Hg.

Hyperventilation should be aggressively used in the suspected event of cerebral herniation and may also be used prophylactically to prevent cerebral herniation. Thus it is reasonable to hyperventilate such patients before endotracheal suctioning, insertion of endotracheal tubes, etc. This therapy, used sparingly, allows this potent intervention to be kept to treat acute spikes in intracranial pressure.

Barbiturates

Barbiturates are highly effective in reducing intracranial pressure and historically have also been proposed in Reye syndrome for the induction of barbiturate coma to prevent intracranial hypertension. Finally, barbiturates have formerly been used after a variety of brain injuries, on the theory that cerebral metabolism was reduced relative to flow, improving the match of flow to demand. This latter application of these anesthetics is not advocated. Since there are no data available to support this mode of therapy in any disease entity, including Reye syndrome. Different conclusions may be drawn about the appropriate use of barbiturates for each of the first two purposes.

For acute reduction of intracranial pressure, barbiturates are highly effective. Thiopental (3–6-mg/kg bolus) is dramatically effective, dropping intracranial pressure within seconds. The arterial blood pressure also drops with such administration, but generally the cerebral perfusion pressure can be improved. Pentobarbital may also be employed (5–10 mg/kg).

Separate from the use of barbiturates for the prevention of intracranial hypertension, the use of barbiturates to produce a protective coma is very controversial and is not now in widespread use. The drug is being used to prevent an event that is ill-defined, and it is difficult to judge whether a good neurologic outcome is a result of the drug therapy. Additionally, barbiturate coma is accompanied by arterial hypotension and hemodynamic instability due to both system vasodilation and myocardial dysfunction. Pressor agents are almost always needed to support the blood pressure. Systemic arterial pressure is just as important a component of cerebral perfusion pressure as is intra-cranial pressure, and therefore this type of therapy carries significant risks.

It is the practice of the authors to use barbiturates for intracranial pressure management in patients who have already demonstrated intracranial hypertension that is impossible to treat adequately with fluid restriction, moderate hyperventilation, and mannitol. In addition, short-acting barbiturates are used to prevent intracranial pressure spikes during suctioning and as short-acting anesthetics during painful procedures. We do not use prophylactic barbiturate coma for "brain protection."

When a decision has been made to use barbiturate drips to control difficult intracranial pressure, the patient should be given a loading dose and then placed on a constant infusion. The apparent volume of distribution (VD) is a function of cardiac index (CI).

$$VD = 0.17 * CI + 0.2$$

where VD is expressed in liters per kilogram. The loading dose (D_{load}) is the product of the desired concentration (($pentobarbital_{serum}$) and VD:

$$D_{load} = VC * (pentobarbital)_{serum}$$

The loading dose should be administered over 2 hours to avoid hypotension.

The subsequent rate of administration ranges from 1 to 5 mg/kg/hr, and this is titrated with serum drug determinations. Target serum levels are 20–30 mg/liter, but higher levels may be needed to control intra-cranial hypertension in some patients. Although serum barbiturate levels are helpful to assess how much drug to administer, there are no rigidly defined effective barbiturate levels for intracranial pressure control. At much higher levels, however, severe hemodynamic instability should be anticipated, with potential adverse effects on cerebral perfusion pressure because of arterial hypotension.

Lidocaine

Lidocaine (0.5–1 mg/kg) as an intravenous bolus prior to suctioning or other noxious stimuli has been shown to be useful to prevent acute rises in intracranial pressure. Higher doses should be avoided, however, since it can cause seizures.

Hypothermia

Hypothermia has been proposed for use on the basis of reducing the cerebral metabolic rate, but its use is associated with complications of hemodynamic instability and increased susceptibility to sepsis. At present, hypothermia has no place in the routine management of Reye syndrome, but further research is needed to assess adequately this mode of therapy.

Decompressive Surgery

Frontal craniectomy has been attempted in patients with Reye syndrome, but the results are dismal. Current therapy without decompression yields good results in stage III, and it is not likely that decompressive surgery offers an advantage over aggressive medical therapy including barbiturates for intracranial pressure control in Reye syndrome.

Ammonia Reduction Therapies

One of the most striking biochemical abnormalities in Reye syndrome is the elevation of serum ammonia concentration. Ammonia is extremely toxic, and peak ammonia levels have been correlated with the prognosis in Reye syndrome. The chemical alters cerebral blood flow regulation and elevates intracranial pressure. Several types of therapy have been designed to lower ammonia levels in children with the disorder.

Dialysis

Peritoneal dialysis was one of the earliest proposed methods for lowering ammonia levels in Reye syndrome, but as experience was gained, it seemed apparent that this modality had no clear-cut benefit. It must be pointed out that no studies were conducted in a randomized fashion, and this modality of therapy was evaluated in the absence of intracranial pressure monitoring. Nevertheless, by 1975, peritoneal dialysis had largely disappeared from the treatment of Reye syndrome. Hemodialysis has not been evaluated in any published study and, to date, has not been carefully evaluated.

Exchange Transfusion

Exchange transfusion has a considerably less sound basis but can be accomplished more easily than can peritoneal dialysis. The theoretical case against the efficacy of exchange transfusion is strong, however, because the efficiency of double-volume exchange for removal of a largely intracellular toxin is not good. The blood must be fresh, as stored blood accumulates high concentrations of ammonia. New concerns about blood transfusion have made this therapy more difficult to justify than ever.

Total Body Washout

The most complete method of washout proposed is called asanguineous total body washout. This procedure has been used in children with severe Reye syndrome. Although the reported results were good, this technique is quite formidable and seems prohibitively expensive and extremely dangerous.

Metabolic Interventions (Fig. 14.1)

The final category of therapies designed to reduce ammonia are metabolic interventions designed to accelerate the detoxification of ammonia or to decrease its rate of production. For example, the administration of sodium benzoate and phenylacetic acid increase two alternative pathways for the excretion of waste nitrogen that do not produce ammonia. Such metabolic interventions have been used in neonatal hyperammonemia syn-

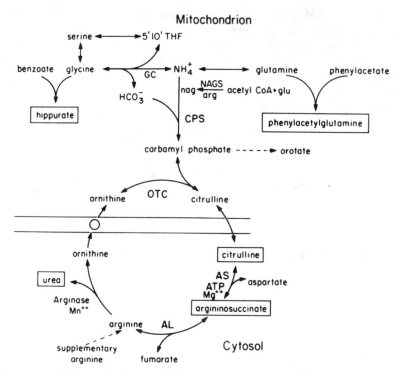

FIGURE 14.1. Pathways of waste nitrogen synthesis in patients with deficiencies of carbamoylphosphate synthetase and ornithine transcarbamoylase, treated with sodium benzoate and phenylacetate. Hippurate and phenylacetylglutamine serve as the waste nitrogen products. *GDH,* glutamate dehydrogenase; *GS,* glutamine synthe-tase; *G,* glutaminase; and α *kg,* α-ketoglutarate. (From Brusilow SW: Inborn errors of urea synthesis. *Butterworths Int Med Rev* 5:140, 1985.)

drome but have not been extensively applied for the treatment of Reye syndrome. It is possible that these types of treatments will have benefit for children with the disorder, but we must await the results of research trials currently underway.

PROGNOSIS

The prognosis for patients with Reye syndrome has been reported to be good, but we would add a qualifier. The prognosis in noncomatose children is excellent; with proper monitoring and therapy, a very low mortality and morbidity rate can be expected. When the mortality and morbidity rates of stage IV and V patients over the past decade are examined, it is difficult to document a dramatic impact.

The long-term outlook for survivors is relatively good, although abnormal anxiety and emotional patterns have been reported, and when survivors are compared with their siblings, minor abnormalities of function can be demonstrated. This probably reflects the global nature of the disease; survivors have a relatively uniform recovery of neurons, whereas patients with severe neurologic injury go on to die or have tremendous neurologic defects. Aggressive neurointensive care has not increased the number of neurologically damaged children and may improve the outlook for patients with Reye syndrome.

CHAPTER 15

Near-Drowning

Drowning is a leading cause of death in childhood, and near-drowning is associated with significant morbidity. The majority of these accidents occur in private swimming pools and, potentially, could be prevented. However, it is inevitable that such children will continue to be seen in emergency facilities and intensive care units (ICUs). The intensive care of these children has received some spectacular publicity because of exceptional recovery after prolonged submersions; hence, this section includes a detailed consideration of brain resuscitative therapies in near-drowning victims.

EPIDEMIOLOGIC ASPECTS

Analysis of adult drowning statistics has identified several risk factors for drowning in this group. (Table 15.1) Significant blood alcohol levels have been found in 33% of drowning victims in studies from Australia, England, and Finland. Alcohol increases susceptibility to drowning in several ways. It increases bravado and lowers acceptable behavior standards, thus producing the carelessness that results in submersion accidents. Furthermore, alcohol depresses coordination and promotes a sense of well-being. People who drown with blood ethanol levels of 0.150 g/100 ml will clumsily try to extricate themselves; those with levels of over 0.3 g/100 ml will frequently remain motionless upon entering the water and will not struggle or attempt to rescue themselves. Ethanol also depresses hepatic

TABLE 15.1. _____
Risk Factors in Drowning

Alcohol ingestion
Drug ingestion
Elective hyperventilation
Myocardial infarction
Epilepsy
Trauma
Child abuse

gluconeogenesis, particularly during exercise and fasting, and hypoglycemia may result. The degree to which this occurs in or predisposes to near-drowning is not known.

Drug abuse has been implicated as an etiologic factor in drowning, but data regarding ts incidence are scarce. Regardless of this fact, in older children and particularly in teenagers, an unobserved drowning warrants a toxilogic screen.

Overestimation of skills and resultant exhaustion are the principal causes of drowning in 70% of those people who drown while swimming. Similarly, exhaustion frequently causes drowning in scuba diving accidents. Among experienced athletes, drowning may occur from hypoxia during underwater swimming after a period of hyperventilation; this has been termed shallow water blackout. Medical illnesses such as myocardial infarction are a cause of death in drowning, but the frequency of this is not known.

Epilepsy has also been implicated as a medical cause of drowning. Epileptic children have been found to have a fourfold increased incidence of drowning for age and account for 3–4% of all drowning victims in some studies. It is frequently difficult to determine whether these children "went under" as a result of the seizures, because histories were generally inconclusive and anticonvulsant levels are often not determined on admission.

Other less common factors in drowning have been found. Carbon monoxide-contaminated air and nitrogen narcosis have resulted in drowning among scuba divers. Trauma, such as that sustained in a boating or diving accident, may present as drowning. Child abuse occasionally takes the form of drowning. Frequently, this is difficult to prove because of the absence of distinguishing skin marks, but it may be suspected when the drowning story is atypical or when other unusual injuries have been noted in the child.

PATHOPHYSIOLOGY

The sequence of events that occurs during drowning has been studied extensively in animal experiments (Fig. 15.1), and several distinct steps were found to occur. After submersion, there is an initial panic and a struggle to surface, during which small amounts of water enter the hypopharynx. This water triggers apnea and laryngospasm, and copious amounts of fluid are swallowed. The animal struggles violently, gasps, loses consciousness, vomits, and aspirates. In approximately 10% of the animals, the initial laryngospasm persists until death from anoxia occurs; there is no aspiration of fluid. This closely coincides with human autopsy data (though it may differ in children).

Electrolyte Abnormalities

The fluid and electrolyte changes that accompany drowning were studied in detail during the 1940s in an attempt to gather data that would guide therapy. It was believed at that time that large volumes of fluid were aspirated by human drowning victims and shifted across the alveolus. Ex-

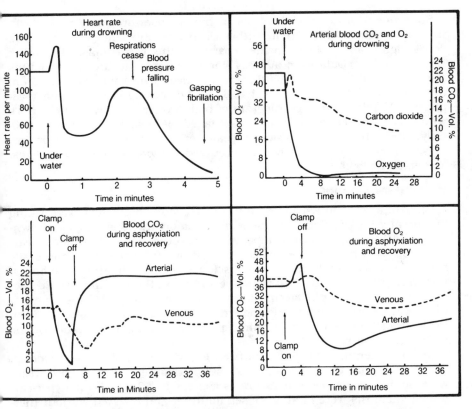

FIGURE 15.1. Sequence of events in acute drowning in dogs. *Graph 1 (upper left)* demonstrates the changes in heart rate during the first 5 minutes after submersion. *Graph 2 (upper right)* shows the changes in blood carbon dioxide and oxygen during drowning. *Graph 3 (lower left)* demonstrates variations of blood oxygen content during clamp-induced asphyxiation with recovery. *Graph 4 (lower right)* demonstrates the alterations in blood carbon dioxide content during clamp-induced asphyxiation with recovery. (From Lougheed DW: Physiological studies in experimental asphyxia and drowning. *Can Med Assoc J* 40:424, 1939.)

perimental models of drowning, using direct intratracheal instillation of large amounts of fluid, reflected this viewpoint. In these models, it was found that large electrolyte, blood volume, and hemoglobin alterations did occur and were dependent on the osmolarity of the drowning medium. Ventricular fibrillation was found to be a common terminal event in these animals. Freshwater drowning was postulated to cause hemodilution, hemolysis, hyperkalemia, hyponatremia, and an elevated circulating volume, whereas seawater (Na = 509 mEq/liter) drowning was postulated to produce hemoconcentration, hypernatremia, and a lower circulating blood volume. Therapy predicated on these findings suggested the intravenous use of hyper-tonic saline for victims of freshwater drowning and hypotonic solutions for victims of seawater drowning.

Subsequent study of electrolytes in human near-drowning patients in the 1960s demonstrated that neither electrolyte imbalance nor hemolysis was a significant problem in these patients; this was confirmed in other clinical studies. Data from autopsy findings in human drowning victims also failed to demonstrate life-threatening electrolyte abnormalities. From this analysis it was concluded that 85% of drowning victims actually aspirate <22 ml of fluid per kilogram of body weight. Experiments in dogs with use of smaller volumes of aspirate failed to cause life-threatening electrolyte disturbances in freshwater, seawater, or chlorinated water drownings, although distinct alterations occurred in blood volume, electrolytes, and arterial blood gases.

Pulmonary Changes

Persistent refractory hypoxemia has consistently been the most striking life-threatening physiologic derangement demonstrated aftrer near-drowning. Additionally, in clinical reports, it has been noted that many near-drowning victims would be pulled unconscious from the water and easily resuscitated with rapid return of consciousness. Within minutes to hours, however, respiratory distress would develop, and these victims would succumb to hypoxia despite facemask or oxygen tent therapy. Microscopic sections of their pulmonary tissue showed alveolar collapse, pulmonary edema, intra-alveolar exudate, and fibrin deposition, resembling infant hyaline membrane disease.

In experimental studies, it has been found that hypercardia, acidosis, and hypoxia routinely occurred after submersion episodes in both freshwater and seawater. Despite aspirates as large as 22 ml/kg, the hyper-carbia and acidosis were mild, were self-limiting, and resolved without therapy within an hour. On the other hand,, hypoxia of life-threatening severity was found after aspirates as small as 2.2 ml/kg, and this persisted unless the animal received mechanical ventilatory support.

In clinical cases and drowning models, the hypoxia produced by fluid aspiration was determined to be due to intrapulmonary shunting and was unresponsive to alternation of inspired oxygen tension. Analysis of tracheal and pulmonary fluid from dogs after drowning demonstrated elevated surface tension activity. After freshwater drowning, this was due to washout and dilution of surfactant; in seawater drowning, the surfactant was shown to be functionally inactive, although still present, in the alveoli. This lack of effective surfactant leads to alveolar collapse. Positive pressure ventilation with continuous positive airway pressure was found to be an extremely effective means of therapy, reversing intrapulmonary shunting and restoring oxygenation both clinically and experimentally. Early deaths from pulmonary disease after submersion are now rare.

Since the advent of positive pressure ventilation, pulmonary disease leading to death or morbidity after near-drowning is infrequent; those that occur are usually related to pulmonary infections or barotrauma. Pneumonia is seen after drowning in contaminated waters or after several days of ventilatory support. Pulmonary interstitial emphysema and pneumothorax frequently occur in patients who drown while scuba diving, although this may also follow mechanical ventilation with high airway pressures.

Current Classification

Currently, we prefer to consider the pathophysiology of near-drowning from four aspects:

1. Asphyxia, cerebral ischemia, and anoxia
2. Fluid overload
3. Pulmonary injury
4. Hypothermia and the diving reflex

Asphyxia, Cerebral Ischemia, and Anoxia

The most important problem, from the standpoint of the long-term outlook for the child, is the anoxic central nervous system (CNS) injury. This primary injury (inadequate delivery of oxygen) is schematically diagrammed in Figure 15.2. Oxygen is obviously required by all tissues, and injury to the brain, lungs, heart, and kidneys would be anticipated. Additionally, gastrointestinal ischemia can be anticipated. The "diving seal reflex" is associated with increased flow to the heart and brain, accompanied by peripheral vasoconstriction. This might increase injury to the kidney and gastro-intestinal system.

The effects of anoxia on the brain are protean. Normal autoregulation of the brain is presumably lost, although there are no human studies that

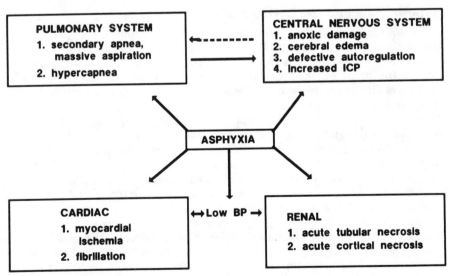

FIGURE 15.2. Pathophysiology of asphyxia in near-drowning. *BP,* blood pressure; and *ICP,* intracranial pressure.

demonstrate this. Cerebral edema occurs, primarily on a cytotoxic basis, and results in an increase in intracranial pressure. Increased intracranial pressure decreases the cerebral perfusion pressure, lowering cerebral blood flow and causing further ischemia.

Fluid Overload

The second major facet of the pathophysiology of near-drowning is water overload (Fig. 15.3). Although investigators have spent much time evaluating the effect of fluid aspiration, few have noted the large amount of water ingested during the drowning process. The victim swallows large amounts of water before aspiration, and the stomach is generally filled with water. Thus several effects can be seen. First and probably most important, the victim will usually vomit, and the potential pulmonary problems from aspiration often outweigh the original pulmonary difficulties arising from the submersion accident itself. Second, fluid is absorbed via the gastrointestinal tract and may result in fluid and electrolyte abnormalities, as already reported. Third, pulmonary edema may result from the ingestion of saltwater. In addition, a severe hypernatremic state may result from saltwater submersion. Finally, fluid overload of any type may exacerbate potential cerebral edema secondary to the primary anoxic neurologic injury.

Pulmonary Injury

The third pathophysiologic process that occurs during a near-drowning accident is pulmonary damage secondary to aspiration of the fluid in which the victim is submerged.

Hypothermia and the Diving Reflex

The fourth process that must be considered is hypothermia (Fig. 15.4). Hypothermia has a variety of effects. Significant hypothermia (i.e., decreases to 30°C or lower) is capable of depressing the neurologic examination to the point of brain death. Although hypothermia may exert some protective effects on the brain because of reduced cerebral metabolism, the clinician can be misled into believing that the child has no brain function. Thus it is critical to maintain support for a near-drowning victim at least until the temperature can be raised toward normal. Another effect of importance is hemodynamic; both the myocardial contractility and the vasomotor tone are decreased by hypothermia. Severe hypothermia may make cardiac resuscitation impossible, and in such instances the physician should continue resuscitation while rewarming methods are instituted.

Many papers have dealt with near-drowning in cold water, and it is important to realize that "cold" generally refers to extremely cold water (i.e., freezing). Even in warm climates, however, it is possible for water beneath ground level (as in private pools) to be significantly colder than the air temperature. Thus it is possible for a small child to become hypo-thermic even in a relatively warm pool in a moderate climate. In the emergency

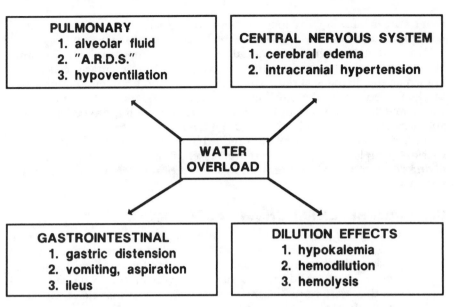

FIGURE 15.3. Pathophysiology of water overload in near-drowning. *A.R.D.S.*, adult respiratory distress syndrome.

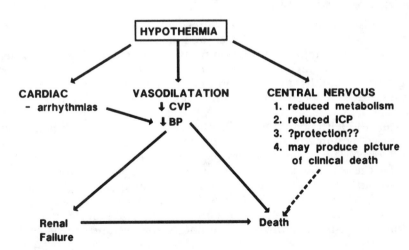

FIGURE 15.4. Pathophysiology of hypothermia in near-drowning. *CVP*, central venous pressure; *BP*, blood pressure; and *ICP*, intracranial pressure.

room and in subsequent management, the child's temperature must be monitored carefully.

Experimentally, it has been noted that many animals undergo profound circulatory pattern changes while submerged. These changes, collectively known as the diving seal reflex, maintain heart and brain circulation while markedly decreasing flow through nonvital organs and skeletal muscle by vaso-constriction. Bradycardia and respiratory inhibition occur during submersion, while the blood pressure is maintained at predive levels.

On the basis of these observations, it has been hypothesized that hypothermia, coupled with the preferential cerebral perfusion pattern from the diving reflex, may contribute to the good cerebral outcome found in some patients.

CLINICAL PRESENTATION AND ASSESSMENT

Children usually present in one of two ways after a near-drowning accident. The majority of children are awake and alert by the time they reach the hospital, and many have probably not suffered a significant injury in the first place. Such children may have gone under the water and sputtered when they were retrieved, but many children were apneic at the scene and received effective artificial ventilation before reaching the hospital facility. The children in this second group suffer cardiac arrest at some point, whether at waterside or during transport to the hospital. These children are the usual population of near-drowning victims who are admitted to pediatric ICUs. It is possible for a child to have minimal neurologic problems and have major pulmonary difficulty, but this is distinctly unusual.

Respiratory Assessment

In the initial assessment of a near-drowned child, the ABCs must be re-emphasized. The airway must be cleared of vomitus, which is extremely common after this injury; ventilation must be secured; and finally, the circulation must be assured and an adequate blood pressure must be achieved. The goals are no different here than in any other emergency stabilization. After the ABCs, a specific evaluation of pulmonary and CNS functions is in order.

In the child with spontaneous ventilation, the pulmonary function can be assessed by numerous means including a blood gas in 40% oxygen and a chest radiogram. Some authors have suggested criteria for intubation based on these parameters, but in the experience of the authors, the decision to intubate is usually clear. These tests simply provide the clinician with an objective handle on the severity of the lung injury. As a general guideline, a child who cannot maintain a $P_aO_2 > 100$ mm Hg in 40% oxygen will require positive pressure ventilatory support and should be intubated.

Radiologically, a wide variety of chest pathologies may develop. Drowning victims have been divided intro "dry" and "wet," based on their chest X-ray findings. Estimates of the incidence of gross pulmonary aspiration have been as high as 90%, but there is no proof of this in the pediatric population. In fact, it is not uncommon to see children with minimal aspiration but fatal nervous system damage. Table 15.2 is a summary of the initial radiologic findings of children referred to the Children's Hospital of Los Angeles between 1978 and 1980. A wide variety of radiologic findings were present, but these findings did not correlate with the eventual outcome of the children. It is also important to consider the definition of "wet"; minor pulmonary edema or a trivial infiltrate is not consistent with massive pulmonary aspiration of fluid. It would appear from these data that the incidence of gross aspiration of water via the trachea is low in children.

Children who have been involved in drowning accidents should be admitted to the hospital for observation. At least one report describes the fatal case of a child who suffered somewhat delayed respiratory distress. It is primarily for respiratory problems that such children are observed, and thus it is important to make a baseline assessment of the pulmonary system with at least a chest radiogram and an arterial blood gas.

Neurologic Assessment

Assessment of the neurologic system may be effectively done with the Glasgow coma scale described in Chapter 12. The use of this scoring system in near-drowning children has been useful, and the score permits fairly accurate identification of children with a high risk of neurologic sequelae. When the Glasgow coma score is >6, no significant neurologic sequelae generally are seen and nearly all of these children survive. It is important to note that this viewpoint is based on the initial hospital examination, not on the examination at the tertiary hospital. Thus if the child has a Glasgow coma score of 7 or 8 at the tertiary ICU but had a score of 3 at

TABLE 15.2.
Initial Chest Radiologic Findings on Admission to Hospital

Radiologic Diagnosis	No. of Children			
	Total	Dead	CNS Damage	Normal
Normal chest	33	2	3	28
Increased perihilar markings	17	3	0	14
Mild pulmonary edema	10	2	0	8
Aspiration	31	8	0	23
Severe infiltrate	3	1	1	1
Pneumothorax	1	0	1	0
Total no. of films	95	16	5	74

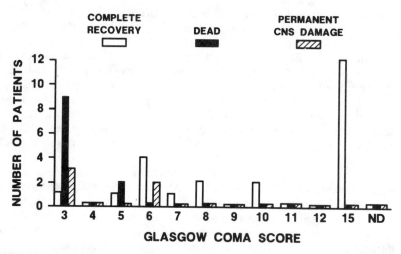

FIGURE 15.5. Glasgow coma score in near-drowning victims at the tertiary hospital. *Open bars* indicate normal survivors; *solid bars* indicate fatalities; and *hatched bars* indicate victims who suffered severe neurologic sequelae (permanent CNS damage). The Glasgow coma score at the tertiary hospital does not adequately prognosticate the patients. (Adapted from Dean JM, Kaufman ND: Prognostic indicators in pediatric near-drowning: The Glasgow coma scale. *Crit Care Med* 9:536, 1981; and from Dean JM, McComb JG: Intracranial pressure monitoring in severe pediatric near-drowning. *Neurosurgery* 9:627, 1981.)

the initial hospital, the child should be prognosticated with a score of 3. The Glasgow coma score when applied at the tertiary center fails to separate normal survivors completely from children who die or suffer neurologic sequelae (Fig. 15.5).

GENERAL MANAGEMENT

Respiratory Support

The most important systems are the pulmonary and cardiac systems because without the adequate function of both, the remainder of the child's body will not be salvageable. Thus it is imperative that there be aggressive take over of these two systems early in the intensive care course of these children. Children who are comatose (i.e., Glasgow coma score of <8 or 9) should be intubated, with particular caution used to avoid gastric aspiration. Arterial blood gas monitoring should be frequent, and if the child does not maintain normocapnia, mechanical ventilation should be employed. A borderline P_aCO_2 is not acceptable in a brain-injured child, and it is critical to be very aggressive in the control of this parameter. Once the decision to ventilate the child has been made, a reasonable range for the P_aCO_2 is between 25 and 30 mm Hg. Oxygenation must be adequate, and until blood gases can be obtained, the child should be placed in supplemental oxygen.

Hemodynamic Support

Hemodynamic management of these children may be difficult because of multiple insults to the cardiovascular system. These injuries include prolonged cardiac resuscitation (which may cause myocardial contusion and dysfunction), hypothermia (with vasomotor collapse, bradycardia and arrhythmias), fluid volume shifts (from fluid restriction, saltwater absorption, and mannitol therapy), and significant metabolic acidosis. Pulmonary arterial catheterization may be very useful in these patients and is particularly recommended after the entertainment of barbiturate therapy for intracranial hypertension.

Fluids and Electrolytes

Fluids and electrolytes should be managed in the same manner as in any other population of critically ill children, with frequent monitoring of laboratory parameters and appropriate consideration of measuring filling pressures. Many of the electrolyte abnormalities reported in drowning models have been overstated, but the intensivist should be aware that virtually any electrolyte abnormality may be seen in multisystem failure. The only safe avenue of management includes frequent monitoring of the patient and laboratory values.

Gastrointestinal Tract and Nutrition

The gastrointestinal system frequently malfunctions after drowning, and the children cannot be effectively fed. Bloody profuse diarrhea may be seen, and hepatic enzymes may be elevated, reflecting an ischemic insult. Although both findings are grim predictors of outcome, conservative management (nothing by mouth and control of gastric pH) usually suffices. To satisfy nutritional requirements, early hyperalimentation may be used. However, it is not clear whether early nutritional support will improve the neurologic outcome of these children.

Other Issues

Two additional issues often arise during discussions of the management of drowning patients. The first concerns the use of antibiotics for aspiration pneumonia. We are unaware of any evidence that aspiration after near-drowning is different from aspiration under any other circumstance, and it remains unclear whether antibiotics should be employed in any aspiration setting. It may be attractive to use antibiotics after a child aspirates dirty water, yet it is likely that those antibiotics will only select the more exotic forms of bacterial life with which the child may become septic. There are no reports that demonstrate the efficacy or requirement for antibiotic therapy in drowning patients. The second issue concerns the use of steroids for cerebral edema after near-drowning. Steroids are beneficial for cerebral edema around brain tumors, but there is no evidence whatsoever that steroids are useful for treating cerebral edema after ischemic or anoxic neurologic injuries. There are seemingly few contraindications to the use of the steroids, but there is little rationale for their use in this setting.

INTRACRANIAL PRESSURE MONITORING

Intracranial pressure has been monitored in drowning patients, and indeed, elevated intracranial pressure is commonly seen in children who die from drowning. In children who never develop intracranial hypertension, the outcome is clearly better than in chidren with intracranial pressure elevation, and this probably reflects less cytotoxic edema formation.

What is not clear is whether intracranial pressure monitoring has any true usefulness in these patients. Various authors recommend intracranial pressure monitoring and suggest that cerebral perfusion monitoring provides a good predictor of outcome. The cerebral perfusion pressure is clearly a worthwhile parameter to maintain. However, it is likely that intracranial hypertension in children after drowning accidents is a reflection of primary neuronal injury (e.g., cell death), and treatment of this "epiphenomenon" is unlikely to provide much improvement in the outcome of these patients.

In fact, brain resuscitative efforts have been made in the pediatric drowning population, but the improvement of outcome is less than spectacular. As a result, although general supportive measures including aggressive hemodynamic and respiratory support are indicated, the role of intracranial pressure monitoring remains controversial in near-drowning. Prudent use of hemodynamic, respiratory, diuretic, and general monitoring support are generally all that is indicated.

CHAPTER 16

Meningococcemia, *Haemophilus influenzae*, Systemic Infections, and Rocky Mountain Spotted Fever

The list of infectious diseases that may require admission to the pediatric intensive care unit (ICU) is nearly endless. Several chapters in the *Textbook of Pediatric Intensive Care* are devoted to the subject. For the sake of a synopsis, we review only the three most prominent systemic infectious diseases that are of interest to the intensivist.

MENINGOCOCCEMIA

Epidemiology

Disease caused by *Neisseria meningitidis* is usually endemic, but there have been reports of epidemics, especially among military personnel. The epidemic nature of the disease was well demonstrated during World War II, when the disease was responsible for more deaths due to infection than any other single microorganism.

Over the past couple of decades, evaluation of endemic disease due to *N. meningitidis* has revealed an overall incidence of approximately 2 cases/100,000 population/yr. Ninety percent of disease occurs in children under 2 years of age, although the mean age of onset is in the mid-teens. In one study from Scandinavia, the incidence in infants under 1 year of age was 15/100,000/yr. Data from the United States are similar, with an incidence in the same age group of 14.4/100,000/yr. Disease is rare in infants under 1 month of age, although reports of neonatal meningococcemia have appeared from time to time. Although neonatal infection has generally been considered a more benign form of disease than that which occurs later in infancy, some cases in the first month of life have been described as fulminant, resulting in death shortly after diagnosis. Attack rates fall dramatically in the 4- to 9-year-old age group.

Nonepidemic systemic infection with *N. meningitidis* occurs sporadically but is more prevalent in the later winter and early spring. Varying sex ratios have been reported, but overall, infection is more common in males

213

than in females. In some series, males make up at least 60% of those affected. Interestingly, the ratios are reversed when acute fulminating meningococcemia is considered, with females making up as much as 70% of those affected with this hyperacute form of disease.

Carriage of the organism in the nasopharynx is common, and most individuals who are exposed become colonized. Development of clinical infection correlates with lack of serum antibody. An elevation of the carriage rate occurs during epidemics, where spread is mostly among household contacts. The rate of carriage in the family group is much higher when the index case is an infant rather than an older child or adult. Upper respiratory symptoms may accompany development of the carrier state and may be related to low-grade infections or to preceding infections by influenza or Echoviruses, which may then result in an accelerated rate of carriage as well as increased risk of actual infection by the meningococcus.

Clinical Manifestations

Initial symptoms of systemic infection usually consist of upper respiratory complaints, fever, joint pains, myalgias, rash, headache, and vomiting. Physical findings include high fever (>40°C in 60%); rash that may be macular, petechial, or purpuric; and meningeal signs when meningitis predominates. Objective diffuse muscle tenderness is generally present. Signs of shock, such as hypotension, tachycardia, diminished perfusion, and cool skin in the presence of elevated core temperature, are present in the cases of fulminant bacteremia. When petechiae are present (50–60%), they are more pronounced in the trunk and extremities. When purpura develops, the lesions are distinct from the petechiae and usually a harbinger of severe disease. In the 80% of patients who have signs of meningeal involvement, alterations in level of consciousness and abnormal pupillary responses may occur, suggesting the presence of elevated intracranial pressure.

Laboratory findings vary with the severity of disease and have been correlated with prognosis in some situations. Factors useful in determining prognosis among pediatric patients with meningococcal infection suggest five factors that, when present, indicate an unfavorable prognosis (Table 16.1). When three or more factors were present at admission, the child had a >85% chance of dying. When two or fewer factors were noted, the fatality rate was <10% (Table 16.2). The laboratory signs often associated with poor prognosis are shown in Table 16.3.

Other factors have also been found to be related to poor prognosis, but in a less predictive way. These include presence of eosinophils and low levels of 17-hydroxycorticoids (both representing relative failure of adrenocortical function), the meningococcal serotype (B and C are more likely to cause death), and age (patients under 2 years of age more likely to have fatal outcome).

Death from meningococcal disease is generally due to intractable shock, even in patients with meningitis. Acute fulminating meningococcemia usually results in death in a matter of hours from the time of admission;

TABLE 16.1.

Unfavorable Prognostic Features in Meningococcal Infections as Defined by Stiehm and Damrosch[a] and Used to Determine the Prognostic Score

1. Presence of petechiae <12 hours prior to admission
2. Presence of shock (blood pressure, 70 systolic or below)
3. Absence of meningitis (<20 white blood cells/mm³) in cerebrospinal fluid
4. Blood leukocyte count normal or low (<10,000 white blood cells/mm³)
5. Erythrocyte sedimentation rate normal or low (<10 mm/hr)

[a]From Stiehm ER, Damrosch DS: Factors in the prognosis of meningococcal infection. *J Pediatr* 68:457, 1966.

mean duration of survival may range from 2 to 20 hours. The pathogenesis of the severe cardiovascular collapse has been a matter of debate.

There is a group of patients who appear to die of profound neurologic deterioration, postulated by some authors to represent elevated intracranial pressure, with or without herniation. Studies that include actual measurement of intracranial pressure are scarce. The ease with which such monitoring is accomplished in the ICU setting and the rarity of adverse sequelae, especially with the use of a subarachnoid screw, make it a reasonable technique in patients with serious disease accompanied by loss of

TABLE 16.2.

Relation of Prognostic Score to Fatality Rate in 63 Cases of Meningococcal Infections from Stiehm and Damrosh[a] and in 15 Cases from the Pediatric Literature

Prognostic Score (Total of Unfavorable Prognostic Features)[a]	Total Cases	Died	Fatality Rate (%)
Cases from Stiehm and Damrosch			
0	21	1	4.7
1	26	2	7.7
2	6	0	0
3	7	6	85.7
4	2	2	100.0
5	1	1	100.0
Cases from the pediatric literature			
1	4	1	25.0
2	6	1	16.6
3	5	4	80.0

[a]From Stiehm ER, Damrosch DS: Factors in the prognosis of meningococcal infection. *J Pediatr* 68: 457, 1966.
[b]Defined in Table 16.1.

TABLE 16.3.
Unfavorable Prognostic Factors in Meningococcal Disease, as Indicated by Niklasson and Coworkers[a]

1. Absence of meningitis (<100 white blood cells/mm^3) in cerebrospinal fluid
2. Presence of low blood pressure (<70 in children under 14 years of age)
3. Presence of petechiae for <12 hours prior to admission
4. Presence of marked hyperpyrexia (rectal temperature, 40°C or above)
5. Absence of marked leukocytosis (<15,000 white blood cells/mm^3)
6. Presence of thrombocytopenia (<100,000 platelets/mm^3)

[a] Adapted with permission from Niklasson P, Lundbergh P, Strandell T: Prognostic factors in meningococcal disease. *Scand J Infect Dis* 3:17, 1971

consciousness, presence of posturing or flaccidity, or evidence of third nerve involvement, which may indicate compression of the brainstem by the uncal portion of the temporal lobes. Third-nerve dysfunction may also represent a localized inflammatory response to the organism, and the decision to monitor intracranial pressure must take into account the entire physical examination. Occasionally, documentation of diffuse cerebral edema on a computed axial tomography (CAT) scan may reinforce the decision to monitor intracranial pressure. The absence of obvious edema, however, should not be taken as a reason not to institute monitoring if clinical signs and symptoms suggest elevated intracranial pressure.

Fulminating Meningococcemia (Waterhouse-Friderichsen Syndrome)

Fulminating meningococcemia is nearly always fatal and represents a hyper-acute form of disease. Petechiae are universally present, purpura generally develops, and the shock state may or may not respond to the fluids and pressor agents generally employed.

The finding of bilateral adrenal hemorrhage in a large percentage of autopsied cases initially led to the belief that the intractable shock was related to adrenal cortical failure. Early attempts at treating this infection with exogenous corticosteroids were promising. Larger studies have failed to demonstrate an effect on mortality, but sporadic reports of success continue to appear in the literature. Evaluations of adrenocortical function have yielded variable results. In many cases, some function is demonstrated, but it is not possible to know whether this function is adequate for the stress of the situation. Stimulation tests with adrenocorticotrophic hormone have, in some cases, resulted in poor response. Replacement therapy or the administration of very large doses of hydrocortisone (40–50 mg/kg) or methylprednisolone has not resulted in reversal of the shock state. Therefore, even if some adrenocortical insufficiency exists, it does not appear to be the sole etiology of the shock.

Several authors have interpreted the pathologic findings in fulminating meningococcemia as consistent with the Shwartzman reaction, which is an experimental condition produced in rabbits exposed to endotoxin and which takes two different forms—local and systemic. In the local Shwartzman reaction, the animal is primed with subcutaneously administered endotoxin, followed 24 hours later by intravenous administration of the same substance. Such treatment results in hemorrhagic necrosis at the site of local injection. In the systemic Shwartzman reaction, both sublethal injections are by the intraveous route and result in bilateral cortical necrosis in the kidneys. Although several authors have attempted to relate the clinical and pathologic finds in fulminant meningococcemia to those seen in the Shwartzman reaction, such arguments have been inconsistent and inconclusive.

The current consensus of medical opinion regarding the pathophysiology of cardiovascular collapse in this disease is that it represents primary response to endotoxin. Indeed, intravenous injection of large doses of meningococcal endotoxin in most animal species results in a syndrome similar to that of fulminant meningococcemia, with significant vasomotor disturbance, high fever or hypothermia, leukopenia, hypoglycemia, and petechial hemorrhage with focal necrosis. Unfortunately, it is not clear why the meningococcal endotoxin produces a more rapidly fatal disease than does endotoxin derived from the enteric Gram-negative organisms or why skin lesions and focal areas of coagulation and bleeding are more prominent in this disesase. Pathologically, the areas of bleeding that are seen may be related to underlying coagulation in capillaries and venules and may also be related to the severity of disseminated intravascular coagulation (DIC) produced by the organism.

Differential Diagnosis

The differential diagnosis of acute meningococcemia includes endotoxin-producing bacterial diseases, such as that produced by *Escherichia coli*, as well as others that can cause general prostration and meningitis, such as *H. influenzae* type B. Enteroviruses may present as fever and petechiae. Even in the absence of an obvious tick bite, the petechiae and purpura of Rocky Mountain spotted fever must make that entity a consideration as well. Noninfectious diseases, such as Henoch-Schönlein purpura, are also possible. Any disease or drug ingestion resulting in inadequate of platelet number or function may be accompanied by intradermal bleeding; such disorders would include DIC of any cause, idiopathic thrombocytopenic purpura, and all the infectious causes listed in Table 16.4. Other bacterial diseases that may prove rapidly fatal include the Gram-negative rods, with that produced by *Pseudomonas* being the most likely.

Routine bacterial tests are imperative and should include blood cultures and, when available, the use of rapid antigen diagnostic testing (countercurrent immune electro-phoresis or latex agglutination). The demonstration of Gram-negative diplococci on blood smear or buffy coat smear has, since 1944, been noted in the disease and may be helpful, as may be the finding of organisms in scrapings from purpuric lesions. Appropriate laboratory tests include white blood cell count with differential, erythrocyte

TABLE 16.4.
Infectious Diseases Associated with Petechiae

N. meningitidis
H. influenzae type B
N. gonorrhoeae
Streptococcus pneumoniae
S. pyogenes
Enteroviruses
Rubella
Rickettsiae
Mycoplasma
Epstein-Barr virus
Cytomegalovirus
Colorado tick fever
Arboviruses
Rat-bite fever
Yersinia pestis

sedimentation rate, platelet count, and evaluation for possible DIC with determination of prothrombin time, partial thromboplastin time, fibrinogen, and fibrin degradation products.

The remainder of the patient's evaluation should follow usual intensive care procedures. Adequacy of airway may be a problem if the mental status is diminished. Additionally, air exchange may be inhibited by the presence of adult respiratory distress syndrome, pulmonary edema, or pneumonia. Increased metabolic demand of the patient in shock may make an otherwise normal level of gas exchange inadequate for the situation. For these reasons, an arterial blood gas and chest X-ray must always be part of the initial and ongoing evaluations.

Detailed evaluation of the central nervous sytem (CNS) is essential. The etiology of an abnormal mental status must be determined. Although it is important to examine the cerebrospinal fluid for evidence of meningeal irritation and to obtain cultures, other causes of altered neurologic function should be considered, some of which preclude the performance of a lumbar puncture. Neurologic dysfunction in a child with meningococcemia may be due to direct effects of local infection and inflammation, diffuse cerebral edema with intracranial hypertension, or diminished cerebral perfusion due to the generalized shock state. If the child's Glasgow coma scale score is ≤7, ongoing bedside measurement of intracranial pressure is indicated and should be instituted prior to performance of the lumbar puncture. If the child's condition allows it, a CAT scan should be obtained prior to placement of an intraventricular catheter or subarachnoid screw. If the patient cannot be safely moved to the radiology department, a subarachnoid screw may be placed on the basis of clinical findings alone. A spinal tap may then be performed if the intracranial pressure reading is <20 mm Hg and there is no evidence of mass effect on CAT scan or physical examination. If the pressure is high, but the ventricles are visible on the scan, a ventricular catheter may be substituted for the screw, and a sample of cerebrospinal fluid may be obtained in that manner. Other contraindications to performance of a lumbar puncture in these children include markedly abnormal clotting studies, thrombocytopenia, irreversible shock, and/or an unstable airway.

Therapy

Specific antibiotic therapy consists of high-dose penicillin, to which the organism is nearly universally sensitive. Since a definitive diagnosis is not usually possible at the time of admission, however, chloramphenicol should be added to cover the other likely organisms. There is no evidence that simultaneous use of an aminoglycoside is harmful, so if there is any reason to suspect an enteric Gram-negative organism, the addition of gentamicin should be considered. In addition, if *Pseudomonas* is a strong possibility, piperacillin offers some theoretical advantages. Wide-scale use of third-generation cephalosporins in therapy for meningococcemia has not been reported.

There is no definitive evidence that corticosteroids are of benefit in changing the outcome of this disease. Administration of systemic corticosteroids can potentiate the Shwartzman reaction, but this adverse effect is only theoretical and has not been shown to apply to the human with bona fide meningococcal infection. Therefore, there is no strong contraindication to the use of steroids and some theoretical benefit to supporting possibly borderline adrenal function in the presence of circulatory failure. Since, in the initial hours of therapy, the pathogen will not be known, it is reasonable to use very high septic shock doses of methylprednisolone (30 mg/ kg), followed by maintenance doses of steroids once meningococcemia is documented, because there may be adrenocortical insufficiency, which may contribute to the hypotension and which may be reversible.

Heparin was once thought to be of potential value because the hemorrhagic findings were correlated with abnormal coagulation. No benefit has been documented from such therapy, but several instances of acute gastrointestinal hemorrhage potentially contributing to patient demise have been reported. The use of heparin, therefore, is contraindicated.

The efficacy of various inotropic and antihypotensive medications has not been documented in shock states related to meningococcal infection. The most widely used drug initially was norepinephrine, which has been sporadically reported to be of benefit even when adrenocortical extract was not. Clinical trials with dopamine, dobutamine, epinephrine, or isoproterenol have not been performed; therefore, there is no information available on which to recommend therapy with any particular agent. Indeed, in many of the published case reports, inotropic agents used singly or in various combinations have not altered the inevitable fatal outcome for some of these patients.

Most authors agree that plasma expansion is the first order of business and that large volumes may be necessary in the presence of endotoxic shock, as it occurs in meningococcal infection. Beyond that, especially with the knowledge that some degree of myocarditis usually exists, it is clear that an inotropic agent may be of benefit. Afterload reduction may be useful in light of the myocardial failure and diminished peripheral perfusion. It is possible that the combination of dobutamine for inotropy and nitroprusside for afterload reduction, with maintenance of adequate preload through the use of volume expansions, may be effective. In the patient with elevated intracranial pressure, however, nitroprusside infusion is relatively contraindicated, as it leads to preferential cerebral vasodilation and may diminish perfusion pressure by increasing intracranial pressure and potentially diminishing arterial blood pressure.

Complications

Patients who survive the first several days of the infection remain at risk for certain complications of meningococcemia, namely arthritis, deafness, gastroenteritis, pneumonia, and pericarditis-myocarditis. The last named are the most important to the pediatric intensivist. Generally, clinically evident myocarditis occurs at 4–7 days into the course of the illness, is probably a hypersensitivity reaction, and is noted in 3–5% of all patients. Some autopsy series have reported a much higher incidence of myocarditis and have suggested that the associated myocardial failure may relate directly to bacterial and leukocyte infiltration of the myocardium and conducting system. Such myocardial involvement may lead to sudden death from a dysrhythmia.

Pneumonia may be severe, requiring respiratory support, and may coexist with pulmonary edema. Pleural effusions may develop, suggesting a possible immunologic reaction in this complication as well.

HAEMOPHILUS INFLUENZAE

H. influenzae type B is the most common cause of bacterial meningitis among children under 5 years of age; the relationship of this organism to the meningitic syndrome is discussed in Chapter 18, "Bacterial Meningitis." *H. influenzae* type B, as well as other types of *H. influenzae*, causes a number of nonmeningitic, potentially life-threatening illnesses including epiglottitis, pneumonia, and sepsis. Other clinical entities that do not usually require intensive care include osteomyelitis, septic arthritis, and facial or periorbital cellulitis. The nontypeable strains are frequently implicated in cases of otitis media.

Epidemiology

The majority of *H. influenzae* type B infections occur in childhood, although a nontrivial percentage continues to occur in the adult population, especially in the elderly. Infection of infants under 30 days of age, although rare, has been reported. The peak incidence with regard to age varies according to the form of systemic disease (Fig. 16.1). The majority of cases

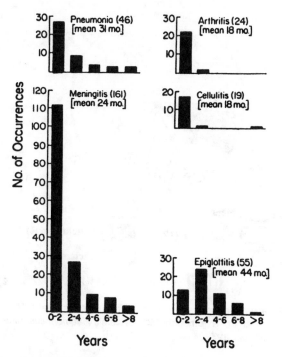

FIGURE 16.1. Age distributions and mean ages for the more common *H. influenzae* clinical entities. (From Dajani AS, Asmar BI, Thirumoorthi MC: Systemic *Haemophilus influenzae* disease: An overview. *J Pediatr* 94:355, 1979.)

of meningitis occur in infants, whereas the majority of cases of epiglottitis occur in older children.

It has been estimated that 20,000 systemic infections attributable to *H. influenzae* type B occur annually. Of these, meningitis accounts for 50%; epiglottitis, for 10–15%; and pneumonia, for approximately 15%. Two to ten percent of children have a primary bacteremia with no discernable site of localization. The overall mortality rate for all types of systemic *H. influenzae* disease is 5–10%, with the majority of deaths occurring in patients with meningitis or pneumonia.

Clinical Manifestations (Fig. 16.2)

As stated previously, the most common clinical presentation of *H. influenzae* type B is an acute meningitis, the diagnosis and therapy of which are discussed in Chapter 18, "Bacterial Meningitis." Epiglottitis is the second most common clinical syndrome produced by *H. influenzae* type B, and its acute management as referable to the upper airway obstruction is covered in Chapter 3. Pneumonia caused by *H. influenzae* type B is not dramatically different from that caused by other microorganisms and re-

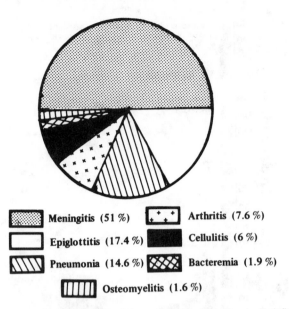

Meningitis (51 %)   Arthritis (7.6 %)

Epiglottitis (17.4 %)   Cellulitis (6 %)

Pneumonia (14.6 %)   Bacteremia (1.9 %)

Osteomyelitis (1.6 %)

FIGURE 16.2. Relative frequencies of different clinical entities due to *H. influenzae* infection. (From Dajani AS, Asmar BI, Thirumoorthi MC: Systemic *Haemophilus influenzae* disease: An overview. *J Pediatr* 94:355, 1979.)

quires the same general approach as any other acute lower respiratory infection.

Acute sepsis secondary to *H. influenzae* may produce some confusion to the clinician, in that it may mimic meningococcemia. *H. influenzae* can present as lethargy, shock, DIC, and a rash indistinguishable from that seen in meningococcemia (Tables 16.5 and 16.6). The death rate for those with meningococcemia was 10%, compared with 75% for those with *H. influenzae*. Additonally, the time from admission to death was shorter for those with *H. influenzae* type B. The deaths seen in *H. influenzae* type B overwhelming sepsis were caused by intractable hypotension and progressive cardiac dysfunction unresponsive to therapy. Over half of the patients who died with *H. influenzae* type B sepsis were treated with penicillin alone because of the clinical impression of meningoccocal disease. This may have contributed to the higher early death rate. Secondary sites of involvement were not significantly different from infections causd by the two organisms, namely there was a similar incidence of meningitis, myocarditis, pneumonia, otitis media, and osteomyelitis.

Therapy

Initial therapy for overwhelming sepsis due to *H. influenzae* type B is not different from that for meningococcemia, and the reader is referred to the previous section for a description of the general approach to this life-threatening infectious disease.

TABLE 16.5.
Demographic Data for Patients with Apparent Meningococcemia: Comparison of Those with Proven _N. meningitidis_ with Those with _H. influenzae_[a]

	N. meningitidis (N = 30)	_H. influenzae_ (N = 12)
Age (months)	23.6 ± 4.7 (16.5)[b]	14.9 ± 3.3 (14.5)[b]
Sex (male/female)	22/8	6/6
Season		
Winter	12	1
Spring	8	3
Summer	6	3
Fall	4	5
Interval between admission and onset of		
Symptoms	2.5 ± 0.6 days (8 hr to 14 days)	1.7 ± 1.2 days (8 hr to 14 days)
Lesions	0.5 ± 0.3	0.6 ± 0.1
Antecedent illness upper respiratory tract infection)	13	4 1 (tonsillitis)
Antecedent therapy	2 (1 given penicillin G; 1 given amoxicillin)	1 (erythromycin)
History of exposure to index case	1	0

[a] Reproduced by permission of Jacobs RF, Hsi S, Wilson CB, et al: Apparent meningococcemia: Clinical features of disease due to _Haemophilus influenzae_ and _Neisseria meningitidis. Pediatrics_ 72:469, 1983.
[b] Values are means ± SE:

Little more need be added regarding treatment, except as it relates to specific antimicrobial therapy. At least 25% of all _H. influenzae_ type B isolates throughout the United States are resistant to ampicillin. Resistance is caused by ability of the microorganism to product β-lactamase and inactivate penicillins. The drug of choice, therefore, is chloramphenicol, although there have been occasional reports of chloramphenicol-resistant _H. influenzae_ type B, primarily from the United Kingdom. Multiply-resistant strains also exist. Some of the third-generation cephalosporins have shown promise with regard to therapy for _H. influenzae_ type B sepsis and meningitis and may be especially useful in young infants who are at higher risk for developing adverse effects from chloramphenicol administration.

Prevention

Close household and day care center contacts should receive chemoprophylaxis with rifampin at a dose of 20 mg/kg/day for 4 days. This should be provided regardless of results of nasopharyngeal cultures, as numerous

TABLE 16.6.
Comparison of Clinical Presentation and Outcome in Patients with
***N. meningitidis* and *H. influenzae* Who Presented wtih Apparent**
Meningococcemia[a]

	N. meningitidis (N = 30)	*H. influenzae* (N = 12)
Fever (≥38°C)	30	12
Irritable but alert	15	2
Lethargy or coma	15[b]	10
Vomiting	14	4
Headache	6	1
Rash	30/30	10/12
Petechial	2	4
Purpuric	3	4
Both	25[c]	2
Maculopapular	1[d]	2[e]
None	0	2
Shock	11	6
DIC	12	5
Adrenal hemorrhage	2/3[f]	5/9
Death	3/30[g]	9/12[h]
Time to death (hours) (mean ± SE)	120 ± 74/4[b]	20.7 ± 4.0

[a]Reproduced by permission of Jacobs RF, Hsi S, Wilson CB, et al: Apparent meningococcemia: Clinical features of disease due to *Haemophilus influenzae* and *Neisseria meningitidis*. *Pediatrics* 72:469, 1983.
[b]$P < 0.05$, compared with that for *H. influenzae* cases.
[c]Six children required skin grafts.
[d]Petechiae were also present.
[e]Both were also purpuric.
[f]Denominator is number of patients examined postmortem.
[g]$P < 0.005$, compared with that for *H. influenzae*; 1 of 14 with meningitis; 2 of 16 without meningitis.
[h]Six of nine with meningitis; 3 of 3 without meningitis.

reports have documented the failure of one-time cultures to accurately detect all carriers. Adult members as well as children should probably receive prophylaxis. The index case also deserves rifampin therapy, since systemic administration of ampicillin and/or chloramphenicol does not eradicate nasopharyngeal carriage of the organism.

Of greater public health significance is the recently licensed *H. influenzae* type B polysaccharide vaccine. Of course, vaccination is not of much use in the pediatric ICU, nor is it especially useful among contacts of an index case, since development of immunity occurs in 2–3 weeks and many of the secondary cases occur within the first 5 days.

ROCKY MOUNTAIN SPOTTED FEVER

Overview and Epidemiology

Of the numerous Rickettsial diseases that affect humans, Rocky Mountain spotted fever is the most important in the United States. It impacts most heavily upon pediatric medical care providers, as most of its victims are children. Its name is misleading, as significantly more cases occur each year in areas east of the Mississippi River, especially in the southeastern and south central states. *Rickettsia rickettsii*, the etiologic agent, is an obligate intracellular parasite that resides in several species of ticks: in the East in the eastern dog tick, *Dermacentor variabilis;* in the West, in the western wood tick, *Dermacentor andersoni.* Humans are only incidentally involved when bitten by an adult tick. Transmission of the agent takes some time, perhaps several hours, so prompt recognition and removal of ticks may be preventive. Transmission may also occur if a breach in the skin is contaminated with the contents of a crushed tick; therefore, care should be used during removal of a tick attached to another person. The remover may acquire the disease, while the bitten person escapes without infection. The highest incidence of disease is among children in the 5- to 9-year-old range. Over half of all cases occur in persons under 19 years of age. Presumably, this finding relates to the prevalence of *R. rickettsii* in the eastern dog tick and to the close association of children and their dogs. In the west, more disease occurs among older people who work out of doors and are exposed to ticks that feed on small wild mammals and rodents. Because transmission of Rocky Mountain spotted fever requires activity of ticks, the incidence is seasonal and peaks in the warm weather months.

Clinical Aspects

The incubation period of Rocky Mountain spotted fever is 2–14 days, with a mean of 7 days between tick bite and onset of symptoms. Less severe disease tends to be associated with the longer incubation periods. The first symptom noted by most patients is fever, often accompanied by headache and generalized malaise, followed shortly by vomiting, myalgias, and photophobia. The fever increases in height, with spikes as high as 105–106°F. There is generally a hectic pattern to the febrile state, and the temperature may fall to nearly normal in the morning, only to rise again in the afternoon. As the disease progresses, headache increases in intensity and may be associated with stiffness of the neck. Some children have shaking chills, abdominal pain, or diarrhea. The mental status eventually becomes clouded, and the youngster may be listless, lethargic, apathetic, or frankly comatose. The rash generally appears 2–4 days after the onset of fever and has been noted in nearly all children with Rocky Mountain spotted fever, although it may be variable in nature. The rash is often the first clue to the etiologic nature of what to this point has been an undifferentiated febrile illness. The eruption begins as discrete erythematous macules, first observed on the ankles and feet and shortly thereafter on the wrists and hands. There is gradual progression with involvement of the limbs and, finally, the abdomen. In some children, it may start on the trunk and move outward to involve the extremities. Regardless of its progression, it is almost always most pronounced over the extremities and almost always involves the palms and soles. In quality, what starts as a rash of discrete blanching macules of several millimeters in diameter becomes morbilliform, then papular, then darkens in hue. Over the succeeding several days, it gradually becomes petechial and sometimes frankly purpuric. The purpura is related to the underlying coagulo-pathy and may become so severe as to result in overt gangrene of the earlobes, scrotum, and digits. In some children, petechiae and purpura do not develop, and the rash remains macullopapular or morbilliform, making the etiologic diagnosis less apparent. Mucous membranes may become involved, conjunctivitis is frequently present, and nonpitting edema of the limbs and periorbital areas is prominent.

Associated findings may include isolated splenomegaly or hepatosplenomegaly associated with mild transient elevation of serum transaminase. Acute tubular necrosis may occur because of hypovolemia; sometimes, renal vasculitis and interstitial pneumonitis and myocarditis may occur, but these are generally without clinical importance. Hemodynamic collapse may occur acutely and is most often related to inadequate intravascular volume. When hypotension fails to respond to fluid administration, the intensivist must suspect the occurrence of myocardial failure secondary to myocarditis.

Neurologic abnormalities may be prominent and severe in some cases. Cortical blindness and deafness may occur but are usually transient. Cranial nerve dysfunction often results in oculomotor palsies. Vascular involvement of the retina and optic nerve may lead to papilledema in the absence of elevated intracranial pressure. The neurologic course may resemble that of acute encephalitis or meningitis, with neck stiffness, lethargy, confusion, disorientation, and coma.

If untreated, the disease reaches its peak in the middle of the second week following initial appearance of the rash. Severe cases progress to deep coma, hemodynamic collapse, respiratory failure, progressive thrombocytopenia, and DIC with overt bleeding into the CNS, lungs, or gastrointestinal tract. Prior to the development of specific antibiotics, the mortality rate was 20–30%.

Laboratory evaluation generally reveals leukocytosis with an increased number of band forms, mild anemia, thrombocytopenia with hypofibrinogenemia, and an elevation of fibrin degradation products. Electrolyte abnormalities are common and consist primarily of hyponatremia and hypochloremia. Serum albumin is often low, and blood urea nitrogen and creatinine are elevated, as are the hepatic enzymes. Examination of the cerebrospinal fluid may be normal or reveal a lymphocytic pleocytosis with elevated protein but normal glucose concentration and absence of organisms on Gram stain.

A complement fixation titer of at least 16 or an indirect fluorescent antibody titer of ≥64 represents confirmation of disease, as does a fourfold rise in either titer. Weil-Felix assay, performed to look for cross-reaction with *Proteus* OX-19 or OX-2 antigens, in unequivocal cases will also show a fourfold rise. Other tests that may be helpful include latex agglutination, microag-glutination, and indirect hemagglutination procedures. Each of these should demonstrate a fourfold rise or an absolute titer of 128. None of these tests are helpful in the acute period of infection, as antibody titers do not peak until 2–4 weeks into the illness.

Entertaining and making a presumptive etiologic diagnosis are essential, as with specific antibiotic therapy initiated early in the course of disease, death should not occur. A springtime or summer febrile illness and unexplained neurologic disease with accompanying rash should spark the clinician to consider, treat, and search for *R. rickettsii*. Muscle biopsy may be a useful evaluative tool and would be expected to show perivascular lymphocyte infiltration. Testing of the specimen by direct immunofluorescence may be positive. The tissue should be Giemsa-stained, which may reveal the presence of coccobacillary forms not observed on Gram stain or hematoxylin and eosin stain.

Differential diagnosis includes the diseases listed in Table 16.7. Many of

TABLE 16.7. _____
Differential Diagnosis of Rocky Mountain Spotted Fever

Other Rickettsial diseases
Murine typhus
Typhoid fever
Colorado tick fever

Bacterial and spirochetal diseases
Meningococcemia
Disseminated streptococcal sepsis
Tularemia
Leptospirosis
Rat-bite fever

Viral diseases
Atypical measles
Enteroviruses
Epstein-Barr virus

Others
Juvenile arthritis
Systemic lupus erythematosus
Henoch-Schönlein purpura
Thrombotic thrombocytopenic purpura
Hemolytic uremic syndrome
Kawasaki disease

the entities to be considered are those that have a prominent vasculitic component, as does Rocky Mountain spotted fever. Indeed, most of the findings in this illness correlate with the underlying disseminated thrombovasculitis. It has been proposed that the vasculitis is due to direct invasion of arterioles and capillaries by *R. rickettsii*, resulting in proliferation of endothelial components and perivascular inflammation. The result is a diffuse vasculitis affecting many organ systems. Origin of the frequently observed thrombocytopenia and DIC is not clearly understood, nor is the microbial proliferation frequently observed at autopsy in the brains of those with fatal disease.

Treatment consists of both specific antimicrobial therapy and supportive care. Most children in whom the disease is recognized early and in whom appropriate antibiotics are administered, will not require the services of the ICU. Antibiotics of choice are chloramphenicol or tetracycline, each at a dose of 100 mg/kg/day. Chloramphenicol is preferred in children. Serum chloramphenicol levels should be monitored throughout the therapeutic course. The recommended length of therapy varies, but most experts believe treatment should continue 6−7 days beyond defervescence. When such treatment is initiated early, the disease often aborts, the patient becomes afebrile in 24−48 hours, and symptoms gradually improve. When antibiotics are withheld until later in the disease, or when the course of illness has progressed very rapidly, the fever may last another week or longer. In the preantibiotic era, patients who did not die began to improve after 2−3 weeks of fever and rash.

Critical care support of advanced disease may include: assisted ventilation necessitated by pulmonary edema that results from the vasculitis and hypoalbuminemia; treatment of pleural effusions or empyema; invasive hemodynamic monitoring and support, especially when the hypertensive patient is also in renal failure; replacement of plasma, platelets, blood, and clotting factors; possible heparinization if thrombotic complications are overwhelming; and neurologic, nutritional, and physical therapy support of the comatose child. As in any disorder involving thrombocytopenia and DIC, great care should be employed during the performance of any procedure such as central line insertion, lumbar puncture, and endotracheal intubation. The nasotracheal approach to intubation should probably be avoided.

Long-term sequelae of mild disease are minimal. When complications such as convulsions or CNS hemorrhages occur, prolonged disability should be expected.

There does not appear to be a role for steroids in any phase of the infection. This issue has not been adequately studied, however.

Summary

Rocky Mountain spotted fever is an easily treatable but sometimes hard to recognize infection primarily affecting children in the summer months. Because the key to prevention of mortality and serious morbidity lies in prompt institution of specific antibiotics, the physician must be aware of the common and rare manifestations of the disease. Therapy should never be withheld awaiting etiologic diagnosis. Appropriate support of vital systems must be provided while waiting for the antimicrobial agents to exert an effect. Occasionally, a patient will have a progressive and fatal course, even in the face of early, appropriate, and aggressive therapy.

CHAPTER 17

Encephalitis

Most children with evidence of acute encephalitis severe enough to significantly alter the state of consciousness should be admitted to the intensive care unit (ICU) for initial evaluation and supportive care. This is especially true in the early phases when the differential diagnosis includes other possibilities, such as cerebrovascular accidents and poisoning, as described elsewhere. Moreover, it is essential to monitor the course closely and to follow the neurologic examination meticulously. Severe encephalitis can result in extensive areas of perivascular infiltrates and diffuse cerebral edema with venous congestion. This process may result in elevation of intracranial pressure (ICP) and cerebral herniation. The infiltrate and immune response may result in seizures, which can be exceedingly difficult to control, and in some cases actual neuronal destruction occurs in the cortex, the basal ganglia, and the brainstem. Such involvement may result in respiratory compromise or hemodynamic instability. Because intensive supportive therapy may be required for these patients, it is therefore mandatory that the first 24–48 hours be spent in an intensive care area.

Indications for initiation of assisted ventilation do not vary from those discussed elsewhere in this book. Of importance regarding intubation and maintenance of ventilatory support is that the clinician avoid the use of long-acting neuromuscular blocking agents, if possible, because of the high incidence of seizures in these patients. If such blockade is necessary to maintain adequate ventilation and oxygenation, then continuous electroencephalographic or cerebral function monitoring should be employed while the patient remains paralyzed, and the patient should be allowed to develop some spontaneous movements prior to administration of each dose of the neuromuscular blocking agent. Failure to recognize and treat ongoing seizure activity in the paralyzed child may lead to profound metabolic acidosis, cerebral ischemia, and brain damage. Another drawback to use of paralysis in such a situation is that it does not permit repetitive performance of the neurologic examination. Therefore, the development of raised ICP may not become clinically apparent until the intracranial hypertension is of such a level as to cause the typical Cushing response and possible herniation. For these reasons, electively monitoring the ICP of any patient

231

with acute encephalitis who requires continued neuromuscular blockade must be considered.

When elevated ICP is documented, therapeutic measures of hyperventilation, dehydration, and routine positioning should be employed. The use of corticosteroids is of no documented value and may prove harmful by causing dissemination of herpes simplex virus. No recommendation can be given concerning the use of barbiturate coma as an adjunctive measure to control intracranial hypertension in this disease, as no systematic studies of this problem have been reported.

SPECIFIC VIRAL INFECTIONS

Arboviruses

The term arbovirus is used to indicate those viruses that are transmitted by arthropods. Although it is no longer an official designation, it is convenient to consider together the group of over 300 separate ribonucleic acid viruses, approximately 60 of which cause disease in humans. The important arboviruses of North America, all of which are transmitted by either mosquitoes or ticks, are presented in Table 17.1. Most of the viruses in this group cause disease that is specific with regard to geographic location and seasonal occurence. They vary in their virulence, with the highest mortality occurring in patients with Eastern equine encephalitis (nearly three-quarters of patients in some series die) and the lowest occurring in patients with Colorado tick fever and Venezuelan equine encephalitis. Those encephalitides borne by mosquitoes (Eastern, Western, St. Louis, California, and Venezuelan) occur strictly in the summer and fall in temperate climates, whereas those carried by ticks may be somewhat more variable. The diseases may be sporadic or epidemic, depending on environmental factors such as weather conditions and the status of the vector population. We are concerned with the more common varieties.

First described during an epidemic in 1933, St. Louis encephalitis is considered the most common arbovirus infection in the United States. Children are likely to be only mildly affected, whereas the elderly tend to have more significant disease. Some unusual clinical manifestations have been described with this disease, including inappropriate secretion of antidiuretic hormone and symptoms and signs suggestive of urinary tract infection (pyuria and dysuria) in the absence of any bacterial urinary pathogens. Overall duration of illness is generally 1–2 weeks. The mortality varies from 5 to 20%, with the higher rates occurring in the older patients. Diagnosis is made by documenting a rise in hemagglutination inhibition and complement fixation titers in blood. It is unusual to culture virus from the cerebrospinal fluid (CSF).

Eastern equine encephalitis is fortunately a relatively rare disease. It preferentially attacks children under 10 years of age, and at least one-quarter of cases occur in infants under 1 year of age. It now chiefly occurs along the eastern coast of both Americas. Clinical infection is characterized by very abrupt onset and severe neurologic signs that progress to maximal

TABLE 17.1.
Important Arboviruses of North America[a]

Family	Genus	Species	Vector	Reservoir	Mortality rate (%)
Togaviridae	*Alphavirus*	Eastern equine	Mosquito	Birds	0–1
		Western equine	Mosquito	Birds	5–20
		Venezualan equine	Mosquito	Horses, small mammals	0–1
	Flavivirus	St. Louis	Mosquito	Birds	0–1
		Powassan	Tick	Birds, small mammals	2
Bunyaviridae	*Bunyavirus*	California	Mosquito	Rodents	Rare
Reoviridae	*Orbivirus*	Colorado tick fever	Tick	Rodents	

[a]From Ho DD, Hirsch MS: Acute viral encephalitis. *Med Clin North Am* 69:415, 1985.

severity within 24–48 hours and is associated with fever as high as 42°C (108°F). Death often occurs within this short time period in up to 75% of cases, and the majority of survivors are left with devastating neurologic sequelae such as cranial nerve palsies, mental retardation, epilepsy, hemiplegia, and asphasia. ICP, when measured as opening pressure during a lumbar puncture, is frequently elevated. Of note, the CSF pleocytosis often consists of at least 50% polymorphonuclear cells, which may persist through the end of the second week of illness.

Western equine encephalitis is found primarily in California and Texas. Inapparent infections are very common, especially among adults. In infants, the disease is abrupt, with clinical evidence of elevated ICP. At least 50% of infants are left with significant sequelae, whereas only 10% of older children and adults have residual effects of the disease. Pathologic findings are striking for evidence of an intense vascular inflammatory reaction, with hyperplasia and occlusion of small vessels, sometimes resulting in multiple infarctions and cystic degeneration of wide areas of cortex. Although viruses can sometimes be grown in culture from CSF specimens, diagnosis depends on measuring a rise in antibody titers.

Herpes Simplex Encephalitis

Herpes simplex encephalitis is one of the most devastating of all central nervous system (CNS) infections, with an untreated immediate mortality rate of over 65%. It is the most common cause of fatal sporadic viral encephalitis in the United States. It does not occur in epidemic form.

CLINICAL PRESENTATION

Although the virus can cause syndromes of aseptic meningitis and myelitis, such illnesses are rare, and the encephalitic picture is by far the most important. This disease generally occurs in previously healthy persons and affects male and female subjects equally. Although it may occur in any season, it is most prevalent during the winter months.

Presenting clinical symptoms and signs vary with the age of the affected child. In younger children and infants, historical information does not generally result in strong support for the specific viral etiology, unless gingivostomatitis or skin lesions are also present. The youngsters are generally febrile with decreased level of consciousness and vomiting. Only rarely is there a prodromal illness. Seizures may be generalized or focal. In older patients, nervous system symptoms follow evidence of preceding upper respiratory involvement in 30% of cases. Onset of fever and headache follows, accompanied by emesis, lethargy or confusion, and (in some cases) hallucinations.

Stiffness of the neck is often noted, as are focal motor seizures. Focal neurologic signs develop in a majority of patients and are thought to represent selective involvement of the temporal or frontal lobes by the infectious particles, sometimes resulting in an erroneous diagnosis of brain abscess or tumor. Brainstem abnormalities that reflect effects of inflam-

TABLE 17.2.
Historical Findings in Suspected Herpes Simplex Encephalitis[a]

	No./Total (%) of Patients Biopsied	
	Positive	Negative
Altered consciousness	27/28 (96)	22/22 (100)
Fever	27/28 (96)	20/22 (91)
Personality change	19/20 (95)	9/16 (56)
Headache	23/28 (82)	15/22 (68)
Vomiting	14/28 (50)	9/22 (41)
Recurrent herpes labialis	6/27 (22)	6/22 (27)
Memory loss	5/28 (18)	1/9 (11)
Photophobia	1/28 (4)	2/22 (9)

[a]From National Institute of Allergy and Infectious Disease Collaborative Antiviral Study Group as reported in Cohen JI: Clinical conference at the Johns Hopkins Hospital: Herpes simplex encephalitis. *Johns Hopkins Med J* 147:157. 1980

mation or cerebral edema develop and are often accompanied by increasing papilledema and other signs of elevated ICP, including transtentorial herniation and cardiorespiratory instability.

The common historical and physical findings in older children and adults at presentation are listed in Tables 17.2 and 17.3 which compare patients with biopsy-proven herpes simplex encephalitis with those who have negative biopsies. It is clear that no specific clinical sign or historical finding distinguishes the two groups. Hence, early diagnosis is difficult.

TABLE 17.3.
Signs of Presentation in Suspected Herpes Simplex Encephalitis[a]

	No./Total (%) of Patients Biopsied	
	Positive	Negative
Disorientation	13/14 (93)	10/12 (83)
Dysphasia	14/16 (87)	7/13 (54)
Autonomic dysfunction	21/28 (75)	13/22 (59)
Ataxia	8/12 (67)	3/9 (33)
Focal Seizures	12/28 (43)	2/22 (9)
Generalized seizures	4/28 (14)	10/22 (45)
Hemiparesis	12/28 (43)	10/20 (50)

[a]From National Institute of Allergy and Infectious Disease Collaborative Antiviral Study Group as reported in Cohen JI: Clinical conference at the Johns Hopkins Hospital: Herpes simplex encephalitis. *Johns Hopkins Med J* 147:157, 1980.

LABORATORY FINDINGS

Laboratory findings in herpes simplex encephalitis are nonspecific. Routine blood studies such as complete blood count and differential may be totally normal or may reflect the presence of an acute infectious process. When the syndrome of inappropriate antidiuretic hormone secretion occurs, these patients may present with hyponatremia, but otherwise the electrolyte pattern is unremarkable.

Evaluation of CSF is essential, although on occasion it may be totally normal. More often, however, abnormalities consistent with the diagnosis of any type of encephalitis are encountered (Table 17.4). These include pleocytosis of variable degree, usually consisting of <200 white blood cells total, which in the first 24–48 hours of illness is generally polymorphonuclear, progressing to a predominantly mononuclear cell count beyond that time.

The particular predilection of the virus for the temporal or frontal lobes has been untilized in employment of various ancillary diagnostic studies, which include the electroencephalogram (EEG), the computerized axial tomography (CAT) scan, the radionuclide brain scan, and brain biopsy.

The classic herpetic EEG shows a diffuse slow-wave background with periodic complexes, sharp waves, and slow waves over one frontal or temporal lobe. When such lateralizing electrical activity is present, it may indicate a severe cerebral insult and predict a foreboding outcome. Similar EEG findings may also occur in nonherpetic encephalitides such as that due to infectious mononucleosis. The EEG, therefore, may provide evidence to support the diagnosis or point to an area of focal damage that should be biopsied, but it is not specific for herpes simplex encephalitis.

Focal abnormalities may also be noted on radioactive brain scan and CAT scan. With the latter type of examination, characteristic findings are unilateral low-density lesions or the suggestion of a mass effect in the temporal lobe or, in some cases, the insular cortex. When hemorrhage is as-

TABLE 17.4.
CSF in Herpes Simplex Encephalitis

Opening pressure	Normal
Color	Clear to xanthochromic
Red blood cells	0 to >500 cells/mm^3
White blood cells	Normal to several hundred
Differential	Early polymorphonuclear predominance, late lymphocytic predominance
Glucose	Normal
Protein	600–200 mg/100 ml
Grain stain	Negative for bacteria
Bacterial culture	Negative
Viral culture	Negative

sociated with the lesion, there is streaked contrast enhancement. Although nearly all patients with biopsy-proven herpes develop abnormal CAT scan findings, they are present on admission in only 64–92%, and sometimes the scan is normal until the fifth day of illness.

Presently, the only means by which to make a definitive diagnosis of herpetic encephalitis is through brain biopsy. During the initial trials of therapy with adenine arabinoside (ara-A), biopsy was required prior to entry into the study population, and the procedure continues to be recommended by most experts because of the need to know the diagnosis in order to make drug therapy comparison valid. There are many other reasons for obtaining a biopsy, but the most important is the fact that in suspected cases of herpes simplex encephalitis that go to biopsy, the diagnosis is substantiated only 50% of the time. A number of other diseases, some of which are treatable, are diagnosed in the other 50% of patients and are listed in Table 17.5. On the other hand, since acyclovir is now the drug of choice for this disease, and is much safer than ara-A, a brain biopsy may not be necessary in all cases.

PATHOGENESIS AND PATHOLOGY

The specific tropism of *Herpesvirus hominis* for the temporal and orbito-frontal lobes has engendered much speculation. The two major hypotheses are that the virus spreads to its most common site of infection via the olfactory bulbs or that it remains latent in the trigeminal ganglion and spreads along the fibers of the fifth nerve to the basal meninges of the anterior and middle fossae. Given current knowledge that the virus normally remains latent in the trigminal ganglion, from whence it travels to the skin of the face or lips in recurrent herpes labialis, and the fact that trigeminal fibers also innervate the base of the brain, the latter hypothesis

---

TABLE 17.5.
Diagnosis in Biopsy-Negative Cases of Suspected Herpes Simplex Encephalitis[a]

Arbovirus encephalitis	Mumps meningoencephalitis
Arteriovenous malformation	Primary brain tumors
Brain abscess	Sagittal sinus thrombosis
Cryptococcal meningitis	Subacute sclerosing pan-
Enterovirus encephalitis	encephalitis
Epstein-Barr virus encephalitis	Subacute bacterial endo-
Focal cerebritis	carditis
Meningovascular syphilis	Toxoplasmosis
Metastatic brain tumors	Tuberculous meningitis

[a]Adapted with permission from Cohen JI: Clinical conference at the Johns Hopkins Hospital: Herpes simplex encephalitis. *Johns Hopkins Med J* 147:157, 1980.

appears most reasonable in patients who possess systemic immunity to the virus. In neonates whose first encounter with the herpes virus results in encephalitis, the classic localization does not occur, and in many of these patients, necrosis of olfactory bulbs is found. Therefore, it may be that the mode of entry into the CNS of the nonimmune host does occur via spread from the nasopharynx, through the cribriform plate and via the olfactory nerves, from whence it progresses to widespread dissemination.

Many of the pathologic findings in herpes encephalitis resemble other acute encephalitides; there is infiltration of lymphocytes and histiocytes, affecting both gray and white matter, and proliferation of microglial cells. Polymorphonuclear cells are usually prominent in the infiltrative process, and there is usually a dramatic vasculitis, more striking than in other types of encephalitis. Intranuclear inclusion bodies are often seen; they resemble those observed in cytomegalovirus, measles, and varicella-zoster infection but are not invariably present.

THERAPY

Supportive aspects of care of the child with suspected or proven herpes simplex encephalitis are not different from those of patients with other acute CNS infections. Appropriate attention must be paid to overall care of the airway and cardiorespiratory system, as well as those aspects of neurointensive care previously discussed. Because of the necrotizing and often focal nature of herpes simplex encephalitis, focal or generalized seizures may be a prominent aspect of disease as exhibited in the pediatric ICU and may require extreme measures to achieve a seizure-free state. In addition, cerebral edema, elevated ICP, and herniation are common occurrences in patients with herpetic encephalitis. Therefore, when signs and symptoms are consistent with intracranial hypertension, rational treatment choices may be more feasible through the use of ICP monitoring.

There are two drugs available for the treatment of herpes simplex encephalitis. The first is vidarabine (adenine arabinoside), and the second is acyclovir (acycloguanosine). Vidarabine has been released for general application and until recently was the therapy of choice for the disease. However, acyclovir is a superior agent, both more potent and less toxic, and has supplanted vidarabine as the agent of choice.

Vidarabine is a nucleoside derivative that blocks deoxyribonucleic acid (DNA) synthesis, exerting a preferential effect on viral DNA synthesis. The drug is metabolized into arabinosyl hypoxanthine, which is also active against the virus, and both compounds are phosphorylated in the cell to active compounds that selectively and competitively inhibit herpes virus DNA polymerase. Vidarabine also causes premature termination of herpes DNA strands.

The plasma half-life of vidarabine is 4 hours in adults, and nearly two-thirds of an administered dose is recovered in the urine. It penetrates the CNS but only achieves levels of about 50% of serum levels. The drug is concentrated in the kidney, liver, and spleen. It is recommended that the drug be used, if at all, with caution in patients with renal failure.

One drawback of this drug is its limited solubility, which requires dilution to <0.7 mg/ml. The dosage required to treat herpes simplex encephalitis is 15 mg/kg/day over 12 hours, and in an adult, this requires nearly 2 liters of solution. Cerebral edema is a concern in herpes encephalitis, and intracranial hypertension is not uncommon. Hence, the requirement to administer large amounts of fluid is a significant problem. Side effects of the drug include nausea and vomiting, and with higher doses, tremors, weight loss, and bone marrow suppression may be seen.

The recommended dose is 15 mg/kg/day for 10 days, administered intravenously over 12 hours. Higher doses have been used in neonates without improving the outcome; toxic reactions are few at this relatively low dose. Occasional relapses occur, and therapy must be reinstituted in such instances.

Acyclovir is a nucleoside analog derivative and is active against herpes virus infections in tissue culture and laboratory animals. It is phosphorylated into active compounds much more rapidly by cells that have been infected with herpes virus than by those that have not. The herpes virus-synthesized thymidine kinase converts the drug into acycloguanosine triphosphate, which inhibits herpes virus-specific DNA polymerase and also causes premature DNA chain termination. The predilection for viral synthetic processes is extreme, and a 3000 times greater concentration of acyclovir is required to inhibit native cellular growth than is required to inhibit viral replication.

Acyclovir is partly excreted by the renal system, but its precise distribution and half-life in humans is not known. Its toxicity is minimal, leading to the current disagreement between American and British investigators concerning the requirement for brain biopsy prior to therapy. The recommended dose is 30mg/kg/day in neonates; 750 mg/M^2/day in children; and 15 mg/kg/day in adults. In all cases the drug is administered over 1 hour, and is given three times a day.

OUTCOME

The outcome from herpes simplex encephalitis has changed with the advent of therapy. Untreated disease, as already pointed out, carries a mortality of nearly 70%, with severe neurologic sequelae in the vast majority of survivors. Vidarabine therapy lowers the mortality to about 30% in non-neonatal disease and drastically lowers the mortality in neonatal herpes.

Several aspects of outcome in relation to therapy need to be pointed out. First, therapy with ara-A is effective in achieving a significant reduction in mortality only when instituted prior to advent of the comatose state, and extremes of age adversely affect outcome.

Documentation that higher doses of vidarabine do not improve the outcome of neonatal disease is consistent with the notion that infected cells are not salvaged by therapy. Instead, drug therapy prevents further viral replication and spread to other neurons. Although therapy with acyclovir may offer promise of better outcome, it is likely that the main avenue to improvement of the outcome from herpes simplex encephalitis is earlier diagnosis and earlier institution of effective therapy.

CHAPTER 18

Bacterial Meningitis

Of all cases of bacterial meningitis, it has been estimated that at least 75% occur in children under 15 years of age. Meningitis is the most common form of bacterial infection of the nervous system in children. It frequently causes life-threatening situations for pediatricians, general practitioners, and emergency room providers engaged in the care of infants and children.

BACTERIOLOGY

The microorganisms responsible for acute bacterial meningitis in children have varied greatly over the past century. Virtually any bacterium is capable of producing infection in the spinal fluid, given the "right" situation, but the single most important variable determining bacterial etiology is patient age. Table 18.1 outlines the etiologic agents responsible for purulent meningitis as related to age. The most frequently implicated organ-

TABLE 18.1.
Etiologic Sources of Bacterial Meningitis as Related to Age[a]

Birth to 2 Months

Main causes	Rare causes
Escherichia coli	*Streptococcus* sp. (non-
Streptococcus agalactiae	type B)
(group B)	*Citrobacter freundii*, *Ci-*
Less frequent causes	*trobacter diversus*
Streptococcus pneumoniae	*Flavobacterium menin-*
Staphylococcus sp.	*gosepticum*
Proteus mirabilis, *Proteus mor-*	*Pasteurella* sp.
ganii	*Neisseria meningitidis*,
Pseudomonas aeruginosa	*Neisseria gonorrhoeae*
Haemophilus influenzae type B	*Campylobacter (Vibrio)*
Listeria monocytogenes	*fetus*
Klebsiella sp.	*Serratia marcescens*
Aerobacter sp.	*Bacteroides fragilis*
Salmonella sp.	*Aeromonas shigelloides*
	Edwardsiella tarda

241

TABLE 18.1.—continued

2 Months to 4 Years

Main causes
  H. influenzae type B
  S. pneumoniae
  N. meningitidis
Less frequent causes
  Mycobacterium tuberculosis
  Staphylococcus sp.
  P. mirabilis, P. morganii
  P. aeruginosa
  E. coli
  L. monocytogenes
  Klebsiella sp.

Rare causes
  Streptococcus sp.
  Haemophilus parainflu-
    enzae
  B. fragilis
  S. marcescens
  Neisseria catarrhalis,
    Neisseria subflava,
    Neisseria sicca
  Pasteurella sp.
  Acinetobacter calcoaceti-
    cus var. lwoffi
  H. influenzae non-type B

4 Years and Older

Mai. causes
  S. pneumoniae
  N. meningitidis
Less frequent causes
  M. tuberculosis
  H. influenzae type B
  Streptococcus sp.
  Staphylococcus sp.
  E. coli
  L. monocytogenes
  Klebsiella sp.
  P. aeruginosa
  P. mirabilis, P. morganii

Rare causes
  N. gonorrhoeae
  Fusobacterium sp.
  N. catarrhalis, N.
    subflava, N. sicca
  Bacillus anthracis (an-
    thrax)
  Pasteurella sp.
  Priopionibacterium (Co-
    rynebacterium) acnes
  E. tarda
  Eikenella (Bacteroides)
    corrodens
  A. calcoaceticus var. an-
    itratus
  A. calcoaceticus var.
    lwoffi
  B. fragilis
  H. influenzae non-type B

[a]Adapted with permission from Bell WE, McCormick WF (eds): Neurologic Infection in Children. Philadelphia, WB Saunders, 1981.

isms in each age group are encapsulated bacteria, a fact that may have some relation to the pathogenesis of the ailment.

Multiple organisms may be involved in meningitis in a single patient, but this is more true for the neonate or for the older child with a foreign body, such as a ventriculoperitoneal shunt. Such children, as well as those with congenital dermal sinuses, are a risk for recurrent episodes of purulent meningitis. Staphylococcus species are the most frequent offenders in children with shunts, whereas in those with dermal sinuses, Gram-negative forms such as *Proteus, Pseudomonas,* and *Escherichia coli,* as well as *Staphylococcus* and *Streptococcus* species, provide the most risk.

PATHOGENESIS AND PATHOPHYSIOLOGY

There are three potential routes by which organisms can gain entry to the central nervous system (CNS) (Table 18.2). In children outside the neonatal period, otitis media is one of the most common abnormalities associated with *Haemophilus influenzae* meningitis and is often seen with meningitis of other etiologies. Cribriform plate entry is seen in children following trauma leading to fractures, but it may also be seen in other patients, such as those who have been in ponds infested wth *Neigleria,* an amebic species. Brain abscesses are relatively rare, and their rupture, leading to ventriculitis and meningitis, is more uncommon.

In general, the most common sequence of events resulting in bacterial entry into the subarachnoid space is colonization of the mucosa of the upper respiratory system, followed by entry of the bacteria into the bloodstream and subsequent seeding of the leptomeninges. Transmission of organisms from the bloodstream to the ventricular system is more common in neonates and may lead to frank pyoventriculitis with dense pus that

TABLE 18.2. ───────────────────────────────
Portals of Bacterial Entry into the CNS[a]

I. Blood Stream
   Most likely pathogens: Pneumococci, *Haemophilus,* meningococci, *E. coli* (infants)
   A. Choroid plexus: May be most common site in invasion
   B. Meningeal blood vessels: Located throughout the subarachnoid space
   C. Arachnoid villi: Located between sagittal sinus and subarachnoid space

II. Transdural
   Most likely pathogens: Pneumococci, Gram-negative enteric bacilli, staphylococci *(Staphylococcus epidermidis), Haemophilus*
   A. Surgery including that for ventriculoperitoneal shunts
   B. Trauma, especially with cribriform plate or petrous bone fractures
   C. Perimeningeal infective focus, such as sinusitis, otitis, osteomyelitis; emissary veins may serve as conduit for spread
   D. Congenital defects including myelomeningocele, spinal dermal sinus

III. Transparenchymal
   Most likely pathogens: Anaerobic bacteria occurs with rupture of brain abscess onto ventricles or subarachnoid space

───
[a]From Kaiser AB, McGee ZA: Central nervous system infections. In Shoemaker W, Thompson L, Holbrook P (eds): *Textbook of Critical Care.* Philadelphia, WB Saunders, 1984.

impairs flow of ventricular contents and is associated with an extremely poor prognosis.

CLINICAL MANIFESTATIONS

In general, most patients present with fever, irritability, and mental status changes, usually associated with vomiting and loss of appetite. Headache is a common complaint in the older child, followed by development of neck rigidity approximately 12–24 hours into the illness.

Neonates and infants under 4 months of age may not reproducibly show signs of meningismus but generally present with nonspecific signs of systemic illness, which may include apnea and convulsions, as well as other signs of sepsis.

Convulsions occur in at least 30% of patients with meningitis at some point in their illness and may be focal or generalized. Focal seizures are more likely in the face of a localized hemorrhagic infarction or in the presence of a subdural effusion, while generalized seizures may be the result of diffuse irritation from inflammation, diffuse ischemia, or hyponatremia that accompanies the development of the syndrome of inappropriate secretion of antidiuretic hormone (SIADH).

Abnormalities clearly present on the physical examination usually include meningismus, or pain associated with neck flexion, and limitation of movement of the neck, as evidenced by eliciting the Kernig and Brudzinski signs. Pathophysiologic correlation of the presence of these signs is presumed to be meningeal irritation due to inflammation, but they have been observed in the absence of striking pleocytosis. In addition, these signs may sometimes disappear with progression of illness and development of deep coma.

Examination of the pupils and retinae are important. As mentioned previously, abnormalities in the pupillary response to light or extraocular movements may occur because of direct irritation of the third and/or sixth nerves. Fourth-nerve involvement is less common but does occur. It is important to determine the cause of such findings, as the subsequent course will be much different if the signs are actually caused by elevated intracranial pressure (ICP) rather than by localized inflammation. Papilledema is not a reliable sign in determining the persence or absence of elevated ICP, but if it is observed, chances are greater that intracranial hypertension exists. It may also be a helpful sign in the differential diagnosis, since papilledema that develops within the first day or two of illness is more likely due to a ruptured brain absess, subarachnoid extension of an intracranial extradural abscess, or other mass-type lesion. Tuberculous and cryptococcal meningitis are more likely to present with focal signs and papilledema than when the disease is caused by the usual bacteria.

Retinal hemorrhages should be sought out, as their presence may be helpful in the diagnosis of cortical vein and sagittal sinus thrombosis, abnormalities of blood clotting mechanisms, and certain types of trauma and child abuse leading to coma or seizure activity.

INDICATIONS FOR ADMISSION TO THE PEDIATRIC INTENSIVE CARE UNIT

The majority of patients with suspected bacterial meningitis are evaluated in the emergency department where the diagnosis is considered and initial therapy instituted. These children are usually sleepy, lethargic, or irritable, but they are rousable and are generally admitted to an isolation room on the general pediatric ward or whatever area is most well suited to care of the individual with a significant infection. As noted, however, the clinical presentation may vary significantly, and some individuals will require intensive care. This is the case for the infant or child who arrives comatose, with abnormal motor response to stimulation, abnormalities of the pupillary response to light, obvious cranial nerve involvement, or other signs potentially indicative of elevated ICP, such as bradycardia and hypertension. Likewise, the youngster who manifests signs of poor perfusion, obvious shock, cutaneous manifestations of disseminated intravascular coagulation (DIC) (petechiae, purpura), or irregularities of respiratory pattern should be admitted to an area where he or she can have constant vigilant nursing care with close monitoring of vital signs. Laboratory data including significant metabolic acidosis, hypoxemia, hypercapnia, neutropenia, significant hyponatremia, anemia, or evidence of renal or liver dysfunction indicate that the particular patient has a more serious illness than most and requires observation in an intensive care unit (ICU). The indications for pediatric ICU admission are listed in Table 18.3.

Even if the individual does not appear critically ill, a relative or absolute nursing shortage in another part of the hospital, which would potentially limit the level of observation provided to the child, should be grounds to bring the youngster to the ICU, even if only for an "overnight" admission. The child whose course has been particularly rapid prior to presentation also deserves special observation and monitoring, as he or she is more likely to develop signs of septic shock or intracranial hypertension and require higher levels of support than are generally available on the usual pediatric floor.

We therefore strongly recommend that in any case in which the clinical or laboratory evaluation (Table 18.4) is complicated (whether from a systemic or a neurologic aspect), the child be admitted to the ICU at least until the course can be determined, the first several doses of antibiotics can be administered, and a tentative bacteriologic diagnosis can be made. It is only through early recognition of complications such as shock or elevated ICP that effective therapy can be initiated in a timely fashion and potentially alter the outcome of fulminant meningitis.

LABORATORY DIAGNOSIS

The definitive diagnosis of meningitis is made by recovery of organisms from culture of the cerebrospinal fluid (CSF). As this may take 24–48 hours for routine bacteria and longer for some of the less common organisms,

TABLE 18.3.
Indications for Admission to the Pediatric ICU[a]

Clinical	Laboratory
Rapid course	Acidosis
Comatose (GCS[b] score, <7)	Metabolic
Abnormal motor response to	Respiratory
stimulation	Hypoxemia
Posturing	Anemia
No response	Thrombocytopenia
Impaired pupillary response	Altered clotting profile
to light	Significant elevation of
Abnormal extraocular move-	Creatinine
ments	Urea nitrogen
Other cranial nerve abnor-	Liver enzymes
malities	Ammonia
Status epilepticus	Lactic acid
Signs suggestive of raised	Hyponatremia
incranial pressure	Neutropenia
Hypertension	Chest radiograph evidence
Bradycardia	of pulmonary edema
Respiratory pattern	
Signs of shock	
Poor perfusion	
Hypotension	
Petechiae and purpura	

[a]Although the presence of any single factor listed in this table may not always be grounds for admission to the ICU, children who present with meningitis and any of the above signs are at risk for disease that is more severe or rapidly progressive than that of the average patient with purulent meningitis.
[b]GCS, Glasgow coma scale.

the culture is of no help in the early stages of disease. Other information can be derived from examination of the spinal fluid obtained by lumbar puncture (LP), which may be of help in making a presumptive diagnosis in the first few hours after presentation. Although the spinal fluid can provide much useful information, it must be remembered that performance of the procedure is not without risks.

The child with fever, headache, and a bit of lethargy who is evaluated in the emergency department for possible meningitis is not in the same category as the patient in the pediatric ICU who is densely comatose, may be seizing, is potentially hemodynamically unstable, and is, therefore, at risk for significant cardiorespiratory compromise when being positioned for the spinal tap. In such a situation the clinician must weigh the relative risks involved and decide whether to initiate therapy before or after the LP has been performed. In the setting of unstable vital signs, it is always better to postpone the tap. Additionally, it must be remembered that the majority of

TABLE 18.4.
Appropriate Laboratory Tests in Suspected Acute Bacterial Meningitis[a]

Potentially Diagnostic	Nonspecific
Lumbar puncture	Complete blood count
Opening pressure	Differential
Appearance	Platelet count
Cell count	Serum electrolytes Na, K,
Glucose, protein	Cl, bicarbonate
Gram stain and culture	Serum/urine osmolality
bacterial, viral (fungal,	Blood glucose
acid-fast)	Blood urea nitrogen/creati-
Rapid diagnostic tests	nine
CIE, LA	Chest X-ray
(Lactic acid)	Electrocardiogram
(Enzymes—CPK, LDH,	(PTT, PT, FDP, fibrinogen)
GOT)	(Sinus, mastoid, skull films)
Blood culture	(Transillumination of skull)
Blood/urine CIE, LA	(Electroencephalogram)
(Tuberculin skin test)	(CAT scan, nuclear medi-
	cine scan)

[a]Parentheses indicate examinations not always indicated in every case of suspected bacterial meningitis. See text for expected results of various tests in bacterial meningitis and indications for performance of bracketed studies. CIE, counterimmunoelectrophoresis; LA, latex agglutination; CPK, creatine phosphokinase; LDH, lactic dehydrogenase; GOT, glutamic oxaloacetic transaminase; PTT, partial thromboplastin time; PT, prothrombin time; and FDP, fibrin degradation products.

patients with meningitis are also bacteremic, thus making possible determination of the etiologic agent by performance of blood cultures alone.

Another situation in which LP is potentially hazardous is in the patient with severely elevated ICP in whom sudden release of fluid from the lumbar space may result in herniation of a portion of the brain, most often the uncal portion of the temporal lobe. Spinal tap should also be avoided in the child with active DIC who may develop a spinal epidural hematoma, which is a catastrophic complication. If the suspicion of intracranial hypertension exists and performance of the procedure is considered absolutely essential, appropriate drugs and methods of resuscitation must be at the bedside. In such a situation, however, the spinal fluid sample may more safely be obtained via ventricular puncture, during placement of a ventricular catheter to measure ICP, and should follow performance of a computerized axial tomography scan and administration of antibiotics. It must be emphasized that intracranial hypertension is exceedingly rare, especially in the first few hours, and those cases in which a tap must be deferred because of potential herniation will not be many. Indeed, the presence of elevated ICP early in the course should encourage the physician to search for another cause of intracranial pathology. For the patient who manifests abnormal clotting parameters, fresh frozen plasma and/or platelets can be administered immediately prior to performance of the procedure.

The critical care physician is often faced with accepting, in transfer, a child with suspected meningitis and mental status abnormalities from another institution. The question of whether or not the tap must be performed prior to transfer is often raised. The same guidelines as discussed previously also apply with regard to patients in whom a tap is contraindicated. In addition, any procedure that delays the administration of antibiotics should never be postponed because of a proposed transfer from one institution to another, regardless of the ability of the referring physician or hospital to obtain appropriate cultures.

There are several aspects of the CSF that must be evaluated once it is obtained. An opening pressure (OP), measured by attaching a sterile manometer to the spinal needle and noting the height in millimeters to which the column of fluid rises immediately after entering the subarachnoid space, is often unfortunately omitted in pediatric procedures. The normal OP in the adult and older child is up to 180 mm H_2O. For the neonate the normal value is assumed to be between 90 and 110 mm H_2O, a value derived from noninvasive fontameter readings that have been correlated with direct intraventricular pressure measurements. The determination of OP must be made with the infant or child horizontal and with his or her back relatively straight. An OP > 200 mm H_2O is cause for concern and should lead the clinician to follow with another form of continuous ICP monitoring.

Appearance of the spinal fluid is the first readily appreciated characteristic, after measurement of the OP. If the fluid is grossly cloudy, evidence for meningitis is strong. In some cases of very advanced meningitis the purulent material may be so thick that it is unable to flow through the spinal needle, and this is sometimes referred to as a "dry tap." The fluid may be xanthochromic in a newborn who is suffering from or has been treated for hyperbilirubinemia, or the yellowish appearance may be subsequent to breakdown of red blood cells (RBCs) from a previous subarachnoid or intraventricular hemorrhage. It will be grossly bloody following an acute subarachnoid or intraventricular bleed or a "traumatic tap," when the needle hits the venous plexus on the posterior surface of the vertebral body. Other causes of hemorrhagic spinal fluid are cortical vein or sagittal sinus thrombosis, herpes encephalitis, anthrax meningitis, and rupture of mycotic aneurysms.

In meningitis the white cell count is generally elevated. Spinal fluid will continue to appear clear with up to 500 white blood cells/mm^3 and does not become grossly turbid until very large numbers of cells are present. In the early stages of meningeal infection or in patients with certain limitations of the immune system, leukocytosis in the CSF may not occur. Occasionally, when the LP is performed very early, the fluid may be clear with few cells, only to turn cloudy after a few hours of continued infection. In bacterial meningitis, granulocytes usually predominate, making up 80–90% of the total number of leukocytes.

In acute meningitis, the CSF glucose and protein are classically deranged. The glucose value is generally much lower than the accepted normal of 50–60% of the serum glucose (in newborns the norm is considered to be at least 75% of serum value), and in many instances the absolute value is as low as 0–20 mg/dl. Because most of the normal data regarding glucose concentration have been reported as percentages of serum values, a blood glucose determination must be obtained. The time of this test is crucial for valid results, yet the "best" interval between determination of blood and CSF glucose values has not been made clear. It is apparent that some period of equilibration is necessary for the CSF concentration to reflect serum values, which may be as long as 2 hours. It is therefore difficult to interpret glucose values in a patient who recently experienced an acute change in serum glucose, such as a seizure, or intravenous glucose administration for hypoglycemia. Under any circumstances, a CSF glucose of <40 mg/dl is considered definitive hypoglycorrhachia unless the preceding hypoglycemia was very severe.

CSF protein values also vary with age. In the adult and older child, values of spinal fluid protein up to 45 mg/100 ml are accepted as being within the normal range, whereas for full-term babies and prematures, levels of up to 150 mg/100 ml and 200 mg/100 ml, respectively, have been measured. The presence of RBCs may raise the protein concentration by 15 mg/100 ml for every 1000 RBCs/mm^3 spinal fluid. Spinal fluid protein concentration is elevated in the presence of bacterial infection, generally to over 100 mg/ml.

Another abnormality in meningitic spinal fluid is elevation of lactic acid level, above the normal of 14 mg/100 ml. Similar elevation is seen in cryptococcal and other fungal meningitides but not in patients with viral disease. Lactic acid levels also rise in ischemic neurologic insults and in patients with intracranial hypertension and brain tumors.

LABORATORY FINDINGS IN PARTIALLY TREATED MENINGITIS

Some interesting issues are raised when diagnosis in the child who receives antibiotics prior to the performance of a LP is considered. It has been estimated that as many as 50% of children with meningitis receive antibiotics in some form prior to diagnosis. Since the majority of patients who are given antibiotics prior to diagnostic LP receive them as outpatients, because of presumed respiratory infection or possible occult pneumococcal bacteremia, these children are generally given some form of penicillin, in a relatively low dose (compared with standard meningitis doses), administered by the oral route.

The major factors that are primarily affected by such treatment are the length of illness prior to hospital admission or spinal tap and the number of bacteria present in the CSF. Because ability to document CSF infection by Gram strain varies with the number of bacteria present, rapid diagnosis by microscopy of CSF is also affected by pretreatment. Although some authors have found the CSF white blood cell count to be altered by oral antibiotics, such that it may more resemble the aseptic meningitis picture, others have not found this to be the case. The majority of evidence indicates that most patients with purulent meningitis will still have a predominance of neutrophils, a low glucose level, and elevated protein. The only bacterium whose growth in culture appears to be significantly altered by prior administration of antibiotics in the meningococcus, with the postulated reason being the exquisite sensitivity of this bacterium to penicillin. Bacteriologic diagnosis of pneumococcal or *H. influenzae* meningitis does not appear to be adversely affected, at least by oral administration of penicillin or ampicillin.

To ensure better diagnostic capabilities in this situation as well as to aid in making a more rapid etiologic diagnosis under any circumstance, counterimmunoelectrophoresis and latex agglutination tests may be performed on CSF, blood, and especially urine to detect antigen from the bacterial capsule. Antigen does not disappear rapidly, even with killing of the bacteria, and may persist for days in the presence of adequate therapy.

Other laboratory abnormalities depend upon the severity of the disease and reflect the body's ability to keep up with the metabolic demands of acute infection nd bacterial dissemination, as evidenced by bacteremia, septic shock, elevated ICP, seizures, coma, and respiratory compromise. Findings to be expected in such a situation are not different from those encountered in sepsis and include metabolic acidosis, increased lactic acid level, hypocapnia or hypercapnia, hypoxemia, alteration of liver and cardiac enzymes, abnormalities of blood urea nitrogen and creatinine, and changes in electrolyte concentrations reflecting the presence of dehydration, SIADH, or diabetes insipidus (DI). Hyperglycemia may reflect response to acute stress, whereas hypoglycemia may represent inadequate stores of glycogen or inability to mobilize such stores, especially likely in a sick neonate.

Patients with concomitant meningitis and bacteremia may exhibit evidence of pneumonia, sinusitis, or involvement of other areas with the offending microorganism that is demonstrable with the use of various radiologic and other laboratory examinations.

COMPLICATIONS

Complications of meningitis are diverse and vary according to a number of factors including age of the patient, infecting organism, rapidity and adequacy of antibiotic therapy, and other parameters not as yet defined. Adverse effects of disease may be acute and temporary or may result in permanent residua of the infection. Children may be left with profound or mild mental impairments, visual and auditory defects, persistent convulsions, communicating hydrocephalus, behavioral abnormalities and impairment of hypothalamic function, or long tract signs such as hemiparesis or quadriparesis.

Temporary problems include development of SIADH, DIC, septic shock, acutely elevated ICP, cerebral vasculitis, and recurrent fevers. Of course, there is some overlap in the two groups of complications, with some problems, such as seizures, hypothalamic injuries, and raised ICP, causing acute management problems and long-lasting sequelae.

SIADH in meningitis has received much publicity, and it is because of the presumed frequent occurrence of this problem that the standard recommendation for fluid therapy in young children and infants with meningitis is to provide approximately two-thirds of calculated maintenance water requirements while providing a normal sodium intake.

In light of the potential significant adverse effects of SIADH, the rationale for treating all children with meningitis with a mild fluid restriction seems reasonable. It must be remembered, however, that fluid restriction of the hypovolemic patient, especialy one with severe infection and sepsis, may lead to serious hemodynamic compromise. Many infants with meningitis have been vomiting for several days, have had elevated body temperature and diminished intake of fluids, and may be significantly dehydrated on admission.

Other forms of dysfunction of the hypothalamic-pituitary axis occur but with much lower frequency than does SIADH. Such abnormalities include DI, loss of temperature control, hyperphagia, and precocious puberty. Of these, the only entity of major concern during the acute stages of meningitis is DI. The excretion of large amounts of very dilute urine creates problems to the opposite extreme than those of SIADH. The patient with DI may rapidly become hypovolemic, with marked hypernatremia and seizures on that basis. Therapy for DI consists of replacement of urine water losses when the disorder is mild, proceeding to supplementation of antidiuretic hormone as a continuous infusion, titrated to control urine output and serum sodium and osmolality values.

DIC and septic shock may occur in meningitis, depending upon the bacterial etiology. Both generally develop only in patients who are bacteremic. This happens most commonly in patients with meningococcemia and, to a lesser extent, in patients with *H. influenzae* meningitis. Neonates with any form of bacterial meningitis are likely to develop DIC and septic shock.

Subdural effusions are more likely to occur beyond the first week of illness but may be noted at any time, including upon admission to the emergency room, hospital, or pediatric ICU. They usually resolve spontaneously, without specific interventions. If they are large or occur in the presence of significant and persistent neurologic symptoms such as seizures, paresis, or evidence of elevated ICP, or if they are suspected of being infected, a burr hole should be made or a needle should be put through an open fontanel, and fluid should be withdrawn by a neurosurgeon.

Subdural effusions are more common in *H. influenzae* type B meningitis than in infection due to other bacteria, but they do occur regardless of the specific bacteriologic etiology. In some series, up to 30–50% of infants and children have been noted to develop this complication.

THERAPY
Nonspecific Care

The usual approach to fluids in the meningitic was alluded to earlier; namely, in anticipation of possible SIADH, the well-hydrated child should be placed on a restricted water intake of two-thirds maintenance fluids made up in a solution containing approximately half-normal saline and dextrose as needed. As many young infants are hypoglycemic, and the majority suffer from hypoglycorrhachia, provision of a 10% dextrose solution may be warranted, with close attention paid to serum glucose values. In the presence of documented SIADH, a more severe fluid restriction may be required.

All of the principles of neurointensive care must be adhered to in these patients. These include: ensuring optimal oxygenation and ventilation, or hyperventilation when intracranial hypertension is documented or suspected; appropriate positioning of the patient to permit maximal drainage of venous outflow; and sedation to an extent that is appropriate for the level of the child's sensorium and perceived degree of pain, discomfort, or agitation. Systematic administration of steroids appears to reduce the incidence of hearing loss in patients with *H. influenzae* meningitis, but steroids have not been shown to affect the course of elevated ICP in the meningitic patient.

The child who has sustained at least one seizure during the course of early therapy, although potentially at low risk for ongoing seizures, is best treated with an anticonvulsant drug such as phenobarbital while in the ICU. The child whose neurologic or cardiorespiratory status is tenuous should be spared the additional metabolic demands and ischemic insults that may accompany an epileptic discharge.

Intracranial Pressure Management and Therapy

It is increasingly common for comatose patients (coma scale score, <7) or for patients who are deteriorating on antimicrobial therapy to have ICP monitors. There is a significant incidence of intracranial hypertension documented in these patients, and more rapid placement of ICP bolts and aggressive therapy of increased ICP clearly have a role in the management of the patients.

Specific Antimicrobial Therapy

For the child admitted to the pediatric ICU, unfortunately, the degree of illness is such that the choice of therapeutic agents must be made on the basis of age alone and before the results of laboratory tests have been reported.

As a result, the reader is again referred to Table 18.1 for a listing of the most common microbiologic etiologies in the various age groups. In the neonate, from birth to 2 months of age, in whom the predominant organisms of Gram-negative bacteria and group B streptococci, provision of an sides penetrate the blood-brain barrier poorly and in light of the sometimes significant incidence of *Listeria monocytogenes*, ampicillin is the penicillin of choice, given in a dose of 150–200 mg/kg/day. Selection of a particular aminoglycoside must be made on the basis of known sensitivity information from the specific community or neonatal nursery. Dosages of the various aminoglycosides vary by age in weeks and are listed in Table 18.5. Because a large number of isolates of *E. coli* demonstrate resistance against kanamycin, starting therapy with gentamicin, until the sensitivities of the offending organism are known, is common.

The major organisms encountered in older infants and children are sensitive to a combination of ampicillin and chloramphenicol. It is essential that the child at risk for *H. influenzae* type B disease *not* receive ampicillin alone, since 20–25% of isolates in many parts of the country have become resistant to the drug by producing an enzyme called β-lactamase. The dose of ampicillin for meningitis is 300–400 mg/kg/day.

Chloramphenicol is usually effective at 75–100 mg/kg/day, and the lower dose may be preferable because of significant toxicity when serum levels are high. Younger children (infants under 2 months of age) should not receive more than 50 mg/kg/day.

In children over 5 years of age, *H. influenzae* is much less common, and

TABLE 18.5.
Aminoglycoside Dose Schedules for Various Age Groups

Drug	Age/Weight (kg)	Dose (mg/kg/day)	Interval (hr)
Amikacin	Under 30 days	15	q. 12
	Over 30 days	15	q. 8
	To adult	Maximum, 1.5 g/day	
Gentamicin	Under 7 days	5	q. 12
	7 days to 1 year	7.5	q. 8
	Children	5–7.5	q. 8
	Adults	3–5	q. 8
Kanamycin	Under 7 days		
	(<2000 g)	15	q. 12
	(>2000 g)	20	q. 12
	Over 7 days		
	(<2000 g)	20	q. 12
	(>2000 g)	30	q. 8
	Over 1 month	30	q. 8
		Maximum, 1.5 g/day	
Tobramycin	Under 7 days	4–5	q. 12
	7 days to 1 year	4–7.5	q. 8
	Children	7.5	q. 8
	Adults	3–5	q. 8

both meningococcal and pneumococcal strains are generally sensitive to penicillin G (dose range, 250,000–400,000 units/kg/day. Because of the small but demonstrable incidence of H. influenzae type B in older children and adults, however, it is preferable also to include chloramphenicol or another drug active against H. influenzae type B in the initial therapy of older children and adolescents. It must be remembered that chloramphenicol use in meningococcal disease interferes with the action of penicillin, resulting in a higher mortality, and is therefore contraindicated. The use of parenteral preparations of trimethoprim-sulfamethoxazole (TMP-SMX) has not been clinically evaluated in this disease, but the TMP-SMX combination has very good in vitro activity against H. influenzae, exhibits excellent penetration into the spinal fluid, and when greater experience in its use is gained, may become useful in therapy for meningitis in the older child and adult at a dose of 10 mg/kg/day for TMP and at a dose of 50 mg/kg/day for SMX, and administered twice daily.

OUTCOME

The clinical course, rapidity of diagnosis, adequacy of therapy, and individual characteristics of host and disease determine the outcome and long-term sequelae for any given patient with purulent meningitis. Untreated cases are almost universally fatal, whereas with current methods of diagnosis and therapy, the mortality rate ranges from 5 to 10% for H. influenzae and meningococcal meningitis, to 20% for pneumococcal and tuberculous meningitis, to nearly 60% in some forms of neonatal disease. Long-term sequelae including hydrocephalus, deafness, cortical or optic nerve blindness, hemiparesis or quadriparesis, or intellectual impairment occur in 30–50% of survivors.

CHAPTER 19

Gastrointestinal and Hepatic Failure

The gastrointestinal tract may complicate care of any child in the intensive care unit (ICU). Some gastrointestinal complications are avoidable, most are treatable if recognized early, and all are potentially lethal. Complications that need to be watched for in all children admitted to ICUs, almost regardless of their primary illness, include bleeding, ileus, diarrhea, pancreatitis, and malnutrition. Survival in all of these cases depends on careful, repeated observations, attention to detail, and rapid intervention.

STRESS BLEEDING

Bleeding from diffuse, erosive stress gastritis can occur in any child admitted to the ICU. The potential becomes even greater if the reason for admission is head trauma, surgery, burns, cancer chemotherapy, renal failure, connective tissue disorders, Reye syndrome, or liver disease (Table 19.1). Stress bleeding may occur in up to 80% of children with these problems and is usually from multiple locations.

Pathophysiology

Stress gastritis occurs when the normal mucosal defense mechanisms of the gastic mucosa become overwhelmed. The integrity of the mucosal cell membrane itself and the adjacent tight junctions are of prime importance in preventing stress gastritis. Decreased cell turnover, hypoxia, and decreased mucosal blood flow impair that integrity.

Ischemia of the mucosa makes it more susceptible to damage by acid. Acid pH also markedly augments the damaging effects of bile salts on mu-

TABLE 19.1.
Factors Predisposing to Stress Gastritis

Ischemia	Bile reflux
Hypotension	Ethanol
Major organ failure	Anti-inflammatory agents
Head trauma	

cosal integrity. Fasting and high concentrations of salt, alcohol, aspirin, and anti-inflammatories such as indomethacin, phenylbutazone, and naproxen also locally decrease the integrity of the cell wall. This results in seepage of hydrogen ion from the lumen through or between mucosal lining cells to the submucosa. Measurement of intramural pH confirms that stress ulceration occurs in those patients whose intramural pH has fallen below the lower limit of normal. Here hydrogen ions cause the release of histamine from mast cells, followed by inflammation and edema. If the process is allowed to continue, local mucosal damage progresses to deeper ulceration into the mucosa and submucosa.

Presentation

The natural history of stress gastritis after thermal burns has been prospectively studied, and lesions developed with 72 hours in three-fourths of patients. Stress lesions can present as hematemesis, melena, hematochezia, or a slow decrease of the hematocrit. Abdominal pain or findings of tenderness on physical examination occur rarely. Nasogastric aspirate will reveal coffee-ground material or bright red blood. The rate of bleeding is variable but may be rapid enough to result in exsanguination.

Prevention

The gastric pH should be maintained at >4.5 to decrease morbidity and mortality. The H_2 receptor antagonists are more effective than placebos in preventing bleeding, but safety and dosage requirements have not been clearly established in the pediatric population. Hourly antacids tend to be more effective than H_2 receptor antagonists alone in preventing bleeding, as intraluminal pH can be more carefully titrated. Early attention to nutrition may also play a role in preventing stress bleeding. Enteral feeding of an elemental diet decreases the incidence of bleeding in patients suffering from severe burns.

Therapy

Once stress bleeding has begun, hemodynamic stabilization is the basic therapeutic modality. Intravenous fluids, colloid, packed red blood cells, and fresh frozen plasma, if needed, should be given until tachycardia and orthostasis are abolished. A nasogastric tube is useful both to monitor the severity of the bleeding and to apply iced lavage.

A team approach is necessary for best treatment of a child with stress bleeding. At a minimum, this team should consist of the physician primarily responsible for the child, a gastroenterologist, a surgeon, and (frequently) a radiologist. Endoscopy should quickly be performed to identify the site of the bleeding. If a discrete ulcer or bleeding site is found, endoscopic therapy is possible, especially in older children, with electrical cautery, laser cautery, or application of topical coagulants.

When endoscopy is unsuccessful in locating the site of the upper intestinal bleeding, arteriography should be undertaken. Upper gastrointestinal series are not indicated in this condition because the yield is low and the presence of barium in the gastrointestinal tract will prevent arteriography from being performed later.

Intravenous cimetidine is frequently administered to help the process from being perpetuated, but there are no data that indicate that intravenous cimetidine or enteral antacids stop bleeding faster than does lavage alone.

Usually, patients with stress gastritis will respond to lavage and correction of underlying hemodynamic problems. Sometimes, bleeding is brisk and persists despite lavage. These patients should undergo arteriography. The ability to suppress bleeding with intra-arterial vasopressors or thromboembolic agents is especially useful in patients with acute processes. Rarely, patients with stress gastritis will bleed so quickly and continuously that hemodynamic stability cannot be maintained and blood transfusions become overwhelming. At this time, surgical intervention with vagotomy (not always permanently successful) or total gastrectomy (successful but with a high mortality and morbidity rate) should be considered.

PARALYTIC ILEUS AND PSEUDO-OBSTRUCTION

Postoperative ileus after abdominal laparotomy is common, with severity inversely worse in younger children. Postoperative ileus is attributed to altered motility within portions of the gut handled during surgery. Alteration of sympathetic neuronal hyperactivity in patients who have undergone surgical procedures even distant from the intestines results in decreased motility due to suppression of the migrating bursts of action potential from the stomach through the small intestine and the colon. In these cases, postoperative inhibition of intestinal activity is more profound and more persistent in the colon, less so in the small intestine, and least in the stomach.

Hypokalemia, hyponatremia, hypomagnesemia, and decreased osmolarity may contribute to the perpetuation of ileus. Other important factors include infections, heart failure, and other metabolic abnormalities. However, anoxic damage should always be considered.

Anoxic damage affects the especially sensitive intramural intestinal ganglia. Regional hypoxia can cause regional paralysis. In shock, disproportionate shunting of blood away from gastrointestinal tract to the brain, heart, and kidneys occurs. Localized area of hypoxia in the small bowel can develop, associated with dilation of the bowel, loss of peristalsis, and functional obstruction. If the anoxic event persists for a prolonged time, permanent destruction of the mesenteric ganglia can be seen.

Localized ileus or pseudo-obstruction can be seen with intraperitoneal inflammation such as cholecystitis or pancreatitis, localized infections and abscesses, and lower lobe pneumonias. It is thought that infection leads to inflammation of afferent nerves, which, in turn, evokes reflex inhibition of peristalsis. Additionally, conditions that alter the parasympathetic (excitatory) to sympathetic (inhibitory) ratio of gut stimulation may lead to ileus.

Anticholinergic drugs can be responsible for the constipation and ileus seen with the phenothiazine-like antidepressants such as chlorpromazine and amitriptyline. Ganglionic blockers, Cogentin, Pro-Banthine, morphine, meperidine, methadone, and other opioids are also frequently found to be the cause of functional obstruction. A good drug history, therefore, is mandatory for patients without obvious reason for the ileus.

Recognition

Most patients with panabdominal ileus will have abdominal distention and decreased bowel sounds. Patients with localized functional obstruction, however, may have abdominal pain, nausea, and vomiting with normal, decreased, or hyperactive bowel sounds. One-third of patients continue to pass flatus.

A plain film of the abdomen can be very useful in demonstrating diffuse ileus. A dilated cecum and transverse colon with no air in the descending colon or rectum is classic for mechanical obstruction but is also seen in functional obstruction. This picture can be differentiated from mechanical obstruction by barium enema or colonoscopy. In general, radiographic evaluation of the colon can be done by using barium, Gastrografin, or metrizamide. Metrizamide is used to image the bowel of neonates and young children when barium is contraindicated because of suspected perforation and when Gastrografin is of concern because of its hypertonicity.

It must be remembered that not all postoperative ileus is functional. Prolonged ileus or ileus that recurs 1–3 weeks postoperatively may, in fact, be mechanical obstruction secondary to intussusception or adhesions. Diagnosis of this problem is difficult because most of the classic symptoms of obstruction are missing or obscured by the nasogastric suction and by pain medicines given postoperatively. Postoperative intussusceptions are usually ileoileal, appear within 8 days of surgery, and require surgical correction. Intestinal adhesions as a cause of postoperative obstruction, on the other hand, tend to occur more than 2 weeks after surgery.

Therapy

Ileus usually resolves with nasogastric decompression, correction of the underlying metabolic, infectious, or inflammatory processes, and intravenous nutritional support. Partial small bowel mechanical obstruction can also be helped in some cases by nasogastric suction, without increasing the risk of surgery should a definitive operation become necessary.

If the cecum has dilated to >12 cm in diameter, a definite danger of perforation exists, even though there is no mechanical reason for the obstruction. If the cecal dilation cannot be reduced by nasogastric decompression, decompression by a long double-lumen colonoscope has been successfully performed. If the cecal dilation cannot be quickly decreased, cecostomy is indicated because perforation carries with it a 35–75% mortality. When functional obstruction is suspected, narcotics, smooth muscle relaxants, and parasympathomimetic agents should be avoided because they can increase the chance of perforation.

Although phentolamine and propranolol prevent postoperative suppression of gastric contractions, they do not prevent small bowel ileus. Edrophonium has been tried and found to be more effective than neostigmine in restoring small bowel function in uncontrolled trials.

OTHER DISORDERS OF MOTILITY

Several other conditions affecting digestive tract motility may cause critical illness in the pediatric patient. These include chronic idiopathic intestinal pseudo-obstruction (CIIP), toxic megacolon associated with ulcerative colitis, and Hirschsprung's disease.

CIIP is a recurring condition characterized by bowel obstruction without organic mechanical occlusion of the lumen. There is no known underlying pathologic etiology. The clinical course in children is characterized by intermittent episodes of abdominal distention, vomiting, abdominal pain, diarrhea, constipation, and malnutrition. Radiographic studies are the mainstay of diagnosis. They demonstrate abnormal esophageal motility, delayed gastric emptying, dilated loops of small intestine, and disturbed colonic motility. Since many children with pseudo-obstruction have esophageal dysmotility, esophageal manometric studies are an aid to diagnosis. The patient with CIIP may require intensive care. Acute attacks may be life-threatening and require nasogastric suction, fluid and electrolyte support, and colonic lavage.

Toxic megacolon, a complication of chronic ulcerative colitis, may also be life-threatening. The features are superimposed on those of fulminant colitis. The condition is characterized by rapid deterioration with abdominal distention, disappearance of bowel sounds, and toxemia. Precipitating factors are thought to be potassium deficiency, opiate treatment, preparation for and performance of barium enema, and mechanical obstruction. Plain films of the abdomen show colonic distention. Since there is a high mortality, the condition demands intensive medical therapy, decompression of the small intestine by intubation, steroids, and consultation with surgery.

An additional disorder of motility which may be life-threatening is Hirschsprung's disease. In infancy, Hirschsprung's disease may be associated with an enterocolitis, either before or after colostomy, that is associated with sudden circulatory collapse and severe mucosal necrosis and ulceration. No specific therapy has been identified. The patient must be sustained with fluid and electrolyte support.

DIARRHEA

Diarrhea in the postoperative or critically ill child occurs principally because of the malabsorption of nutrients or secondary to infection, as is

TABLE 19.2. ⎯⎯⎯⎯⎯⎯⎯⎯⎯⎯⎯⎯⎯⎯⎯⎯⎯⎯⎯⎯⎯⎯⎯
Common Causes of Diarrhea

Malabsorption
Intraluminal problems
  Pancreatic insufficiency
  Severe liver failure—Biliary atresia
  Bacterial overgrowth secondary to dysmotility
Enterocyte damage or brush border enzyme depletion
  Postinfection
  Hypoxia
  Necrotizing enterocolitis
  Surgical resection
  Inflammatory bowel disease
  Lymphatic obstruction

Infection
Antibiotic-associated colitis—*Clostridium difficile*
Viral infections—Frequently nosocomial
Bacterial infections
  Nonbloody—*Salmonella* and *Escherichia coli*
  Bloody—*Shigella, Yersinia,* and *Campylobacter*

shown in Table 19.2. Although the mucosal phase of absorption is critical to all macronutrients, injury or dysfunction of the intestinal mucosa becomes clinically evident chiefly by the resulting effect on carbohydrate absorption. Malabsorption of carbohydrates, in turn, causes an osmotic diarrhea. In addition, bacterial fermentation of a portion of the carbohydrate reaching the colon results in the formation of short-chain fatty acids. This contributes to the osmostic load presented to the colon with decreased water reabsorption in the colon. Short-chain fatty acids also stimulate peristalsis. Abdominal distention ensues because of the large fluid loads in the lumen and the production of gaseous products of fermentation.

Complete digestion and absorption of sugars require the action of brush border carbohydrases including lactase, sucrose-α-dextrinase, and glucoamylase. Thus injury to the villus surface on which these enzymes reside will impair sugar absorption. Depletion of carbohydrases may occur as a result of a variety of viral, bacterial, or parasitic injuries. Enzyme depletion is also noted in the critically ill child who is significantly malnourished and in children with impaired blood flow to the gut or even following generalized hypoxia.

Necrotizing Enterocolitis

Necrotizing enterocolitis (NEC) is a frequent gastrointestinal emergency in the neonatal ICU. The disorder predominantly affects premature infants, and its etiology may be multifactorial. Mortality appears to be associated with low birth weight and perinatal complications. However, hypoxic injury to the intestinal mucosa is critical to most hypotheses. Under these conditions, sugar malabsorption occurs. Malabsorption of carbohydrates is so typical of NEC that it has become a screening test for the development of NEC in many nurseries.

Data from animal experiments indicate that hypoxia may affect transport of simple sugars. Weanling rats exposed to high nitrogen environments suffered a loss of intestinal transport capacity for carbohydrate by sodium-dependent mechanisms in the absence of changes in histology, ultrastructure of the small intestinal mucosa, or disaccharidase levels.

The mucosal phase of absorption is also compromised by intestinal resection. Diarrhea in the postoperative infant or child who has had major resection of the small intestine results principally from decreased surface absorptive area available to luminal contents. Diarrhea may be worsened in these patients by (a) gastric acid hypersecretion, (b) entry of bile salts into the colon, causing a cholorrheic enteropathy with contraction of the bile salt pool, and (c) abnormalities in gastrointestinal motor activity. Elevated levels of vasoactive intestinal polypeptide have been reported in patients with short bowel syndrome, but the significance of these observations is unclear.

Infectious Causes of Diarrhea

Infectious causes of diarrhea in the intensive care patient are common and may cause malabsorption of nutrients. Diarrhea occurring in patients on antibiotics may be caused by *Clostridium difficile* infection. Antibiotic-associated colitis is thought to be rare in children. The most common antibiotics causing pseudomembranous enterocolitis, the severest form of *C. difficile*-induced diarrhea, are penicillins and clindamycin. Bloody diarrhea associated with pseudomembranous colitis is rare, and abdominal tenderness may not be marked until the terminal events ensue.

Nosocomial infection is a likely cause of diarrhea in the ICU. Rotavirus and rotavirus-like infections are particularly incriminated. Viral infections result in diarrhea due to the impairment of absorption and the initiation of water and electrolyte secretion from the mucosa to the lumen. Bacterial infections include *Salmonella* and *Escherichia coli* may cause fever, crampy abdominal pain, watery diarrhea, and associated hypovolemia and electrolyte problems.

Diagnosis

Since diarrhea in critically ill children is generally attributable to malabsorption and/or infection, the diagnostic approach is focused on these possibilities. Stool examination can be performed by the unit personnel, or alternatively, the sample can be sent to the laboratory. The following examinations should be performed.

Screening Tests for Infection

Blood

Bright red blood in the stool is frequently indicative of colonic inflammation secondary to infectious causes. Thus the presence of visible blood in diarrheal stools should trigger further investigation for enteric pathogens such as *Shigella, Yersinia,* and *Campylobacter.* Alternatively, the presence of bright red blood in the stool may indicate idiopathic inflammatory bowel disease or allergic colitis. Allergic colitis may be induced by intolerance to dietary proteins, especially in the infant. In addition, bright red blood may indicate ischemic injury. The infant with NEC may occasionally have visible blood in the stool. Stools containing no visible blood should be tested for occult blood. A variety of methods, including guaiac-impregnated filter paper (Hemoccult), are available for this purpose.

Fecal Leukocytes

Examination of the diarrheal stool for white cells is useful in identifying infectious or inflammatory causes of diarrhea. A stool sample should be smeared on a glass slide and stained with methylene blue or Wright stain. The presence of neurophils in the stool suggests *Shigella, Yersinia, Campylobacter,* or invasive *E. coli* as a possible cause. The presence of leukocytes generally eliminates viral or toxigenic bacterial causes of diarrhea.

Culture

If a bacterial cause is suspected as the basis for the patient's diarrhea, stool culture for enteric pathogens is appropriate. The presence of *C. difficile* can be detected by culture or by assay for *C. difficile* toxin.

Virus Identification

Diarrhea induced by virus can be detected by enzyme-linked immunosorbent assay (ELISA) for viral antigens. The ELISA test for rotavirus has been shown to be extremely sensitive. ELISA may also be available for other enteritides such as adenovirus.

Screening Tests for Carbohydrate Malabsorption

The screening tests for carbohydrate malabsorption, using freshly passed feces, are meaningful only if the child being tested is currently being fed a potentially offending carbohydrate. These fecal screening tests include the measurement of pH (fecal pH) and reducing substances in the stool. Release of organic acids by bacterial fermentation of malabsorbed sugar forms the basis for utilizing this measurement as a screening test for carbohydrate malabsorption. The fecal pH test is performed by dipping Nitrazine paper into the most liquid part of a fresh stool. The resulting color on the paper is compared with a provided chart. A fecal pH below 5.5 is abnormal. Sugar that escapes small bowel absorption and is excreted in the stool may be detected by placing a small amount of fecal material in a test tube and diluting it with twice its volume of water. Fifteen drops of the resulting suspension are then placed in a second test tube with a Clinitest tablet. The resulting color is compared with a chart provided in the Clinitest kit used for testing of urine. Positive results are considered to be 0.5%. A result of 0.25% is considered equivocal. Since sucrose is not a reducing sugar, an accurate test for sucrose malabsorption requires the use of 1 N HCl instead of water.

Other Tests

Breath Hydrogen Test

Hydrogen (H_2) in breath results when carbohydrate that escapes small intestine absorption is fermented by colonic bacteria. A fixed portion of the H_2 produced is absorbed into the portal circulation and excreted in breath. The choice of sugar substrate for testing is dependent on the nature of the carbohydrate malabsorption suspected. Thus lactose is the substrate used when lactose malapsorption is suspected. The test is commonly performed after an overnight fast, but fasting may be shortened in the smaller infant. Methods for breath H_2 testing are available in the literature.

Sigmoidoscopy

Sigmoidoscopic examination is valuable if inflammatory bowel disease or pseudomembranous colitis is suspected. Flexible sigmoidoscopy can be conveniently performed even in small children, and biopsies can easily be obtained. Pseudomembranous colitis is described by excrescences and raised yellow pseudomembranes with areas of ulceration. It should be kept in mind that pseudomembranous colitis induced by *C. difficile* is only one end of the spectrum of *C. difficile*-induced diarrhea. That is, the most common clinical presentation of this infection is self-limited diarrhea.

Therapy

Acute self-limited diarrhea such as that attributable to viral agents requires a short period on a clear liquid diet, followed by gradual advancement in feedings. More intensive supportive care may be necessary to correct fluid and electrolyte disturbances.

Malabsorptive conditions require modification of the child's enteral feedings. Whenever possible, changes in feedings should be based on identification of the nutrients malabsorbed by the patient. Therapy of severe intestinal injury and short bowel syndrome frequently requires intravenous hyperalimentation. Total parenteral nutrition has dramatically improved the survival after massive small bowel resection and may permit normal infant growth and development. Short bowel syndrome may gradually improve as the bowel adapts by hypertrophy of the bowel lumen, lengthening of villi, and slowing of motility. During this adaptive time, dilute tube feedings of elemental diet should be administered to the degree tolerated. Enteral administration of elemental diet may increase enterocyte hyperplasia while improving the negative nitrogen balance of the patient and repleting missing nutrients. Complete parenteral therapy is discussed in Chapter 28 of the *Textbook*.

Therapy of infectious diarrhea is dependent on identifying the offending agent. Exterotoxic *E. coli* rarely needs to be treated with antibiotics but usually responds to Bactrim if necessary, while *Campylobacter jejune* may respond to erythromycin if needed. There is no evidence that "antidi-arrheal" agents such as Lomotil or Kaopectate help to cure infectious diar-rhea, and there is good evidence that they may prolong and worsen the severity of the disease.

PANCREATITIS

Pancreatitis should be suspected in the child with the acute onset of abdominal pain, nausea, vomiting, and localized ileus. Although it occurs in the epigastrium, the pain of pancreatitis differs from that of peptic ulcer disease, in that it is usually band-like rather than crampy, with referral of the pain straight through to the back. If the tail of the pancreas is in-volved, there may be localized inflammation of the diaphragm and phrenic nerve, with pain referred to the left shoulder. Occasionally, the left shoul-der pain may be greater than the abdominal discomfort, leading to distrac-tion of the physician from the etiology of the disease process.

Fever is commonly in the 100–103° range. Tachycardia and tachypnea are frequent. Usually, the blood pressure is normal, although profound or-thostatic hypotension may be seen. The abdomen is usually mildly to mod-erately tender, rarely with board-like stiffness or rebound. Bowel sounds are decreased but present in all but the most severe cases.

Leukocytosis in the 12,000–18,000 range is seen along with hemocon-centration of the hematocrit.

Serum amylase is usually elevated, although the height of elevation does not correlate with the severity of the clinical disease process. Where the amylase is only mildly elevated and if the patient does not have renal fail-ure or severe burns, urinary clearance of amylase may be helpful in dem-onstrating increased renal clearance of amylase to creatinine. Other pro-cesses associated with hyperamylasemia include parotitis, esophageal perforation, acute renal failure, pregnancy, and bowel infarction. Serum lipase is also elevated in most cases of pancreatitis and can be ordered where there are other reasons to expect hyperamylasemia.

Laboratory findings that suggest a poor prognosis include serum cal-cium of <7.5 mg/dl, leukocytosis of >20,000, PO_2 of <60, and azotemia. The hypocalcemia of fatal pancreatitis is probably multifactorial in etiol-ogy, including extraskeletal calcium sequestration, hypersecretion of glu-cagon, hypomagnesemia, and saponification of fatty acids.

During pancreatitis, any organs that come in direct contact with the pancreas may exhibit dysfunction secondary to localized inflammation. Thus localized areas of ileus are frequently seen in those loops of bowel that have possibly come in contact with the pancreas. This results in such radio-graphic findings such as "sentinel loop," if the small bowel is concerned, and "colon cut-off," if the transverse colon and descending colon are in-volved. Through a similar mechanism, red blood cells and white blood cells may be seen on urinalysis if the tail of the pancreas involves the left kid-ney. When the head of the pancreas is swollen and edematous and there is inflammation of the common bile duct, mild cholestasis may be seen. At these times the alkaline phosphatase or 5′-nucleotidase may be 2–4 times normal, and the serum bilirubin will be in the 2–5-mg/dl range.

Therapy

At this point, there are no magic medicines that treat pancreatitis more effectively that "pancreatic rest." This usually entails keeping the patient on a nothing-by-mouth diet. Of particular importance is the need to keep fat and protein out of the proximal bowel because these food products cause the release of cholecystokinin, which, in turn, results in pancreatic enzyme release. This is more destructive to an already-inflamed pancreas than any other single manipulation that could be made.

Intravenous fluids can be lifesaving, as third spacing of fluid becomes a major problem in pancreatitis. Fluid and colloid should be given quickly enough to decrease the tachycardia and correct the orthostasis. Central venous pressure or Swan-Ganz monitoring may be necessary because of the combined hypovolemia plus pulmonary complications. Careful restitution of serum calcium, magnesium, and potassium are necessary in the more severe cases.

Pulmonary problems occur in as many as 40% of patients with pancreatitis, although this complication is frequently underappreciated. When it occurs, pulmonary effusion is usually on the leftside, although bilateral sympathetic effusions can be seen. The loss of intrapulmonary surfactant through release into the serum of pancreatic lipase and phospholipase can result in severe atelectasis. In these cases, endotracheal intubation and the use of positive end-expiratory pressure are indicated.

Abdominal pain can be severe, requiring narcotic analgesics for relief. This needs to be remembered, especially in the older child who may have taken illicit drugs previously and who, when complaining of pain, may be viewed with skepticism.

For those patients with gastric atony secondary to localized inflammatory response, large volumes of gastric secretion will accumulate. These patients will feel more comfortable with nasogastric decompression. The nasogastric tube also serves to remind the patient and family that the nothing-by-mouth order is to be taken seriously.

LIVER FAILURE IN THE PEDIATRIC INTENSIVE CARE UNIT

Etiologies

Liver failure in the pediatric ICU is most frequently associated with toxins or drugs, viral hepatitis, or Reye syndrome (Table 19.3). However, accidental ingestion of toxic amounts of either iron, acetaminophen, or vitamin A can cause acute hepatic failure. Idiosyncratic hypersensitivity to isoniazid, α-methyldopa, and some antibiotics and anticonvulsants can also cause acute hepatocellular fulminant hepatic failure. If the child does not die of the liver failure itself or the associated complications, recovery will be complete, as there is rapid regeneration of the injured hepatic tissue after toxic damage.

TABLE 19.3. ————————————————————————
Common Etiology of Liver Failure in the Pediatric ICU

Viral hepatitis	Iron intoxication
Reye syndrome	Acetaminophen
Trauma	α-Methyldopa
Aspirin	Isoniazid

Although hepatitis A is the kind that most frequently affects children, hepatitis B is the one most likely to cause fulminant hepatic failure, representing as much as 75% of some series. People exposed to hepatitis B who then develop fulminant failure tend to have an enhanced antibody response because there is earlier appearance of antibodies to hepatitis B surface antigen (anti-HBs) and e antigen (anti-HBe), with more rapid clearance of hepatitis B surface antigen than is found in patients who do not develop fulminant hepatitis. Work with the recently discovered δ-agent indicates that the frequency of δ-agent markers is higher in patients with fulminant hepatitis B than in patients with acute uncomplicated hepatitis B. If the child can be maintained throughout the hepatic failure, recovery can be complete, without chronic liver scarring or damage. Recovery, however, occurs less quickly after viral hepatitis than after toxic hepatitis, because of suppressed regeneration associated with viral exposure.

Clinical Features and Complications of Acute Hepatic Failure

Mild to moderate nausea, anorexia, and fatigue are common with acute hepatitis (Table 19.4). The presence of protracted vomiting, altered behavior, bruisability, or ascites should warn the clinician that this case may be associated with acute hepatic failure. Behavioral alterations seen with hepatic failure range from euphoria to belligerence and the unexpected use of foul language. Sleep patterns may be altered, with the child sleeping all

TABLE 19.4. ————————————————————————
Complications of Hepatic Failure

Nutritional	**Respiratory failure**
Hypoglycemia	Pulmonary edema
Hypokalemia	
Hyponatremia	**Hepatorenal syndrome**
Amino acid abnormalities	
	Infections
Bleeding	
Indicates factor V, VII, or X	**Hepatic encephalopathy**
Stress gastritis	Cerebral edema
Variceal bleeding	Neurotransmitter abnormalities

day and being up all night. Confusion may range from altered spatial orientation (the basis for the Reitan trail test or the five-pointed star test) to slurred speech and complete disorientation. Asterixis may be present. Hyperventilation, hyperthermia, and hyperreflexia also reflect central nervous system involvement. The child may be lethargic, poorly arousable, or unarousable or may demonstrate decerebrate posture. Throughout its course, the depth of hepatic encephalopathy is one of the most reliable means of assessing and following the severity of the hepatic failure. Although the more severe grades of encephalopathy are associated with more severe hepatic failure and poorer prognosis, if life can be sustained long enough, recovery can be complete and frequently without permanent neurologic sequelae.

Liver function tests are usually drawn at the time of admission. This battery of tests usually includes transaminases and alkaline phosphatase. Transaminases become elevated with altered hepatocellular membrane integrity. The absolute height of transaminase elevation does not correlate with the severity of the disease; however, it is usually elevated 10- to 100-fold in fulminant hepatic failure. The pattern of change in transaminase levels with time can be useful in following the activity of the disease as long as the liver is still capable of producing transaminase. Sometimes in acute hepatic failure there will be such rapid destruction of hepatocytes that the transaminase will seem to fall precipitously as a premoribund event.

As alkaline phosphatase is produced in the bile canaliculus in response to increased pressure within the canaliculus, alkaline phosphatase of liver origin rises with any extrahepatic or intrahepatic obstruction to bile flow. Inflammation, hydropic degeneration of hepatocytes, or hepatocytes enlarged by fat or metabolites may lead to intrahepatic causes for alkaline phosphatase elevation in acute hepatic failure. As alkaline phosphatase is expected to be high in children because of bone growth, 5'-nucleotidase may be useful to differentiate bone from liver alkaline phosphatase and is better than heart fractionation for this purpose.

Neither transaminases nor alkaline phosphatase defines liver function, however. This can be best appreciated by carefully monitoring serum bilirubin, albumin, and prothrombin time, all of which require hepatocyte metabolism and thus reflect "function." With severe deterioration of liver function, there will be a mixed hyperbilirubinemia in the range of 15–40 mg/dl, the albumin will decrease to <3.0 mg/dl over several days, and the prothrombin time will become more than 3 seconds beyond control.

Therapeutic Guidelines

Mortality rates are high for this disease, being almost 60% in the Fulminant Hepatic Failure Surveillance Study and rising to 80% when grade IV encephalopathy is present. Survival can occur only when continuous attention to detail is combined with frequent small interventions designed to keep the child as close to normal metabolically as possible.

Basic monitoring should consist of hourly observations of blood pressure, pulse, respiration, mental status, urine output, and central venous pressure. Arterial blood gases should be drawn on admission to rule out other treatable causes of coma. Serum ammonia levels (preferably arterial) are useful in confirming a hepatic origin to coma and in monitoring progress. Serial electroencephalograms may likewise be useful. Intracranial pressure monitoring is done in some units when grade III encephalopathy ensues.

The mainstays of therapy are to keep the child normovolemic with normal electrolytes. Profound hypoglycemia is found in as many as 40% of children with acute hepatic failure and must be vigorously treated. Profound alterations in serum sodium and potassium are also frequent. Patients with acute hepatic failure may require large doses of intravenous potassium to maintain a normal serum level because of the kaliuresis associated with secondary hyperaldosteronism. Decreased serum sodium, because of an antidiuretic-like activity, is combined with increased total body sodium and fluid retention due to a hyperaldosterone-like activity. In addition, there is a shift of sodium into intracellular compartments in some patients. A delicate balance needs to be developed whereby as little sodium as possible is administered to present fluid overload, while serum sodium is carefully monitored to see that it does not begin to fall below 130 mg/dl.

Adequate caloric intake is essential. Since most children with acute hepatic failure have severe hepatic encephalopathy, total parenteral nutrition should be started at once if oral nutrition cannot safely be maintained. Hypertonic glucose is usually necessary because the ability of the liver to store glycogen has been significantly impaired. Some researchers have recommended maintaining serum glucose in the range of 100–300 mg/dl to help prevent cerebral edema. Protein administration should continue to the maximum tolerated level. Attention must be given, however, to adding those amino acids most needed by the body and avoiding those that tend to make encephalopathy worse. Branched-chain amino acids have been suggested to correct relative deficiency and to decrease muscle catabolism, thus decreasing the production of aromatic amino acids and ammonia. α-Keto analogs of branched-chain amino acids have also been used to pull nitrogen from glutamine, act as a nutritional source, and clear encephalopathy.

Although fatty acid emulsions are usually given to patients on total parenteral nutrition as a quick and easy method for delivering calories and essential fatty acids, this may not be appropriate in patients with liver diseases who cannot metabolize the fatty acids quickly. It is postulated that intrahepatic accumulation of fatty acids may further compromise hepatic function and that nonesterified fatty acids may compete with tryptophan for binding on albumin, thereby increasing the chance for encephalopathy.

There are no specific medications to improve liver failure at this time. Adrenocorticosteroids have been used in the past. However, results of a more recent study indicate that steroids are not helpful and may be mildly deleterious in patients with fulminant viral hepatitis. Vitamin K is, of course, commonly given for the associated coagulopathy.

Gastrointestinal Bleeding

As many as 70% of patients with acute hepatic failure may experience gastrointestinal bleeding, and as many as 30% will die from this complication. Bleeding occurs for a number of reasons, including stress gastritis and portal hypertension. Both of these problems are exacerbated by the coagulopathy of liver disease.

Coagulopathy occurs from inadequate synthesis of factors V, VII, and X. In chronic liver disease, hypersplenic sequestration of platelets may occur. Vitamin K should be administered, but frequently the coagulopathy does not respond. Diffuse intravascular coagulopathy also exists in most patients with acute or chronic liver disease, with exacerbation during stress induced by bleeding or infection. Trasylol, heparin, and ϵ-aminocaproic acid are not recommended prophylactically but have been used when bleeding from disseminated intravascular coagulation develops.

The incidence of stress gastritis in patients with hepatic failure can be reduced by maintaining the pH of the gastric contents at ≥ 4.5. This has been associated with a dramatic decrease in severe bleeding and a decrease in mortality. This can be accomplished by H_2 receptor antagonists and/or antacids and gentle nasogastric suction.

Respiratory Failure

Neurogenic pulmonary edema, fluid overload from the antidiuretic-like activity seen in patients with liver failure, and intrapulmonary shunting due to the release of vasoactive products in liver failure may be responsible for the hypoxia seen in 40–60% of patients with hepatic failure. Increasing the concentration of inspired oxygen may be all that is necessary in some patients to correct the hypoxia. Others may benefit from positive end-expiratory pressure, whereas others may require endotracheal intubation.

Hepatorenal Syndrome

Evidence of renal failure occurs in as many as 70% of patients with acute hepatic failure. The term hepatorenal syndrome connotes previously normal kidneys that decompensate in the presence of severe liver disease. Although the precise cause of hepatorenal syndrome is unknown, proposed theories include the effect of increased serum bile acids on renal membrane function and the effect of endotoxemia on renal function.

Great care should be taken to prevent precipitous drops in intravascular volume in the incipient hepatorenal syndrome. This includes avoiding large-volume paracentesis and strong diuretics, which could decrease intravascular volume.

Infections

The three sites of infection in children with liver diseases are: (a) bacteremia of gut organisms, due to poor hepatic clearing of organisms seeded from the edematous bowel of portal hypertension; (b) urinary tract infections; and *(c)* aspiration pneumonias. There is ample evidence that prophylactic antibiotics are not of value. Worsening of encephalopathy, sudden development of hepatorenal syndrome, and new onset of leukocytosis or fever, however, should raise the possibility of infection. Hygenic precautions, attention to avoiding activities likely to cause sepsis, such as drawing blood from the femoral area, and swift administration of antibiotics, should signs of infection appear, may contribute to increased survival.

Hepatic Encephalopathy

As liver failure increases, the stage of hepatic encephalopathy will increase. Precipitating factors that will also make encephalopathy worse include excessive protein load, hyperammonemia, respiratory alkalosis, hyponatremia, hypokalemia, hypoglycemia, infection, upper intestinal bleeding, azotemia, hypoxia, and administration of medications that suppress the sensorium.

Encephalopathy is, therefore, a multifactorial problem resulting in synergistic depression of mental status. A great deal of research has been devoted to further understanding of this complex problem, often with conflicting or nonreproducible results. A theory that encephalopathy is due to depression of neural energy metabolism has been suggested because oxygen extraction by the brain is reduced in animals with liver failure. Histologic evaluation of animals and humans dying of liver failure, however, shows little ultrastructural changes of neurotoxicity.

The mechanism by which ammonia may precipitate encephalopathy is not well understood. One theory is that ammonia converts glutamate, a powerful neuroexcitatory compound, to glutamine, a compound lacking or blocking effective excitatory transmission. Ammonia is also known to depress cerebral blood flow and oxygen consumption and may have a direct effect on the neuronal cell membrane; however, its specific roll in encephalopathy is yet to be determined.

Alteration of neurotransmission across neurons may be a more likely explanation of the reversible deficits seen. Ammonia, amino acids, short-chain fatty acids, octopamine, and other compounds that interfere with the normal flow of information from one neuron to the next have been described. Acetylcholine, norepinephrine, dopamine, serotonin, and histamine are the "classic" neurotransmitters. The more recently described gut peptides of vasoactive intestinal polypeptides, somatostatin, bombesin, and the enkephalins can also act as neurotransmitters. Agents that interfere with transmission or bind or displace neurotransmitters from receptor sites are believed to be present in liver failure and may be thought of as "false" neurotransmitters.

Monitoring of the patient with hepatic encephalopathy is best performed by the crude clinical criteria for grade scoring of encephalopathy. A system for classifying encephalopathy uses a scheme of 0–IV:

Grade 0 Normal
Grade I Altered spatial orientation, sleep patterns, and effect

Grade II Drowsy but arousable, slurred speech, confusion, and asterixis
Grade III Stuporous but responsive to painful stimuli
Grade IV Unresponsive, with decorticate or decerebrate posturing possible

Treatment of hepatic encephalopathy includes the prevention and therapy of processes known to precipitate encephalopathy, reduction in protein intake (especially aromatic and straight-chained amino acids), and reduction of serum ammonia levels by the addition of neomycin plus a laxative or lactulose. Neomycin has successfully been used as an antibiotic that is poorly (< 1%) absorbable and effective, at least acutely, against urea-splitting gut flora. Lactulose, a nonabsorbable synthetic disaccharide, causes a watery diarrhea of low pH. This results in loss of the normal colonic flora and overgrowth of non-urea-splitting organisms. The low pH may also prevent the absorption of ammonia and aromatic amino acids. Neomycin and lactulose are approximately equally effective. There is some evidence that the combination may be more effective than either one alone. Although lactulose is more expensive than neomycin, it has been suggested for patients with renal impairment or for those patients who fail to respond to neomycin. When the patients is on parenteral antibiotics for other reasons, there is no evidence that additional neomycin is necessary; however, lactulose to induce frequent as well as low pH bowel movements is probably indicated. Lactulose or lactose enemas may also work well in this situation to reduce the encephalopathy.

Addition of branched-chain amino acids to hypertonic (20%) glucose may help improve nutritional status and reduce the concentration of aromatic amino acids but has not consistently been shown to improve cerebral function better than the conventional therapy described earlier. Because it is clear that many children with hepatic failure and encephalopathy require nutritional support, branched-chain amino acids plus hypertonic glucose may be appropriate and well tolerated for nutritional support.

Cerebral Edema

Cerebral edema is the cause of death in as many as 40% of patients with hepatic failure. The etiology for cerebral edema is as poorly understood as the etiology for encephalopathy, but both appear to be related, since patients who develop progressively deeper levels of encephalopathy eventuate into cerebral edema if the process is not stopped.

Intracranial pressure monitoring is suggested once stage III encephalopathy has occurred. Steps to reduce vigorously intracranial pressure include elective intubation and hyperventilation, increasing the osmolarity of the serum, hypothermia, and phenobarbital. To be effective, these techniques must be initiated early enough in the course of the disease that fixed neurologic changes from cerebral edema have not occurred. Concepts of cerebral edema care are not unique to hepatic failure and are covered elsewhere in this book.

CHAPTER 20

Renal Failure

PRINCIPLES OF DIAGNOSIS AND MANAGEMENT OF ACUTE RENAL FAILURE

Diagnosis

Acute renal failure (ARF) is characterized by loss of the function of the kidneys in the regulation of water, electrolyte, and acid-base balance, with the accumulation in the blood of nitrogenous wastes.

The adult literature on the incidence, etiology, mortality, and morbidity of renal failure is more voluminous than the pediatric literature and allows greater predictability of prognosis based on the factors of age, pre-existing illness, and precipitating cause of renal failure.

Over the past 15 years, an increasing recognition of the frequent occurrence of nonoliguric renal failure in adult patients (up to 50% in some series) has been reflected in the internal medicine literature. This has been attributed to more generalized use of nephrotoxic drugs, such as the aminoglycosides, the conversion of oliguric to nonoliguric renal failure through use of potent diuretics, and improved resuscitation and survival of trauma victims. In most reported series of renal failure in children, either oliguria is used as a criterion by which the diagnosis is made, or a very low incidence of nonoliguric renal failure, most commonly in postoperative patients, is reported. In pediatric patients, nephrotoxic drugs and surgery may lead to nonoliguric renal failure, but the majority of cases do seem to be oliguric. Oliguria is defined as a urine output of <0.5 ml/kg/hr of <300 ml/m^2/day.

The mortality of children for all renal failure is much less than that of adults. The majority of cases of ARF occurring in children are potentially reversible with optimal management.

The etiologies of renal failure seen in a particular institution depend greatly on demographic and socioeconomic characteristics of the population served. In the pediatric intensive care unit (ICU) of The Johns Hopkins Hospital from July 1982 to June 1984, 39 patients with ARF were seen. The distribution of etiologies leading to ARF is presented in Table 20.1.

The presence of only one patient with primary renal parenchymal disease in this 2-year series does not reflect a low incidence of these problems in our patient population but, rather, reflects the success of conservative management of most cases of glomerulonephritis on the regular pediatric ward. There were no cases of hemolytic-uremic syndrome (HUS) seen in these 2 years.

The distribution of etiologies of ARF seen in the pediatric ICU is not fully representative of the distribution of etiologies in the institution as a whole, as neonatal renal failure is managed in the neonatal ICU; therefore, etiologies particular to the neonate, such as asphyxia, congenital anomalies, and renal venous and renal arterial thrombosis, are not represented. In addition, oncology patients not requiring dialysis during this period were likely to be managed in the oncology center. Most patients listed as having ARF after cardiac arrest were victims of multiple trauma, and most patients with sepsis had shock and sepsis complicating a primary infectious disease such as gastroenteritis, meningitis, or pneumonia.

In most series of ARF in children, mortality is associated with the irreversible nature of the underlying disease rather than with the renal failure itself. This has been especially true following cardiac surgery, in which

TABLE 20.1.
Etiologies of ARF in The Johns Hopkins Hospital Pediatric ICU (July 1982 to June 1984)

	Total	No. Dialyzed (%)
Postcardiac surgery	12	4 (33)
After cardiac arrest	6	3 (50)
Sepsis	8	1 (12)
Acute poststreptococcal glomerulonephritis	1	0 (0)
Autoimmune (SLE, JRA)[a]	3	2 (67)
Cancer and sepsis	4	4 (100)
Oxalosis	1	1 (100)
Sepsis after bone marrow transplant	1	0 (0)
Reye syndrome	1	1 (100)
Sickle cell disease and sepsis	1	1 (100)
Uric acid nephropathy after chemotherapy	1	1 (100)
Total	37	18 (50)

[a]SLE, systemic lupus erythematosus: JRA, juvenile rheumatoid arthritis.

setting death is usually associated with cardiac failure refractory to medical management.

Postoperative Renal Failure

Although renal failure occurs relatively rarely after cardiac surgery in adults, the incidence is higher in children (6–8%), with mortality reported to be at 10–89%. The risk of renal failure is much higher in infants than in older children and is still higher in neonates (up to 29%). Factors increasing the risk of postoperative renal failure include complex congenital heart diseases, especially those associated with cyanosis and/or polycythemia, left-sided obstructive lesions with low preoperative renal perfusion, or low postoperative cardiac output due to myocardial dysfunction. Preoperative cyanosis leads to some degree of baseline renal cortical hypoxia, and associated polycythemia may contribute further to decreased renal blood flow. Existence of preoperative renal impairment should alert the clinician to the possibility of increased risk of postoperative renal failure.

Other risk factors include perioperative use of aminoglycosides and the X-ray contrast administered for angiography. The intraoperative factors that make renal failure more likely include hypotension, hypoxia, arrhythmias, administration of α-adrenergic vasopressors or high-dose dopamine, and prolonged cardiopulmonary bypass (>90 minutes). The latter is important, not only because of alteration of renal blood flow but also because of the possible occurrence of hemolysis, with free hemoglobin possibly resulting in renal damage.

Neonates are at higher risk not only because of the increased proportion of patients with complex cardiac lesions but also because of their lower baseline total renal blood flow and, in particular, their comparatively low outer cortical blood flow.

If oliguria or anuria occurs postoperatively in the patient who has had cardiac surgery, the increased blood volume due to decreased water clearance can be difficult to manage with fluid restriction alone, especially if multiple inotropic drugs and antibiotics must be administered. The excess intravascular volume can further strain a myocardium compromised by surgical trauma. In addition, the metabolic consequences of renal failure—hyperkalemia and acidosis—are poorly tolerated by the postoperative patient and can lead more rapidly to arrhythmias and further circulatory compromise.

Because of the difficulty in managing these problems by conservative means, several groups have attempted early peritoneal dialysis in patients with postoperative renal failure and borderline myocardial function. Peritoneal dialysis is chosen because of the high incidence of hypotension when hemodialysis is used in patients with unstable hemodynamics on inotropic support. Peritoneal dialysis avoids rapid shifts in osmolarity that could exacerbate postanoxic cerebral edema. Some have wondered whether patients with low cardiac output might have low mesenteric blood flow and, therfore, low peritoneal clearance which might hamper the efficiency of peritoneal dialysis, but this does not seem to be the case. In most cases in these series, dialysis was performed for hyperkalemia (at lower levels than in patients with primary ARF) or for fluid overload. Blood urea nitrogen (BUN) was usually only mildly elevated, as dialysis was most commonly started <48 hours postoperatively. Fluid removal by dialysis allows for more liberal fluid administration and hyperalimentation if indicated.

These patients also frequently have severe neurologic damage secondary to persistent hypotension. Renal failure is also associated with higher mortality in the neonatal population, as it often occurs in the settings of asphyxia, prematurity, sepsis, and a profound catabolic state. Children over the age of 2 have a much better outlook with meticulous medical management, early detection and treatment of complications, and dialysis if necessary.

The presenting clinical picture of ARF that is seen most commonly in the ICU is one of oliguria in a patient with hemorrhage, burns, or cardiopulmonary arrest or after cardioulmonary bypass for cardiac surgery in whom urine output cannot be re-established with the correction of volume status. A careful review of the history, physical, and urine and other laboratory studies should reveal any other predisposing conditions, such as exposure to nephrotoxic drugs, the possibility of urinary tract obstruction, recent administration of radiotherapy or chemotherapy for tumor, or the presence of hemoglobinuria or myoglobinuria. Etiologies of oliguria, such as antidiuretic hormone (ADH) secretion due to pulmonary disease, mechanical ventilation, or central nervous system (CNS) disorders, should be considered and ruled out. It is also essential early in the course of investigation of oliguria to assure that the urinary catheter is functioning properly.

It is important to identify quickly the prerenal and postrenal causes of oliguria, as they are usually readily reversible with correction of the underlying abnormality (i.e., fluid replacement, treatment of congestive heart failure, and relief of urinary tract obstruction). Much work has been done to provide laboratory criteria for the differentiation of oliguria due to prerenal causes from true ARF. This is important so that prerenal oliguria can be recognized early and treated vigorously to prevent progression to true ARF. Another cause of oliguria in ICU patients is ADH secretion (appropriate or inappropriate) which can occur in some of the same clinical settings as ARF (e.g., postoperative, trauma). Inappropriate ADH secretion is triggered by pulmonary disease when decreased venous return to the heart is caused by mechanical ventilation or when increased negative intrathoracic pressure causes relative distention of the atria and great vessels through stimulation of atrial baroreceptors. CNS hemorrhage or other causes of increased intracranial pressure can also result in ADH secretion. Drugs such as narcotics, antihistamines, and anticonvulsants can stimulate ADH secretion and cause transient oliguria. Excess ADH secretion should be thought of in patients with inappropriately high urine osmolality in the face of low serum osmolality and, often, low serum sodium, as it is important not to give these patients a fluid load to try to generate urine output. The laboratory studies that enable differentiation of these various causes of oliguria are present in Table 20.2. Urinary studies should be performed on a 1-hour collection, with the serum samples being obtained at the end of the hour. In some cases, results will fall in an intermediate range, not being clearly compatible with either prerenal causes or ARF. In these cases, calculation of the renal failure index (RFI) often helps to place the patient clearly in one category or the other. The urinary elements of all of these measurements of renal function are altered by the prior adminis- tration of diuretics, and samples should be obtained, if possible, before these agents are given. In the neonate, there is limited availability of urea due to the anabolic state of the neonate, and perhaps immature tubular function limits maximum concentrating ability. These facts should be re- membered for the interpretation of these studies in neonates. Fractional extraction of sodium (FE_{Na}) may rise postoperatively in the absence of renal failure in cardiac patients who were in congestive heart failure preopera- tively, if hemodynamics improve and excess body sodium is urine output.

Determinations of serum urea nitrogen and creatinine are helpful in dis- cerning the existence of renal insufficiency. They will usually be in the normal range if ADH secretion is the cause of oliguria. In patients with a normal metabolic rate, with the new onset of renal failure the urea nitro- gen and creatinine will usually rise at the rate of 10–20 mg/dl in 24 hours and 0.5 mg/dl in 24 hours, respectively, but there are many factors that can alter the rate of rise (Table 20.3). In patients with fever, sepsis, trauma, or burns, the rate of rise may be 40–50 and 2–5, respectively, whereas

TABLE 20.2.
Laboratory Differentiation of Etiology of Oliguria

Test	Prerenal Oliguria	Oliguric Renal Failure	ADH Secretion
Urine			
Sodium (mEq/l)	<20 (<40)[a]	>40 (>40)	>40
Specific gravity	>1.020 (>1.015)	<1.010 (<1.015)	>1.020
Osmolality (mOsm/l)	>500 (>400)	<350 (<400)	>500
Urine/plasma ratios			
Osmolality	>1.3	<1.3	>2
Urea nitrogen	>20	<10	>15
Creatine	>40 (>20)	<20 (<15)	>30
RFI[b]	<1 (<3.0)	>1 (>3.0)	>1
FE_{Na}[c]	<1 (<2.5)	>1 (>3.0)	Close to 1

[a]Numbers in parentheses are for neonates.
[b]RFI (renal failure index) = $(U_{Na} \times 100)/U_{cr}/P_{cr}$.
[c]FE_{Na} (fractional excretion of sodium) = $(U_{Na}/P_{Na})/(U_{cr}/P_{cr}) \times 100$.

TABLE 20.3.
Factors That Alter the Serum Levels of Urea Nitrogen and Creatinine[a]

	Urea Nitrogen	Creatinine
Increased	High protein diet	Rhabdomyolsis
	Gastrointestinal hem-orrhage	Dehydration
	Dehydration	
	Steroid administra-tion	
	Hypercatabolic states (fever, trauma, post-operative)	
Decreased	Low portein diet	Decreased muscle mass (malnutrition)
	High fat and carbohy-drate diet	Burns
	Liver disease	Hyperlipidemia
	Hyperlipidemia	

[a]From Ruley EJ, Bock GH: Acute renal failure in infants and children. In Shoemaker WC, Thompson WL, Holbrook PR (eds): *Textbook of Critical Care Medicine*. Philadelphia, WB Saunders, 1984, p 606.

patients with rhabdomyolysis have acceleration of creatinine accumulation alone. Creatinine clearance can be determined from timed urine collections.

Other laboratory studies to be obtained in the patient admitted with primary oliguria are listed in Table 20.4. The presence of hematuria, proteinuria, and casts with edema and hypertension may lead to a diagnosis of glomerulonephritis. In infants or young children, oliguria in the setting of vomiting, diarrhea, and, possibly, bloody stools may represent HUS. The peripheral blood smear should be examined carefully for signs of hemolysis and adequacy of platelet count. The admission of an oliguric child with growth retardation or X-ray signs of osteodystrophy may lead one to suspect the deterioration of a previously stable state of chronic renal insufficiency. In such children, urinary tract obstruction should be carefully ruled out by utilizing sonography or, if necessary, intravenous pyelography. It is better to avoid the latter, if possible, because of the problems of (a) inability of the compromised kidneys to excrete the dye, with its retention causing intravascular volume overload, and (b) the possibility of X-ray contrast agents further compromising renal function via renal vasoconstriction. In addition, if the renal function is very poor, the dye will not be sufficiently concentrated by the kidneys to permit visualization.

An unusual situation in which the clinician should be alert to the possibility of the development of oliguria is the patient in whom there is increased intra-abdominal pressure. Effects on urine output are more likely to occur when the increase in pressure is acute and severe, as in closure of gastroschisis or omphalocele in the neonate. Anuria has been reported in adult patients with increased intra-abdominal pressure due to

TABLE 20.4. _____

Ancillary Studies in the Patient with Oliguria[a]

Hematologic

Hemoglobin, hematocrit	Anemia
White blood count	
Platelet count	In HUS, after cardiopulmonary bypass, renal vein thrombosis
Peripheral smear	Burr cells, helmet cells in HUS

Coagulation

Prothrombin time	May be prolonged in sepsis, disseminated intravascular coagulation (DIC)
Partial thromboplastin time	
Fibrin split products	

Stool

Guaiac	May be positive in HUS
	Gastrointestinal hemorrhage may cause elevated BUN

Urine

Culture sediment	Red cells—Consider acute glomerulonephritis (AGN), Henoch-Schönlein purpura, systemic lupus erythematosus (SLE)
	Red cell casts—AGN
	Tubular casts—Tubular injury
	Uric acid crystals—May be significant, status after chemotherapy
Labstix	If positive for heme, examine fresher urine for red cells; if absent, consider myoglobinuria or hemoglobinuria
	Protein

Radiology

Chest X-ray	? Cardiac enlargement, pulmonary vascular engorgement, pulmonary edema
	? Osteoporosis—Consider chronic renal failure

Electrocardiogram

Signs of hyperkalemia
    Peaked T waves
    Wide QRS
    Absent P wave
Signs of hypocalcemia
    Prolonged Q-T
Voltage changes consistent with left ventricular hypertrophy, strain

Electrolytes

Sodium (usually normal or $\downarrow$)
Potassium (normal or $\uparrow$)
Calcium ($\downarrow$)
Phosphate ($\uparrow$)
Bicarbonate (may be $\downarrow$)

TABLE 20.4.—*continued*

Serologic

C_3 complement	AGN
Streptococcal serologies	AGN
Antinuclear antibody	SLE

Other

Haptoglobin	Transfusion reaction
Creatine phosphokinase	Rhabdomyolysis
Uric acid	May be etiologic (tumor lysis) or secondary

bleeding and tight abdominal closure. The patients with high intra-abdominal pressure due to bleeding had apparently adequately replaced intravascular volume, and brisk diuresis ensued after operation to relieve the pressure with no change in cardiac output, central venous pressure (CVP), or peripheral resistance. The oliguria does not, therefore, seem to be due to a decline in cardiac output because of decreased venous return. It is believed, however, that intrarenal redistribution of blood flow may play an important role in this syndrome.

It is important to recognize increased intra-abdominal pressure as a cause of postoperative oliguria or anuria, for in the postoperative setting it is easy to assume that oliguria is due to third-space volume loss or intraoperative blood loss, but volume replacement will not alleviate the decline in renal function, whereas prompt surgery to relieve increased intra-abdominal pressure is associated with rapid diuresis. In infants with abdominal wall defects the development of this problem is best averted by direct measurement of intra-abdominal pressure through use of intraoperative pressure measurements via either the esophageal route or gastrostomy. Preliminary results indicate it is inadvisable to close the abdominal wall if pressure exceeds 20 mm Hg. If this is the case, a silo is best employed, with delayed closure to allow time for the compliance of the abdominal wall to increase.

Management

Once the diagnosis is made, it is essential to take great care in managing all aspects of the patient with ARF, as spontaneous recovery is likely to begin in 1–3 weeks and survival and return of renal function is likely to occur if the patient does not die of the underlying disease process or suffer infectious, metabolic, or hemorrhagic complications of ARF or its treatment. The keys are: (a) careful monitoring of fluid and electrolyte balance, (b) nutritional management directed at preventing a catabolic state, and (c) meticulous care to avoid infection. The physiologic consequences of ARF are listed in Table 20.5.

The first step in managing an oliguric patient is to ensure the adequacy

TABLE 20.5.
Physiologic Consequences of ARF

Cardiovascular
Hypervolemia
  Pulmonary edema
  Hypertension
  Peripheral edema
Cardiac arrhythmias related to hyperkalemia
Pericarditis (rare)
Pleural effusion

Metabolic
Hyperkalemia
Hyponatremia
Hypocalcemia
Hyperphosphatemia
Hyperuricemia
Hypermagnesemia
Azotemia
Acidosis

Hematologic
Anemia
  Dilutional
  Decreased erythropoietin (minor effect)
  Hemolytic
  Gastrointestinal (GI) bleeding
Thrombocytopenia—HUS or abnormal platelet function
Coagulopathy

Gastrointestinal
Nausea, vomiting
GI bleeding
Catabolic state—Poor nutrition

Neurologic
Irritability
Sedation
Seizures
Coma

Infectious
Urinary tract
Sepsis
Pulmonary
Peritonitis

of intravascular volume. Careful physical examination may indicate the presence of hypovolemia (dry mucous membranes, "tenting" of the skin, postural changes in heart rate and blood pressure) or fluid overload (peripheral edema, rales, liver enlargement, gallop, hypertension). A chest X-ray should be done to look for signs of pulmonary edema or cardiomegaly. An electrocardiogram (ECG) should be obtained with subsequent rhythm strips followed at frequent intervals, to look for changes associated with hyperkalemia (Fig. 20.1). In the absence of evidence of hypervolemia, a

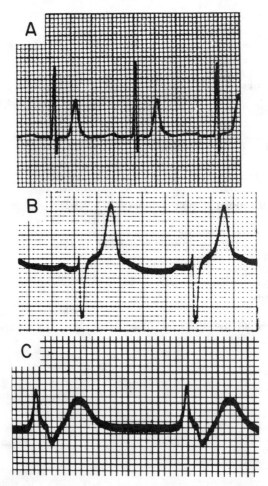

FIGURE 20.1. ECG signs of hyperkalemia. *A:* First-degree atrioventricular block and peaked T waves, mild hyperkalemia. *B:* Peaked T waves, slightly widened QRS (K-6.1). *C:* Absent P waves, peaked T waves, wide QRS (K-8.1). (From Chung EK: *Electrocardiography.* New York, Harper & Row, 1980 *(A)*; and Marriott HJL: *Practical Electrocardiography.* Baltimore, Williams & Wilkins, 1972 *(B* and *C).)*

fluid challenge of normal saline of 20 ml/kg should be given. This volume load should always precede diuretic administration in the oliguric patient, lest diuretics decrease renal perfusion by exacerbating pre-existing dehydration. A CVP catheter is invaluable in this situation for assessing the state of intravascular volume and the response to therapeutic maneuvers. The hypotensive patient who may be relatively hypovolemic due to decreased resistance must be adequately volume loaded, as injudicious attempts to raise blood pressure through the use of α-adrenergic sympathomimetic agents such as Neo-Synephrine, norepinephrine, or high-dose dopamine (> 10 μg/kg/min) may actually further compromise renal blood flow even in the face of increasing systemic blood pressure. The answers to these questions of adequacy of perfusion, volume status, and peripheral resistance are certainly more easily ascertained through use of a pulmonary artery catheter if the size of the child permits its use. In postoperative cardiac patients, a left atrial catheter provides much useful information and is easily removed when no longer needed. Cardiac output can also be determined by using a central venous catheter and arterial line with the dye dilution technique. In patients thought to have fixed renal failure who have stable hemodynamics and do not require inotropic support, central venous catheters should be removed as soon as possible to avoid infectious complications.

If there is no response to fluid challenge, some authors have suggested the use of mannitol or furosemide to distinguish prerenal oliguria from fixed renal failure or to convert oliguric to nonoliguric renal failure. The rapid intravenous administration of mannitol at 0.5g/kg should result in a urine output of > 0.5 ml/kg within 1 hour if the cause of the oliguria is prerenal or if fixed ARF has not occurred. This mannitol test may be falsely negative if the patient is dehydrated, so assurance of normal volume status prior to its use is essential. There is some concern about the hazard of this test causing hypervolemia and possibly pulmonary edema in patients who cannot excrete the mannitol. The risk of mannitol administration probably outweighs its benefit if there is any question of incipient volume overload or congestive heart failure.

The use of furosemide may be beneficial early in the course of ARF as a provocative test to generate urine production, since its vasodilating and natriuretic properties may attenuate ARF to some degree. Furosemide should be given to euvolemic patients in an intravenous dose of 1 mg/kg. If there is no response in 30 minutes, incrementally higher doses of up to 10 mg/kg may be used, although at such a dose level there may be concern about its ototoxicity. If there is no response to fluid challenge, low-dose dopamine at 2.5–5.0 μg/kg/min should be added. If these drugs are successful in generating urine output, improvement in glomerular filtration rate does not necessarily parallel increased urine volume, but increased urine flow simplifies fluid management and drug administration in these patients.

If these initial therapeutic maneuvers do not improve urine output or if, despite increased output, BUN and creatinine continue to rise, the reality of fixed ARF must be addressed and managed. Meticulous supportive care is essential to avoid complications during the period prior to recovery of renal function, which usually begins in 5–10 days. The possible consequences of ARF that must be guarded against are: (a) derangements of fluid and electrolyte balance, (b) hypertension, (c) infection, (d) gastrointestinal (GI) hemorrhage, (e) encephalopathy, and very rarely, (f) uremic pericarditis. The patient should be weighed, and the weighing should be repeated twice daily under standardized conditions, to assess fluid balance. The basic principles of conservative management, once fixed renal failure occurs, are: (a) to normalize intravascular volume, systemic blood pressure, and renal blood flow; (b) to maintain normal sodium, potassium, and acid-base balance; and (c) to minimize accumulation of nitrogenous wastes by restricting protein intake while at the same time providing adequate caloric intake to prevent a catabolic state and promote resolution of the primary disease and renal repair. In addition, special care must be taken to avoid infectious complications. Prophylactic measures for GI bleeding, such as the administration of cimetidine (4 mg/kg orally) or ranitidine (2 mg/kg orally) and antacid, should be instituted. In most cases, these simple measures are sufficient to support the patient until renal function begins to recover spontaneously.

Fluid

Fluid administration, both oral and parenteral, should be restricted to the sum of insensible losses (300 ml/m^2) plus measured urine output and any other losses (e.g., GI, respiratory, increased evaporative loss due to burns). Table 20.6 shows the usual electrolyte content of these fluids as a guide to replacement. Burns represent a special problem in fluid management which is dealt with in detail in Chapter 24. Evaporative loss in the burned patient is gauged by the formula:

$$\text{Volume loss (ml/hr)} = (25 + \% \text{ body surface burned}) \times \text{body surface area (m}^2)$$

if renal failure occurs, although ordinarily in burned patients, fluids are administered to maintain urine output at >1 ml/kg/hr. Patients with ARF and extraordinary losses may become hypovolemic and must be followed carefully, to look for signs of dehydration and orthostatic changes in vital signs. It is imperative that hypovolemia be detected and appropriately corrected, as failure to do so can cause recurrent renal vasoconstriction with resultant exacerbation or prolongation of ARF. Patients who are hypovolemic without electrolyte imbalance may benefit from the administration of the needed volume as blood or colloid, whichever is indicated clinically. Colloid preparations available for use include 5% human serum albumin, Plasmanate, and Hespan (6% hydroxyethyl starch). The volume administered should be determined by CVP measurement or the disappearance of orthostatic changes, with 10–20 ml/kg given initially.

Insensible loss may be <300 ml/m^2 in patients who are hypothermic, in barbiturate coma, or on mechanical ventilation with humidified gases. Paradoxically, hypercatabolic patients may need less water because of water

TABLE 20.6.
Electrolyte Composition of Body Fluids[a]

Fluid	Electrolyte (mEq/l)		
	Na	K	Cl
Gastric	20–80	5–20	100–150
Pancreatic	120–140	5–15	40–80
Bile	120–140	5–15	80–120
Small intestine	100–140	5–15	90–130
Ileostomy	45–135	3–15	20–115
Diarrhea	10–90	10–80	10–110

[a]From Cole CH (ed): *The Harriet Lane Handbook*, ed 10. Chicago, Year Book Medical Publishers, 1984.

produced endogenously through catabolism which may reduce the requirements for exogenous water by one-third. This hidden water production amounts to 3 ml/g protein catabolized. Electrolyte content of urine should be monitored daily, with measured sodium losses being replaced. Potassium losses should be measured but not replaced unless hypokalemia occurs. Twice daily weights are helpful in assessing volume status. A breakdown of body mass should result in a loss of 0.5–1% of weight per day; stable or increasing weight indicate fluid retention which can be addressed by further fluid restriction and administration of furosemide and/or dopamine infusion. Another sign of fluid retention is decreased serum sodium concentration. Conversely, a large daily weight loss or elevated serum sodium may indicate inadequate fluid replacement. Some have advocated the removal of fluid through the induction of diarrhea by the administration of sorbitol by mouth or rectum (70% and 20% solutions, respectively).

It may be difficult to limit fluid to 300 ml/m^2 in critically ill patients receiving multiple intravenous drugs such as pressors and antibiotics. If fluid overload persists or develops in this situation, it may be better to opt for early dialysis rather than continue to battle circulatory overload in the face of low or absent urine output, especially in postoperative cardiac surgery patients. Results of recent studies in children have shown early peritoneal dialysis to be effective and without excess morbidity in postoperative cardiac patients.

Sodium

The usual sodium abnormality seen in ARF is hyponatremia due to water retention. If hyponatremia is present during the oliguric phase of ARF, fluid administration should be reduced below 300 ml/m^2 to allow correction of the serum sodium, unless sodium falls below 120 or seizures occur, in which case dialysis is necessary. If diuresis is induced with furosemide and/or dopamine, urinary sodium losses may increase and should be measured and replaced. Urinary sodium excretion may be elevated in the absence of diuretic administration in cases of nonoliguric renal failure or may increase suddenly during the recovery ("diuretic") phase of oliguric renal failure. This must be watched for or hyponatremia may occur. In patients who are not hypervolemic, hyponatremia may be corrected by calculating the sodium deficit and administering one-half this amount as 3% saline. The volume administered should be $\{[(140 - P_{Na}) \times 0.6 \times$ weight (kg)]/0.45\} ml 3% saline containing 340 mEq of sodium per liter.

Hypernatremia rarely occurs in ARF unless water in excess of sodium is removed by dialysis against a hypertonic solution, or ongoing (water) losses are inadequately replaced.

Potassium

Patients with ARF accumulate potassium because the kidney is responsible for elimination of 90% off the potassium that must be excreted daily, with the remaining 10% being lost in the intestine. Patients with chronic renal failure compensate over time for the kidney's decreased ability to excrete potassium by increasing losses in the gut. With ARF, there is not time for such compensation to occur.

Although most critically ill patients are in a catabolic state, patients with an intrinsic cause for their renal disease have a lower level of metabolic demand than patients with burns, rhabdomyolysis, recent surgery, or trauma. In addition to having an increase in serum potassium because of a decline in the kidney's ability to excrete potassium in exchange for sodium, these latter patients have increased release of intracellular potassium due to accelerated protein catabolism and/or direct tissue damage or hemolysis. The difference can be dramatic, with serum potassium rising 0.3–0.5 mEq/l/day in afebrile noncatabolic patients with renal failure and 0.5–1 mEq/l/day in patients with rhabdomyolysis. Patients with fever, trauma, or burns can have increases of > 1 mEq/l/day. The catabolic state also leads to increased acidosis due to release of tissue phosphate. Serum bicarbonate declines approximately 2 mEq/day. Acidosis accelerates the rate of development of hyperkalemia by causing a shift of potassium from inside cells into the extracellular and intravascular spaces, with an increase of 0.5 mEq K^+ for each 0.1-unit decline in pH. For these reasons, patients with ARF should receive no exogenous potassium from any source unless hypokalemia occurs. It is important to remember to avoid giving cold, stored blood which can contain up to 30 mEq potassium per liter. Drugs that contain potassium, such as aqueous penicillin G (1.7 mEq potassium per million units penicillin), should not be administered. Serum potassium and serial ECGs should be followed closely especially in the setting of hypercatabolism, tumor lysis, or trauma, even in patients in whom frank renal failure has not yet developed.

When the electrophysiologic effects of hyperkalemia on cardiac excitation and conduction are considered, the necessity and basis for the emergency treatment of hyperkalemia can be better understood. Treatment should be instituted for serum potassium of >6.0 mEq/l and at lower levels if the potassium is rising rapidly in the setting of tissue breakdown and refractory oliguria. Measures to be taken can be categorized as *(a)* antagonizing the electrophysiologic effects of hyperkalemia, (b) driving potassium intracellularly, and (c) removing potassium from the body (Table 20.7). Immediate protection of the myocardium against the effects of slowed conduction and diminished contractility can be afforded through the use of intravenous calcium, which acts in two ways. It causes an increase in potassium conductance even in face of decreased transmembrane potential gradient, which results in an increase in phase 0 slope and amplitude; and it increases calcium entry through calcium channels, which increases contractility. The intravenous administration of calcium can cause bradycardia, and the ECG must be monitored continuously.

The measures that drive potassium into cells include the administration of glucose, insulin, and sodium bicarbonate. This would serve to re-establish the normal transmembrane potential. While their administration is being instituted, the ECG should be followed continuously, and equipment for emergency dialysis should be readied, because if the potassium does not stabilize or decline, cardiac arrest refractory to resuscitative efforts may ensue, even in the absence of premonitory ECG changes. Dialysis must be instituted if the potassium is over 6.5 mEq/1 or, even earlier, if there is continued accelerated release of intracellular potassium, as these conservative measures, by not reducing the total body potassium, cannot be effective. The administration of the ion exchange resin sodium polystyrene sulfonate (Kayexalate) is the only measure available, short of dialysis, that reduces the total body potassium burden. Combining the resin with sorbitol induces increased GI potassium loss due to the resultant diarrhea. The sorbitol is also essential to prevent bowel obstruction due to inspissation of resin, especially when given by mouth. It must be remembered that Kayexalate works by exchanging equal milliequivalent amounts of sodium for potassium, and if the patient's intravascular volume is already increased, this added sodium intake could lead to the development of congestive heart failure. In this situation, proceeding to dialysis expeditiously is advisable. While dialysis is being prepared, Kayexalate should be continued, as it can remove up to 1 mEq of potassium per gram of resin administered.

Hypokalemia, though rare, may occur in patients on dialysis or in patients who attain an anabolic state through hyperalimentation as a result of potassium being incorporated into new cells.

Calcium-Phosphate

Hyperphosphatemia and associated hypocalcemia may develop rapidly after the onset of ARF due to (a) decreased ability of the kidney to excrete phosphate, (b) increased tissue release of phosphate secondary to catabolism, (c) decreased absorption of dietary calcium because of diminished production of 1,25-dihydroxy-vitamin D, and (d) decreased release of calcium from bone due to resistance to parathyroid hormone. In cases of rhabdomyolysis or massive tumor lysis, hyperphosphatemia in the absence of hyperuricemia may actually be the inciting factor leading to renal failure. Mitigating against the occurrence of symptomatic hypocalcemia is the acidosis

TABLE 20.7.
Therapy for Hyperkalemia

Drug	Dose and Route	Onset (Duration)	Mode of Action	Comments
I. Calcium gluconate, 10% (100 mg/ml)	20 mg/kg i.v. over 5 min. May repeat ×2	Immediate (30–60 min)	Counteracts electrophysiologic effects of hyperkalemia	Monitor ECG for bradycardia; stop infusion if heart rate <100.
II. Sodium bicarbonate, 7.5% (1 mEq/ml)	1–2 mEq/kg i.v. bolus or infusion over 20 min	20 min (1–4 hr)	Causes movement of K into cells	Assure adequate ventilation; do not administer simultaneously with calcium gluconate; will precipitate
Glucose +	1–2 g/kg (5–10 ml of 20% dextrose)	15–30 min (3–6 hr)	Same	
Insulin	0.3 unit/g glucose; administer by infusion together over 2 hr			Monitor blood glucose
III. Sodium polystyrene sulfonate (Kayexalate)	1 g/kg p.o. in 70% sorbitol or p.r. in 30% sorbitol every 6 hr		Removal of K from body	Removes 1 mEq Kg resin; 1 g resin = 4.1 mEq Na; watch for volume overload due to NA; do not administer with Mg- or Al-containing antacids, since it may cause obstipation
IV. Dialysis				Do not ignore I, II, and III while preparing for IV

that raises the level of ionized calicum. Caution, therefore, must be exercised in the correction of acidosis, as an abrupt rise in pH can precipitate a rapid fall in the level of ionized calcium with the onset of tetany, laryngospasm, or seizures. In the absence of frank tetany, exogenous calcium should not be administered, because in the presence of high serum phosphate, it could result in calcium deposits in the kidney with worsening tubular obstruction which would exacerbate pre-existing renal failure. Instead, treatment should be directed at lowering serum phosphorus concentration by decreasing phosphorus intake and by use of phosphate-binding agents such as calcium carbonate or calcium lactate. The past practice of using aluminum hydroxide has been abandoned due to the problem of aluminum intoxication which has already been described in infants with renal failure.

Dialysis

Indications for adding dialysis to the medical management outlined above include:

1. Volume overload with evidence of pulmonary edema or hypertension, which is refractory to pharmacologic therapy, or in the setting of impaired myocardial function after cardiopulmonary bypass
2. Hyperkalemia of >6.0 mEq/l, if hypercatabolic, or >6.5 mEq/l despite conservative measures
3. Metabolic acidosis with a pH of <7.20 or a HCO_3 of <10.
4. BUN of >150, or lower if rising rapidly
5. Neurologic symptoms secondary to uremia or electrolyte imbalance
6. Calcium/phosphorus imbalance—hypocalcemia with tetany or seizures in the presence of a very high serum phosphate

Some authors have reported improved survival and recovery of renal function by utilizing very early peritoneal dialysis in the setting of anuria in postoperative cardiac patients, attributing the improved outcome to prevention of hyperkalemia and volume overload which may further compromise a myocardium functioning precariously with maximal inotropic support. The deaths in these series were all due to intractable myocardial failure in patients with complex cardiac anomalies.

Acute dialysis is less likely to be necessary in the setting of intrinsic renal disease due to acute glomerulonephritis, as BUN and creatinine rise more slowly in the absence of increased catabolism. Conservative management of fluid and electrolyte status is more likely to be adequate in this setting than in hypercatabolic states due to burns, trauma, sepsis, or surgery. In primary renal disease, however, dialysis may be necessary to reduce fluid overload, to reduce hypertension, and to sustain the patient through the acute phase of the disease. Some intrinsic renal diseases such as HUS may benefit from early dialysis despite failure to meet the above criteria, but this is controversial.

In obstructive nephropathy associated with renal failure, if volume overload precludes the correction of severe acidosis prior to surgery or if hyperkalemia is present, dialysis may be indicated prior to surgery, after which it may no longer be needed. Careful fluid and electrolyte management to compensate for postobstructive diuresis in the postoperative period is essential to avoid dehydration and any further renal compromise due to hypovolemia.

Peritoneal Dialysis

The principle upon which peritoneal dialysis is based is that the peritoneum is a semipermeable membrane across which water and solutes diffuse along their concentration gradients. In adults, peritoneal dialysis is only 20% as efficient as hemodialysis in removing urea from the blood, as the time to achieve equilibrium across the peritoneum generally far exceeds the "dwell" time employed. In children, however, the higher ratio of peritoneal surface area to body mass results in an efficiency 50% as great as hemodialysis, which is sufficient to achieve the desired objective in most situations, with the exception of some poisonings. The efficiency of peritoneal dialysis is greatest in the infant. For a description of the technique of peritoneal dialysis, see pages 1026–1029 in the *Textbook of Pediatric Intensive Care.*

Principles of Hemodialysis

The principles of hemodialysis are basically the same as those of peritoneal dialysis, in that solutes diffuse across a semipermeable membrane from blood to dialysate or from dialysate to blood along their concentration gradients. For example, urea, creatinine, and potassium travel from blood to dialysate and acetate from dialysate to blood, with the latter helping to correct the metabolic acidosis. The rate at which this diffusion occurs is dependent upon the surface area and permeability of the membrane and the rate of blood and dialysate flow. These characteristics are all readily known, and the rate at which urea and water removal occurs can be much more precisely predicted in hemodialysis than in peritoneal dialysis. Elegant mathematical formulae are available to enable calculation of a dialysis prescription for urea clearance in terms of duration and blood flow. These are not easily applied in the situation of ARF, as they assume a steady state of urea generation, metabolic rate, and protein intake. For a full discussion of hemodialysis, see pages 1029–1032 in the *Textbook of Pediatric Intensive Care.*

Nutritional Management of Acute Renal Failure

The goals of nutritional management in ARF are (a) to control water and electrolyte intake to avoid fluid overload and electrolyte imbalance as described previously, and (b) to provide adequate calories to maintain body protein stores as near normal as possible while restricting protein intake, to minimize azotemia and the accumulation of the byproducts of catabolism that lead to acidema and hyperkalemia. Meeting these goals is more difficult in patients with acute, as opposed to chronic, renal failure because of low or absent urine output and the high frequency of hypercatabolic states in the clinical situations that predispose to ARF versus the usually normal metabolic demand in patients with chronic renal failure. In addition, loss of renal function in ARF occurs so suddenly that little adaptation is possible.

Caloric and Protein Supplementation

Patients with ARF who are catabolic have a high rate of accumulation of potassium, phosphate, and urea and therefore might need dialysis sooner. It has clearly been shown that calories supplied in the form of carbohydrates, fat and amino acids, sparing the breakdown of endogenous proteins, is effective in reducing the rate of rise of urea, creatinine, and potassium levels, thereby delaying the need for dialysis and making it necessary less often.

In patients with functioning GI tracts who can be fed by mouth or nasograstic tube, part or all of nutrient intake can be given via this route, eliminating the risk of infection attendant upon the use of hyperalimentation lines. Frequent small feedings are better than infrequent large feedings to avoid large swings in blood glucose levels. In oral as well as intravenous alimentation, fluid intake should be minimal to avoid fluid overload and hyponatremia. Carbohydrate intake should be approximately 3–5 g/kg/day and can be given as food supplemented with hard candies. Tube-fed patients may receive glucose polymers such as Polycose, which contains 3.8 cal/ml. Commonly available amino acid mixtures such as Aminaid may be used. Further caloric supplementation can be given in the form of fat, such as medium-chain triglycerides added to food or in tube feedings.

Parenteral nutrition is often necessary in patients with ARF because of the nature of their underlying illness or because ARF itself can cause anorexia, nausea, and vomiting. In addition, patients on peritoneal dialysis often cannot tolerate feeding due to increased intra-abdominal pressure. Peripheral hyperalimentation can supply carbohydrates as 5–10% dextrose, fat as 10–20% lipid, and protein as amino acids, but the amount of calories supplied may be insufficient to prevent endogenous protein breakdown, due to constraints on the volume that can be administered. If early recovery is anticipated and the patient does not have increased caloric requirements due to hypercatabolic nature of the underlying disease, central hyperalimentation should be avoided because of the risk of catheter-related sepsis.

In patients who are hypercatabolic and have need for increased caloric supplementation, central hyperalimentation is essential not only for protein sparing but also to allow for tissue repair of the underlying insult. The administration of hypertonic glucose solutions often leads to hyperglycemia and requires careful monitoring of blood sugar status. Administration of insulin may be necessary to avoid ketoacidosis. Special care should be taken with vitamin C, since it is metabolized to oxalate which can be deposited in the kidney.

HYPERTENSION IN ACUTE RENAL FAILURE

Hypertension is a common concomitant of ARF. Its occurrence may be due to volume overload, especially in patients with primary parenchymal renal disease as a cause for the renal failure. Alteration in the renin-angiotensin system and autonomic neuropathy also result in vasomotor instability. The generally used approach to hypertension in the patient with ARF is briefly discussed below.

Moderate hypertension in patients with ARF can usually be controlled via careful fluid management as previously outlined. Furosemide may be efficacious in initiating a diuresis that may relieve fluid overload. Mannitol should be avoided in patients with oliguria and hypertension due to obvious fluid overload, as inability to excrete the mannitol and failure to initiate a diuresis may result in further expansion of the vascular volume with the precipitation of congestive heart failure and pulmonary edema. If diuresis cannot be provoked and significant hypertension persists despite fluid restriction, management sould progress to the use of parenteral medications which have the advantage of being both predictable in their onset and duration of action and titratable to their effect on blood pressure.

Rapidly acting parenteral agents efficacious in the management of hypertension in patients with ARF are diazoxide, sodium nitroprusside, and trimethaphan. The choice is, in part, determined by the monitoring capabilities available. Diazoxide is a nondiuretic thiazide with direct arterial vasodilating effects. Diazoxide may be the safest drug to use in the emergency situation in which intra-arterial monitoring is not available, as the time of peak effect is 5 minutes after administration with a duration of action of 4–12 hours, which allows time for invasive monitoring and other drugs to be instituted. The standard method for administering diazoxide is a dose of 5 mg/kg injected rapidly as an intravenous bolus. Rapid bolus injection is necessary because the drug is highly protein bound, with only the free drug being active. This may be repeated in 30–60 minutes if the first dose is only partially effective. An alternative method of administration consists of "mini-dose" boluses of 1–2 mg/kg every 5 minutes until the desired effect is achieved or a maximum of 300 mg is reached, but this may not be as effective as a larger single bolus, due to the protein binding. Diazoxide can exacerbate sodium and water retention and should be used in combination with furosemide. In addition, diazoxide can result in reflex sympathetic stimulation, causing an elevation of heart rate with increased cardiac work, which may be undesirable in children who have undergone cardiac surgery. Trimethaphan, a ganglionic blocker, and sodium nitroprusside, a direct-acting vasodilator, are both potent and rapidly acting and mandate the use of continuous intra-arterial pressure monitoring to facilitate titration of the drug to its effect. Trimethaphan is more variable in its onset with a possibly greater lag between change in dose and blood pressure response. In addition, as it is a ganglionic blocker, it may result in urinary retention which is most undesirable in the setting of ARF. It is rarely used in pediatrics.

Sodium nitroprusside has the advantage of being immediately effective. For greatest reliability and safety of administration, an infusion pump is mandatory. The drug is titratable to effect, which ceases within 1–2 minutes of discontinuation of the infusion. Sodium nitroprusside may be preferable to diazoxide in the setting of volume overload and/or myocardial compromise because of its venodilation properties with reduction in preload in addition to arterial dilatation.

Nitroprusside is inactivated by the liver and kidney enzyme, rhodanese, through the transfer of the cyanide ion to the sulfur donor, thiosulfate, to form thiocyanate. The rate of detoxification is contingent on thiosulfate availability. Lower cyanide levels can be achieved by infusing exogenous thiosulfate, although there are no reports of its use in children. Nitroprusside toxicity is associated with prolonged infusion or infusion rates of > 10 μg/kg/min. Actually, thiocyanate toxicity is more common than cyanide toxicity and is manifested by nausea, sedation, irritability, dizziness, and tinnitus, which may be seen when thiocyanate levels exceed 10 mg/dl.

Hydralazine may be used intramuscularly or intravenously as a first-line agent in moderately severe hypertension, or it may be started as the patient is weaned from nitroprusside. It is not as satisfactory as an initial agent, as its onset is slow (10–20 minutes). The reflex tachycardia that occurs with hydralazine as well as nitroprusside partially compensates to maintain the blood pressure and usually requires the addition of a β-adrenergic blocker such as propranolol, which initially may be given intravenously and later orally. The β-adrenergic blocker is also beneficial, in that it blocks the production of renin and, therefore, aldosterone release, in addition to lowering heart rate. Its use is not recommended in patients whose cardiac output is marginal or who are requiring inotropic agents to maintain output. The new β-adrenergic blocker, labetalol, may prove most useful in the treatment of pediatric patients with hypertension and ARF, as this drug has, in addition, a vasodilating effect due to α-adrenergic blockade.

It was initially thought that only patients with elevated plasma renin levels would benefit from the angiotensin-converting enzyme inhibitors, such as captopril therapy. It is true that the magnitude of the initial response is greater if the plasma renin activity is high, but with continued administration, patients (including children) with normal or even low renin levels respond equally well.

The most distressing side effect of captopril reported has been the deterioration of renal function, even to the point of oliguric renal failure in both adults and children with pre-existing compromised renal blood flow due to renal artery stenosis, either bilateral or in a solitary native or transplanted kidney, or associated with hypovolemia or sodium depletion.

The effect of captopril on renal function in these situations of compromised renal blood flow does not represent drug "toxicity" but rather is the predictable hemodynamic consequence of captropril's interference with the physiologic mechanism for sustaining glomerular filtration in the face of fixed reduction of perfusion pressure.

As a result, the dose of captopril should be started at a low level and increased slowly. This is especially important in neonates who are very sensitive to very low doses and who may have decreased clearance of the drug. As the drug is excreted only by the kidney, a lower maximum dose should be used in cases of renal insufficiency. Doses may be as high as 4 mg/kg/day when creatinine clearance is near normal, but they may be as low as 0.5 mg/kg/day when creatine clearance is below 10.

SPECIAL CONSIDERATIONS IN THE PATHOPHYSIOLOGY AND TREATMENT OF HEMOLYTIC-UREMIC SYNDROME

HUS is the occurrence of hemolytic anemia, thrombocytopenia, and renal failure. It commonly occurs following gastroenteritis, due to either viral agents or *Shigella*. In some parts of the world (India, Argentina), HUS is endemic and is the most common cause of renal failure in infants. In other areas, the disease is sporadic and a less common cause of renal failure.

Early thinking about the pathophysiology of HUS related to the presence of microthrombi in renal vessels, with a peripheral blood picture resembling disseminated intravascular coagulation (DIC). This suggested to some investigators the possible etiologic role for endotoxin, producing a Shwartzman-like reaction in the renal microcirculation, leading to decreased glomerular perfusion and ARF. The proposed mechanism entailed infectious damage to vascular endothelium with the initiation of fibrin deposition, trapping of platelets, and mechanical fragmentation of erthrocytes with resultant obstruction of renal vessels and renal failure. Although many clinical studies have failed to demonstrate endotoxin in patients with HUS, a prospective study of patients with shigellosis demonstrated by use of the limulus test the presence of endotoxin prior to the onset of hemolysis in one-half of the children who subsequently developed hemolysis. Not all of these children developed frank renal failure, although all had some elevation in urea nitrogen and creatinine. Very few patients without hemolysis had positive limulus tests. To explain the failure of other investigators to detect the presence of endotoxin, the authors proposed that endotoxin was only intermittently released or quickly cleared by the liver. The possible role of a DIC-like syndrome in the pathogenesis of HUS led in the early 1970s to the therapeutic use of various anticoagulants, such as streptokinase and heparin, or antiplatelet agents, such as aspirin and dipyridamole. Use of these agents did not result in improved outcome and, in the case of heparin, was associated with a possibly increased incidence of hemorrhagic complications. In light of increased morbidity with no clear efficacy, the use of these agents declined. Currently accepted management is conservative and supportive, as described previously for renal failure of any etiology, with dialysis performed for indications discussed earlier. This management has produced fairly good outcomes with regard to mortality and recovery of renal function. About half of patients require dialysis, most commonly peritoneal. Long-term sequelae are infrequent and consist of hypertension, chronic renal failure, and neurologic sequelae.

Seizures, when they occur in patients with HUS, may be related to hyponatremia associated with volume overload, hypertension, uremia, or fluid shifts related to dialysis. In some cases of HUS, CNS disturbance and/or seizures may be caused by vascular lesions similar to those seen in the kidney. If focal neurologic findings persist, a computed tomography scan should be performed, to look for cerebral infarction. It is becoming more widely recognized that microangiopathic changes in HUS may not be confined to the kidney; the clinician should be alert for signs of myocardial or CNS involvement or the occurrence of mesenteric thrombosis. The outcome and long-term morbidity of endemic HUS may be worse than the sporadic form, as is demonstrated in a series from Argentina.

HUS has much in common with thrombotic thrombocytopenic purpura (TTP), and similar pathogenesis is likely. TTP occurs more often in adults, and HUS occurs more often in children, but crossover does occur. The two syndromes differ mainly in the extent and distribution of thrombotic lesions, with HUS involving primarily the kidney and TTP involving many organs, including the brain. Some authors have struggled with the differential diagnosis of HUS versus TTP in children with significant neurologic involvement unresponsive to dialysis alone and therefore not explained solely by uremia or electrolyte abnormalities. It is probably not necessary to definitely label a child as having TTP rather than HUS, although plasma exchange has been more often successful in patients with TTP than in those with HUS. The presence of encephalopathy unresponsive to correction of uremia and electrolyte abnormalities by dialysis is a possible indication for trying plasma exchange.

Although the role of endotoxin in HUS seems plausible in terms of the infectious antecedents and the pathologic similarities to DIC, there is a significant difference between the two, in that in HUS, platelet consumption is increased without corresponding increase in fibrinogen turnover or coagulopathy. In addition, a study in animals showed increased rather than decreased vascular prostacyclin activity following the administration of endotoxin. In recent years, attention has been directed away from endotoxin and toward the role of prostaglandins in the pathogenesis of HUS, as patients with this syndrome have been shown to lack a plasma factor that stimulates prostaglandin I_2 (PGI$_2$) activity. PGI$_2$ is a potent vasodilator.

The platelet antiaggregatory effect of PGI$_2$ is probably mediated by an increase of cyclic adenosine monophosphate (AMP) levels within the platelets. Increased cyclic AMP results in immobilization of calcium ions, the release of which is essential for platelet aggregation. Deficiency in PGI$_2$ in the setting of endothelial damage could therefore allow the formation of platelet thrombi. Some authors suggest that the patients who develop HUS and TTP may have a underlying defect in PGI$_2$-stimulating activity and are therefore unable to respond to the vascular endothelial damage by increasing PGI$_2$ synthesis. This theory is bolstered by the occurrence of some familial cases of HUS in whom PGI$_2$-stimulating activity was persistently low. This, however, has certainly not been found in all cases.

The clues regarding prostacyclin-stimulating factor deficiency have led to experimental use of plasma exchange and/or plasma infusion for this syndrome. The efficacy of these new modes of therpay has yet to be shown, as no controlled studies have been done.

Aspirin and dipyridamole are drugs that interact with platelet prostaglandin production and thus affect platelet aggregation. Dipyridamole has an antithrombotic effect that occurs via inhibition of phosphodiesterase, which results in delayed degradation of cyclic AMP. Aspirin prevents platelet aggregation by irreversible inhibition of platelet cyclo-oxygenase which normally is involved in the formation of the potent aggregatory prostaglandin, thromboxane A_2. In humans, a single dose of 325 mg aspirin decreases platelet cyclo-oxygenase activity by nearly 90%, and this inhibition persists for 48 hours. Aspirin at low doses (5 mg/kg) potentiates the action of dipyridamole by inhibiting platelet cyclo-oxygenase, but at high doses aspirin also inhibits vessel wall prostacyclin synthesis and, via resultant decreased levels of PGI_2, increased cyclic AMP level.

In adults with HUS it was found that a large dose of aspirin (1200 mg/day) increased the platelet count, whereas decreasing the dose to 300 mg/day was associated with a decline in the platelet count. This has not been duplicatable in children. These findings indicate that there may be more than a single mechanism leading to PGI_2 deficiency involved in the pathogenesis of HUS.

As a result of experimental studies, it has been speculated that there is an imbalance between plasma oxidants and antioxidants in HUS. Increased lipid peroxidation with decreased levels of antioxidants (e.g., α-tocopherol) could, itself, inhibit PGI_2 synthetase, and in the presence of a trigger for endothelial damage (e.g., endotoxin) the balance between the thromboxane and prostacyclin pathways of arachidonic acid metabolism would be upset in favor of thromboxane synthesis, resulting in increased platelet aggregation. Illnesses such as HUS and TTP may occur because of such a trigger and/or the presence of either a congenital or acquired decrease in antioxidant activity.

Parenthetically, it is fascinating that in patients with axotemia due to chronic renal failure the opposite imbalance of platelet-vascular prostaglandin synthesis occurs. These patients have prolonged bleeding times due to decreased platelet aggregation, and this seems to be due to a plasma factor that inhibits platelet thromboxane A_2 production while augmenting vascular PGI_2 production.

The response to plasmapheresis or plasma infusion (usual dose of 30 ml/kg the first day, followed by 15 ml/kg daily thereafter) in reported studies has often been dramatic with respect to the normalization of platelet counts, but the improvement in renal function is not as rapid and may not occur at all. Choice between plasmapheresis and plasma infusion may depend on level of renal function and volume status as the volume of plasma used may precipitate volume overload, hypertension, and/or congestive heart failure if not combined with fluid removal by dialysis. Actually, it has been reported that plasma infusion was associated with a reduction in blood pressure, allowing antihypertensive therapy to be reduced.

HUS is a syndrome of diverse etiologies, not a single disease. It may not be true that there is a single pathogenesis and, therefore, a single optimal therapy for HUS. Deficiency of a factor that stimulates PGI_2 activity has been present in some, but not all, patients. Other mechanisms, which have not been looked for in all patients, may be operative, such as the presence of an inhibitor of PGI_2 activity, increased degradation of PGI_2, or deficiency of PGI_2-stabilizing factor. Meticulous supportive management is of primary importance no matter what the etiology ultimately found. Further controlled studies are necessary to establish whether plasma infusion or exchange truly alter the course of the disease. At the present time the methods for identifying deficiency of PGI_2 activity are too complex and unavailable to guide day-to-day management decisions.

CONCLUSION

ARF occurs as a result of diverse etiologies in the critical care setting, but the management is fairly uniform no matter what the etiology. It is evident that despite the large number of elegant experimental models, the pathophysiologic mechanisms of ARF remain controversial.

Despite the recent advances in dialysis for children and even neonates and despite the increasing sophistication in monitoring and treatment, ARF as a complication of other illnesses can lead to increased morbidity and mortality. Indeed, in the ICU, ARF is probably better prevented than treated. Prevention involves awareness of clinical situations that place patients at high risk for the development of renal failure, such as trauma, sepsis, and cardiac surgery. In these situations, it is mandatory to meticulously avoid the accumulation of multiple insults that, when added to the primary problem, make renal failure more likely. Precautions should be taken to avoid hypovolemia and hypotension, maintain cardiac output, and limit exposure to nephrotoxic drugs and vasoconstrictors. Careful attention to such details, especially maintenance of adequate intravascular volume and solute diuresis, has reduced the incidence of renal failure in adults after cardiovascular surgery and X-ray contrast studies and should be of benefit in children at risk.

CHAPTER 21

Diabetic Ketoacidosis

Diabetic ketoacidosis (DKA) is certainly among the most frequently discussed, if not the most frequently seen, metabolic disorders in intensive care units (ICUs). Despite advancing knowledge on the pathophysiology and treatment of diabetes mellitus, DKA remains a significant source of morbidity and mortality in all age groups.

PATHOPHYSIOLOGY—INSULIN

Glucose metabolism is the result of a complex interaction of a number of factors, including glucagon, cortisol, growth hormone, and insulin (Fig. 21.1). Diabetes mellitus arises from inadequate insulin effects and, in pediatrics, almost always from inadequate amounts of insulin. Insulin must be considered in terms of both its facilitative and inhibitory effects. Insulin stimulates anabolism and, therefore, the storage of glycogen, protein, and fat in muscle, liver, and adipose tissue. Conversely, it inhibits glycogenolysis, gluconeogenesis, proteolysis, lipolysis, and ketogenesis.

In the liver, with a falling insulin/glucagon ratio, there is increased hepatic gluconeogenesis from pyruvate. Additional glucose is released through unimpeded glycogenolysis.

In muscle, insulin accomplishes three essential anabolic functions. First, it enhances cellular entry of glucose. Second, it promotes glycogen synthesis. Third, it promotes amino acid transport and protein synthesis. In diabetes, these processes are impaired.

In fat, insulin inhibits intracellular lipolysis, enhances lipoprotein cleavage to allow fat absorption, and enhances glucose entry to provide for production of glycerol in order to form triglycerides. With insulin lack, lipolysis continues unabated, and reciprocal fat absorption and triglyceride synthesis are blocked.

CAUSES OF ACIDOSIS

Depressed insulin levels permit lipolysis to accelerate in adipose tissue, releasing long-chain fatty acids. In the liver, these fatty acids are shunted toward β-oxidation and ketone production rather than transported out as

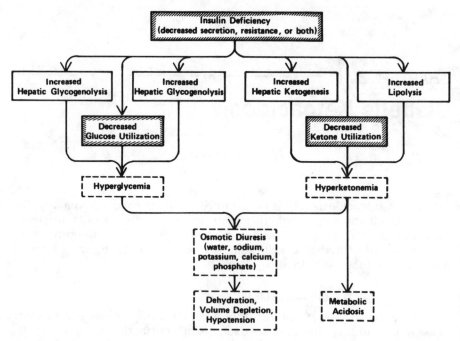

FIGURE 21.1. Physiologic consequences of insulin deficiency. (From Barrett EJ, DeFronzo RA: Diabetic ketoacidosis: Diagnosis and treatment. *Hosp Pract* p. 89, 1984.)

triglycerides; this path is determined by the increased glucagon/insulin ratio. Ketones normally stimulate insulin release and thereby inhibit lipolysis—the lack of this feedback permits extreme lipemia and ketonemia and prevents triglyceride synthesis in adipose tissue.

The commonly used tests for serum ketones employ the nitroprusside reaction, which reflects acetoacetate levels as well as acetone less well (about 20 moles of acetone react the same as 1 mole of acetoacetate). β-Hydroxybutyrate does not react at all. This fact is key in knowing how loosely to interpret the reported "ketone levels," since the relative proportions of the three compounds may vary greatly, influenced by acid-base and redox states.

Lactic Acid

Lactic acidosis in DKA may rise, in part, from anaerobic glycolysis in hypoperfused tissues during hypovolemia caused by osmotic diuresis. This anaerobic state increases the ratio of NADH to NAD, favoring the formation of lactate as the hydroxy acid of pyruvate. Likewise, a greater proportion of acetoacetate is converted to its hydroxy acid, β-hydroxybutyrate. Measuring lactate and acetoacetate gives a crude indication of the relative proportions of ketoacids.

FLUID AND ELECTROLYTE CHANGES

Hyperosmolality

The hyperosmolar state induced by insulin deficiency is responsible for at least as much physiologic mischief as is the ketoacidosis (Fig. 21.1). The osmolality can be estimated by the well-known formula:

$$\text{Osmolality} = [\text{Glucose (mg/dl)}]/18$$
$$+ [\text{SUN (mg/dl)}]/2.8$$
$$+ 2([\text{Na] (mEq/1l)} + [\text{K] (mEq/l)})$$

Thus, both hyperglycemia and dehydration contribute to the hyperosmolality. In fact, the values generally reported suggest that in a typical child with DKA, glucose is elevated by about 400 mg/dl, and serum urea nitrogen (SUN) is elevated by about 15 mg/dl, therefore contributing about 22 and 5 mOsm/l, respectively. The volume of fluid loss for this typical child in DKA represents 15% of body weight. The fluid loss is, of course, due to the osmotic diuresis induced by glucose.

Alterations in Sodium, Chloride, and Water

Chloride is retained in exchange for ketone salts, especially in patients maintaining large volumes of fluid and salt intake during the development of DKA. The resultant hyperchloremia may be worsened, prolonging recovery from acidosis, if normal saline is used in large volumes during resuscitation. A good solution for this problem should be one containing a small portion (10–30%) of the sodium as bicarbonate. The currently common practice of supplying potassium as a 50/50 mixture of chloride and phosphate salts should also be of benefit in this regard.

Hyponatremia is usually reported by the laboratory when sera from DKA patients are analyzed, and quite commonly the reportedly low value is an artifact. Extreme lipemia can decrease the measured sodium value simply by decreasing the aqueous phase of blood, in which sodium is found.

Alterations in Potassium

Hyperkalemia is commonly found at presentation with DKA and is commonly presumed to have occurred as a consequence of the elevated extracellular hydrogen ions being exchanged for the major intracellular cation, potassium. According to the theory, the protons from the increased amount of ketoacids travel down their concentration gradient into the intracellular fluid (ICF). This then alters the transmembrane electrical potential, to favor release of cations from the ICF. Potassium, as the major ICF cation, moves down this electrical gradient into the extracellular fluid (ECF). This theory has been challenged, but the importance of the hyperkalemia remains.

Alterations in Phosphate, Calcium, and Magnesium

Profound hypophosphatemia, presumably due to osmotic diuresis, and depressed levels of red blood cell 2,3-diphosphoglycerate have been described in DKA. Clearly, in the treatment of DKA, exuberant replacement of phosphate can result in astonishingly depressed serum levels of calcium and magnesium. As a result, there has been some controversy over phosphorus replacement. In the treatment of DKA with calcium, phosphorus, and magnesium, the consensus would seem to be that phosphate replacement is of theoretical, if unproved, benefit. Its use must be approached with caution, and careful monitoring of calcium and magnesium levels is warranted. The chief advantage to using potassium phosphate may be in helping to avoid hyperchloremic acidosis during therapy.

CLINICAL PRESENTATION

DKA is present when a child presents with a serum glucose concentration above 300 mg%, a positive nitroprusside (Acetest) reaction at 1:2 dilutions or greater, a blood pH below 7.3, and a serum bicarbonate below 15 mEq/l. Approximately 30% of newly diabetic children will present with DKA, and 10% of patients with DKA are admitted in a comatose state. The mortality rate for patients with DKA is about 9% for all ages (chiefly the elderly). About 75 deaths from DKA occur per year per 100,000 diabetics under age 15 in the United States.

The child with DKA presents often with the history familiar to every medical student, that of polyuria, polydipsia, polyphagia, and weight loss. These signs are followed by headache, bellyache, vomiting, lethargy, and hyperpnea. The physician's first moment of contact is sufficient to reveal an acutely and gravely ill child with lethargy, dehydration, hyperpnea, and (assuming intact olfactory capabilities on the part of the physician) the smell of acetone on the child's breath.

If the history is vague or unavailable, and the child is unresponsive, immediate differential is quite broad and includes intoxications (especially salicylates and alcohols), Reye syndrome, inborn errors of metabolism, sepsis, meningoencephalitis, and of course, DKA, nonketotic hyperglycemic coma, or hypoglycemia coma.

MANIFESTATIONS REQUIRING INTENSIVE CARE

The child with DKA who arrives in the emergency room (ER) with a clear sensorium and good peripheral circulation is likely to have a gratifyingly smooth course of therapy and may not require admission to the pediatric ICU following stabilization in the ER. However, the presence of shock, dysrhythmias, or coma indicates a need for prompt admission to the pediatric ICU.

Cerebral Edema

Central nervous system (CNS) changes seen in DKA really consist of two clinically distinct patterns. The first is the very uncommon progressive cerebral edema seen generally during treatment for DKA. The second is the altered sensorium seen commonly in DKA and loosely characterized as diabetic coma. Diabetic coma has been amply described as correlating with serum osmolality better than with any other blood chemistry value. This state would seem to differ little from the clouding of consciousness seen in other hyperosmolar states. Serial electroencephalograms have been seen to track both the level of consciousness and the hyperosmolality. There is considerable individual variation, however, in some patients with DKA retaining consciousness despite serum osmolalities in excess of 350 mOsm/l. It is not clear what the mechanisms are for production of altered consciousness in the diabetic hyperosmolar state.

On rare occasion, the treatment of DKA may be accompanied by progressively deepening coma and death due to cerebral edema. This unusual course of events has been well recognized for many years. Retrospective clinical reviews have failed to characterize any typical patterns of biochemical findings at presentation of therapies, or of biochemical changes during therapy, such as would allow prediction and prevention of this calamitous problem. Deepening coma during treatment for DKA does appear to be more likely to occur in the pediatric diabetic and is almost always fatal.

In addition, nonfatal elevation of cerebrospinal fluid (CSF) pressure has been seen. In the first several hours of standard therapy, CSF pressure rises during isotonic saline rehydration from acute hyperglycemic hyperosmotic diuresis, and cerebral edema follows acute hyperglycemia corrected by insulin (but not by dialysis), without rehydration.

In the literature, the indications for and against lumbar puncture and monitoring in DKA are unclear but should be carefully considered in each case. In the child, especially the infant, with DKA who presents with fever and a clouded sensorium, concerns should always be raised about sepsis or meningoencephalitis. This then begs the question of whether a lumbar puncture should be performed. The indication would be to prove the existence of infected CSF before antimicrobial therapy is initiated. The contraindications are twofold. First, positioning the child with pre-existing shock and acidosis for lumbar puncture embarrasses both chest excursion and venous return to the heart. Second, the child might well have significant cerebral edema, such that a sudden withdrawal of lumbar CSF could produce downward herniation of the intracranial contents. For these reasons, in the case of a child with DKA in whom meningoencephalitis is considered likely, antibiotics should be given during the initial resuscitation. Lumbar puncture later, if still deemed important, could produce Gram stain or antigenic evidence of the more common bacterial infections.

Intracranial pressure (ICP) monitoring need not be instituted for every child with DKA who presents in coma. In the vast majority, the sensorium will clear with correction of the metabolic abnormalities. If coma is deep enough to warrant intubation (Glasgow coma score of ≤7), preparation should begin for ICP monitoring. Once the hyperglycemia is being corrected, if the patient's neurologic status worsens or fails to improve in the first few hours, computed axial tomography scanning and ICP monitoring need to be done.

Pulmonary Edema

Another decidedly unusual finding in DKA, possibly in part related to osmolality changes, is pulmonary edema. The observation of increasing oxygen requirements with or without radiographic changes consistent with pulmonary edema has been made by several authors. Abundant theories are available as explanations, including myocardial failure, low plasma oncotic pressure, increased pulmonary capillar permeability, and neurogenic pulmonary edema with raised ICP.

Cardiac Dysrhythmias

Life-threatening disturbances in cardiac rhythm can be caused by hyperkalemia, hypokalemia, or hypocalcemia, and since these electrolyte changes are all seen in patients being treated for DKA, such patients should be considered at risk for fatal cardiac dysrhythmia. On admission of the child with DKA to the ER, an electrocardiographic monitor should be applied and continued until the child is clearly responding to therapy, with normalizing blood chemistries and neurologic status. Early in the course of treatment, an electrocardiogram (ECG) may provide the earliest evidence of hyperkalemia (T waves are large), before any laboratory could provide the serum potassium level (Fig. 21.2). In our experience, lead II provides

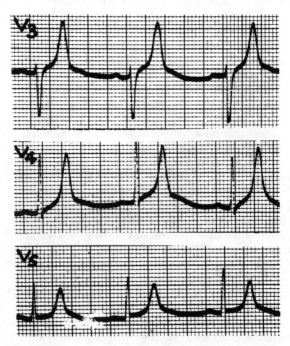

FIGURE 21.2. ECG in hyperkalemia. Note the tall peaked T waves. (From Marriott HJL: *Practical Electocardiography*, ed 7. Baltimore, Williams & Wilkins, 1983, p 469.)

reliable information in patients of all ages, whereas in infants the precordial leads may be misleading.

MANAGEMENT

The physician directs the care for the critically ill child with DKA most effectively when he or she has a clear set of priorities forming the framework for the therapeutic plans. In descending order of importance, these priorities are: (a) establishment of the airway, breathing, and circulation (ABCs), (b) consideration of differential diagnosis, (c) provision of insulin, (d) fine tuning of the biochemistry, and (e) care to avoid complications of therapy. This rationale for care is outlined in Table 21.1.

As with any gravely ill child, the first priorities lie in making certain that the airway and breathing are adequate. If the child is comatose (Glasgow coma score of <8), the trachea is intubated to prevent aspiration and in anticipation of possible respiratory failure. Barbiturates and opiates (other than fentanyl) produce hypotension in these hypovolemic patients and are not used as adjuncts in intubation. Fentanyl ($5\mu g/kg$ intravenously) and lidocaine (1.5 mg/kg intravenously) are reasonable alternatives, if indicated. Since cerebral edema and raised ICP are probably not issues before insulin and fluid resuscitation are begun, ketamine (1.0 mg/kg intravenously) may also be useful, if indicated. In most cases, the drugs of choice for intubating the comatose child in DKA are atropine (0.01 mg/kg intravenously), pancuronium bromide in a defasciculating dose (0.01 mg/kg intravenously) and succinylcholine (1 mg/kg intravenously). There are two reasons for the defasciculating dose of pancuronium to be of special importance in the child with DKA. First, since succinylcholine is known to elevate serum potassium and is purported to raise ICP, its use must be approached warily in a disorder such as DKA, where hyperkalemia (at presentation) and intracranial hypertension (after initial resuscitative measures) are already potentially grave problems. Pancuronium at a dose of 0.01 mg/kg reduces some of the membrane effects of succinylcholine and should reduce the risks inherent in its use in the patient with DKA. Pancuronium may not be needed before use of succinylcholine in infants and toddlers, as fasciculations are not likely in these age groups.

Next, needs for effective circulating blood volume and (in view of the differential diagnosis list) for glucose should be met. A large-bore intravenous catheter is inserted quickly and by whatever route is most expeditious for the given institution and clinical situation. For the child in shock, normal saline or Ringer's lactate (both readily available and isotonic) is started immediately, with volumes of 20 ml/kg being administered as rapidly as possible, and as often as necessary, until blood pressure, heart rate, and evidence of perfusion begin to return to normal. With the initial venipuncture, blood is withdrawn for blood count, glucose, SUN, electrolytes, calcium, magnesium, phosphate, ketones, lactate, osmolality, PCO_2, and pH, and a few drops are withdrawn for a reagent-strip glucose determination and a capillary-tube hematocrit (this last will not only produce a rapid clue to hemoconcentration but will also allow gross examination for li-

TABLE 21.1. _____
Initial Treatment for Suspected DKA

Goal	Time	Approach
1. ABCs	First minutes	Intubate if patient is comatose and assure adequate breathing and circulation
2. Differential diagnosis and begin monitoring	First minutes	*Brief* history Venipuncture (large bore i.v.) and complete blood count, SUN, glucose, electrolytes, osmolality, ketones, pH, PCO_2, Ca^{2+}, Mg^{2+}, PO_4, Chemstrip, and spun hematocrit Give dextrose (0.5 g/kg i.v.) and ECG—monitor rhythm strip (check T waves)
3. Volume repletion	First minutes	Assess blood pressure, heart rate, and skin perfusion Give 20 ml normal saline or LRS per kilogram repeatedly p.r.n. to reverse shock
4. Reverse hyperglycemia and ketosis	After no. 2 is in progress	Give regular insulin at 0.1 unit/kg/hr i.v.
5. Fine-tune biochemistry	After nos. 2 and 3 are in progress	Change volume replacement to 0.45% saline with 25 mEq KCl and 20 mEq K_2HPO_4 liter Adjust solution according to monitored ECG, electrolytes, and pH
6. Avoid hypoglycemia	When glucose ≤ 300 mg/dl	Add 5% dextrose to intravenous fluid and reduce insulin infusion to 0.05 μ/kg/hr
7. Avoid excessive bicarbonate	1–2 hours	Remove $NaHCO_3$ from intravenous solutions

pemic serum). Depending on the magnitude of diagnostic dilemma at this point, blood might be sent for toxicology screen, prothrombin time, ammonia, liver enzymes, or culture. One team member changes the initial crystalloid as soon as possible to 0.45% NaCl with, added to each liter, 25 mEq of $Na-HCO_3$, 25 mEq NaCl, 20 mEq KCl, and 20 mEq K_2HPO_4. This is slightly hypertonic (i.e., probably isotonic for the patient in DKA), but potassium and phosphate will enter ICF rapidly, leaving a slightly hypotonic solution with adequate sodium (127 mEq/l) and without excessive chloride (122 mEq/l) so as to reduce the development of hyperchloremic acidosis. The theoretical advantages of this solution over lactated Ringer's solution (LRS) are two. First, for a patient with already-elevated lactate levels, bicarbonate is preferable to lactate as an exogenously supplied base. Second, LRS contains only K^+ at 4 mEq/l and no phosphate and so needs further modification for use in DKA. These advantages may be outweighed in situations were dextrose-free 0.45% NaCl is not readily available, but LRS is. In such situations, of course, LRS with added K^+ might be the better option.

As the initial volume of fluid is infusing, the child is given intravenous dextrose at 0.5 g/kg (2 ml of 25% dextrose in water per kilogram), unless hyperglycemia is certain. There is really no reason to use 50% dextrose in children, given the risks of phlebitis, skin slough, and ischemia (with accidental intra-arterial use) which are magnified by the miniscule vessels available. Also, 50% dextrose in water should always be diluted with an equal volume of water. Concerns about aggravating the hyperosmolar state are not warranted, since the extremely hyperglycemic child might have a serum (glucose) of 1000 mg/dl (10 g/l), throughout an ECF = 0.6 l/kg × body weight, giving him an ECF glucose load of 6 g/kg, so that 0.5 g/kg raises the glucose load by 8% and, hence, total serum osmolality by about 1%. The risk, therefore, is minimal, and the benefit to a hypoglycemic brain may be all-important.

As soon as the hyperglycemia and ketosis are certain, a continuous intravenous infusion of regular insulin is established, at a rate of 0.1 unit/kg/hr, through a separate intravenous line. There has been no evidence to establish the need for an initial bolus of intravenous insulin. When the serum glucose falls to 300 mg/dl, the insulin infusion is reduced by 50%, and 5% dextrose is added to the intravenous fluids. This therapeutic protocol represents the commonly, if not universally, held belief in continuous infusion as the best method of insulin delivery in treating DKA. The continuous infusion has previously been preceded by an intravenous bolus of 0.1 unit/kg, but review and study have failed to demonstrate theoretical or practical need for this protocol, and the intravenous bolus is no longer a universally standard part of intravenous insulin therapy for DKA, although many authors still recommend its use.

After the initial phase of fluid resuscitation in which adequate circulating blood volume is re-established (i.e., shock is reversed), fluid therapy is planned for the ensuing 24 hours. The fluid volume allows for maintenance needs, ongoing losses (vomiting, osmotic diuresis), and correction of the initially estimated deficit. This deficit, generally equal to at least 10% of body weight, will have been partly made up by resuscitation fluids, is 50% corrected within 8–12 hours, and is completely replaced in the next 24 hours. As noted earlier in this chapter, measurements of serum electrolytes are misleading until acidosis, hyperglycemia, and lipemia have cleared.

The use of sodium bicarbonate in the care of the child with DKA remains controversial, largely because the putative benefits and risks remain unproved theories. When acidosis is severe (pH of <7.1), bicarbonate therapy has been proposed to improve myocardial function, reduce the potential for dysrhythmia, diminish insulin resistance, reduce the work of breathing, hasten recovery from coma, and avoid the hyperchloremic state that can prolong acidosis. Stated risks include increased hemoglobin-oxygen affinity (thus risking increased tissue hypoxia), paradoxically increasing CNS acidosis (by more rapid diffusion of CO_2 than HCO_3 across the blood-brain barrier), reducing the ionized fraction of calcium, and producing hypokalemia. None of these concerns (pro or con) has been demonstrated by prospective reproducible study to be of practical significance in children with DKA. Applying the maxim "Primum non nocere" would lead to the conclusion that bicarbonate use would best be reserved for those patients with a pH of <7.2, and this argument would find few detractors. Rapid injection of bicarbonate should be avoided. The preferable means of infusion is probably by inclusion of bicarbonate in the first 2 hours of volume-repleting crystalloid, in a concentration of 25 mEq/l (up to 50 mEq/l in those patients with a pH of <7.0), as described earlier.

Monitoring

Initial laboratory tests may include various tests to exclude diagnoses from the differential list, as noted earlier. The initial tests specifically necessary to begin monitoring the course of therapy for DKA should include blood gases, pH, electrolytes, SUN, glucose, creatinine, osmolality, ketones, lactate, calcium magnesium, and phosphate. Hourly determinations should follow for pH, PCO_2, Na^+, K^+, glucose, and ketones, with the interval lengthened only when stable control has been reached. The full initial panel should be repeated every 4–6 hours during the first 24 hours of treatment.

The ECG should be continuously monitored and displayed. Additionally, a lead II strip should be run and saved hourly at first, to aid in detecting severe alteration in K^+ and Ca^{2+} (Figs. 21.3 and 21.4). Urine output must be carefully followed, and the patient in shock should have a bladder catheter in place. Neurologic status should be assessed at least hourly, and in the obtunded patient, a method of quantitation (such as the Glasgow coma scale) is helpful. Clearly, such a patient requires frequent monitoring of vital signs through the individual attention of a nurse skilled in pediatric intensive care.

TREATMENT IN THE PEDIATRIC INTENSIVE CARE UNIT
Shock

The child with shock from DKA should have continued aggressive fluid therapy as described previously. Careful monitoring is essential, including central venous pressure, arterial pressure, and urinary output. An arterial catheter should be placed in order both to permit continuous measurement of blood pressure and to provide a means for rapid blood sampling for monitoring acid-base, electrolyte, and glucose status. A catheter in the

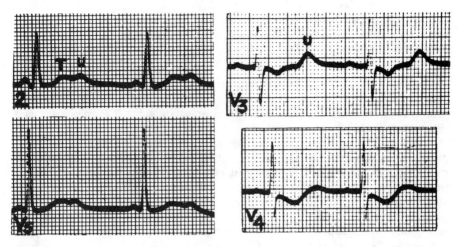

FIGURE 21.3. ECG in hypokalemia. Note the flattened T and the presence of the U wave. (From Marriott HJL: *Practical Electocardiography,* ed 7. Baltimore, Williams & Wilkins, 1983, p 467.)

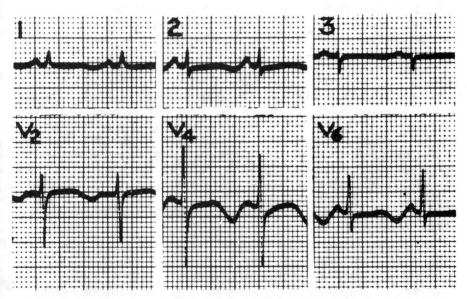

FIGURE 21.4. ECG in hypocalcemia. Note the prolonged Q-T interval. (From Marriott HJL: *Practical Electrocardiography,* ed 7. Baltimore, Williams & Wilkins, 1983, p 468.)

urinary bladder is essential to monitor ongoing losses and to promptly detect renal failure from the antecedent hypoperfused state.

Cerebral Edema

The child with DKA who presents in coma (Glasgow coma score of ≤ 7) cannot adequately protect his or her airway and should be intubated promptly. Preparations should begin immediately for ICP measurement. (Should the child's sensorium begin to clear, the preparations can be aborted, but impending cerebral edema must be assessed and managed promptly.) Computed tomography scanning should precede ICP monitoring, as coma may be due to CNS infarction from hyperviscosity or to other unsuspected intracranial pathology. In all stages, caution is essential to avoid rapid correction of serum hyperosmolality or acidosis, as either event could theoretically potentiate cerebral edema. Once ICP monitoring has been established, the approach to the management of any intracranial hypertension is the same as in other CNS cytotoxic states.

Pulmonary Edema

Pulmonary edema in DKA is rare, but when it occurs, care should be taken to ensure that adequate arterial blood oxygenation continues, to avoid further tissue injury (especially CNS) and prolonged acidosis. Low plasma oncotic pressure should be avoided, and any potential neurogenic cause for pulmonary edema should be promptly treated. The standard blood gas indicators for intubating the patient with acute respiratory failure ($P_aCO_2 > 50$ torr, $S_aO_2 < 90\%$ with $F_IO_2 < 0.60$) are not strictly applicable in DKA. In the face of metabolic acidosis, respiratory failure may occur well before the P_aCO_2 rises to 50 torr; poor cardiac output makes otherwise "borderline" P_aO_2 and S_aO_2 values wholly inadequate for tissue oxygenation; sustained hyperpnea results in fatigued respiratory muscles, and the development of electrolyte disturbances potentiates this; and the patient in deepening coma must have a controlled airway. For these and other reasons, intubation of the child in DKA must be considered early and in anticipation of rapid multisystem failure. If >5 cm H_2O positive end-expiratory pressure is employed, the clinician needs to consider that the cardiac output suffers most from positive end-expiratory pressure in the hypovolemic patient, and the presence of coma, implying elevated ICP, accentuates the importance of this consideration.

Transition from Care in the Pediatric Intensive Care Unit to Ward Care

When acidosis has resolved, mental status is normal, and interest in food has returned, the patient may be advanced to oral feeding and subcutaneous insulin. Since intravenous insulin has a half-life of only a few minutes, it is an error to discontinue the intravenous insulin before subcutaneous insulin has been given. The subcutaneous insulin should only be given when a meal both precedes it and stays in the patient. The proper sequence, therefore, is to allow a meal or snack at an appropriate time, then to give 0.25 units of regular insulin subcutaneously per kilogram (more or less may be indicated by the preceding drip requirements), and then to discontinue the intravenous drip of insulin. At this juncture, it is appropriate to discontinue any central venous or arterial catheters and arrange to transfer the patient out of the pediatric ICU.

CHAPTER **22** _____

Poisoning

Although poisoning is a common cause of admission to the pediatric intensive care unit, the drugs and their symptoms as well as the respective treatments are so varied as to be impossible to cover in a single review. Nearly a hundred pages of the *Textbook of Pediatric Intensive Care* (Chapter 32) are devoted to the subject.

As a result of the space limitations of a synopsis, only a brief overview of the drugs involved in common serious poisonings in childhood (Table 22.1) and sure elements in the differential diagnoses (Table 22.2) are covered. Toxidromes or classes of drugs involved with a constellation of symptoms (Table 22.3) and classic laboratory tests used in the differential diagnosis of toxicologic emergencies (Table 22.4) are also covered.

After this, a table for specific intoxicants and their antidotes (Table 22.5) is included. Next, there is a brief review of general techniques for hasten-

TABLE 22.1. _____
Drugs Involved in Serious Childhood Poisonings[a]

Drugs	Others
Acetaminophen	Alcohols (ethyl, isopropyl, methyl)
Antiarrhythmics	Ethylene glycol
Anticonvulsants	Caustics
Antihistamines	Herbicides
Antihypertensives	Organophosphates
Aminophylline	Petroleum distillates
Aspirin	
β-Blockers	
Digoxin	
Hallucinogens	
Iron	
Opioids	
Theophylline	
Tricyclic antidepressants	

[a]From Kilham HA: Hospital management of severe poisoning. *Pediatr Clin North Am* 27:603, 1980.

313

TABLE 22.2.
Clinical Manifestations of Poisonings[a]

Sign or Symptom	Poison
Odor	
Butter almond	Cyanide
Acetone	Isopropyl alcohol, methanol, acetylsalicylic acid
Coal gas	Carbon monoxide
Pungent aromatic	Ethchlorvynol
Oil of wintergreen	Methyl salicylate
Pear	Chloral hydrate
Garlic	Arsenic, phosphorus, thallium, organophosphates
Alcohol	Ethanol, methanol
Petroleum	Petroleum distillates
Skin	
Cyanosis (unresponsive to oxygen—Methemoglobinemia)	Nitrates, nitrates, phenacetin, benzocaine
Red flush	Carbon monoxide, cyanide, boric acid, anticholinergics
Sweating	Amphetamines, lysergic acid diethylamide (LSD), organophosphates, cocaine, barbiturates
Dry	Anticholinergics
Bullae	Barbiturates, carbon monoxide
Jaundice	Acetaminophen, mushrooms, carbon tetrachloride, iron, phosphorus
Purpura	Aspirin, warfarin, snakebites
Temperature	
Hypothermia	Sedative hypnotics, ethanol, carbon monoxide, phenothiazines, tricyclic antidepressants (TCAs), clonidine
Hyperthermia	Anticholinergics, salicylates, phenothiazines, TCAs, cocaine, amphetamines, theophylline
Blood pressure	
Hypertension	Sympathomimetics (especially phenylpropanolamine in over-the-counter cold remedies), organophosphates, amphetamine, phencyclidine (PCP)
Hypotension	Nacotics, sedative hypnotics, TCAs, phenothiazines, clonidine, β-blockers
Pulse rate	
Bradycardia	Digitalis, sedative hypnotics, β-blockers, ethchlorvynol
Tachycardia	Anticholinergics, sympathomimetics, amphetamine, alcohol, aspirin, theophylline, cocaine, TCAs

Sign or Symptom	Poison
Arrhythmias	Anticholinergics, TCAs, organophosphates, phenothiazines, digoxin, β-blockers, carbon monoxide, cyanide
Mucous membranes	
Dry	Anticholinergics
Salivation	Organophosphates, carbamates
Oral lesions	Corrosives, paraquat
Lacrimation	Caustics, organophosphates, irritant gases
Respiration	
Depressed	Alcohol, narcotics, barbiturates, sedative/hypnotics
Tachypnea	Salicylates, amphetamines, carbon monoxide
Kussmaul	Methanol, ethylene glycol, salicylates
Wheezing	Organophosphates
Pneumonia	Hydrocarbons
Pulmonary edema	Aspiration, salicylates, narcotics, sympathomimetics
Central nervous system	
Seizures	TCAs, cocaine, phenothiazines, amphetamines, camphor, lead, salicylates, isoniazid, organophosphates, antihistamines, propoxyphene
Pupils, meiosis	Narcotics (except Demerol and Lomotil), phenothiazines, organophosphates (late), Valium, barbiturates, mushrooms (muscarine types)
Mydriasis	Anticholinergics, sympathomimetics, cocaine, TCA, methanol, glutethimide, LSD
Blindness, optic atrophy	Methanol
Fasciculation	Organophosphates
Nystagmus	Diphenylhydantoin, barbiturates, carbamazepine, PCP, carbon monoxide, glutethimide ethanol
Hypertonus	Anticholinergics, strychnine, phenothiazines
Myoclonus, rigidity	Anticholinergics, phenothiazines, haloperidol
Delirium/psychosis	Anticholinergics, sympathomimetics, alcohol, phenothiazines, PCP, LSD, marijuana, cocaine, heroin, methaqualone, heavy metals
Coma	Alcohols, anticholinergics, sedative hypnotics, narcotics, carbon monoxide, TCAs, salicylates, organophosphates
Weakness, paralysis	Organophosphates, carbamates, heavy metals
Gastrointestinal system	
Vomiting, diarrhea, abdominal pain	Iron, phosphorus, heavy metals, lithium, mushrooms, fluoride, organophosphates

[a]From Guzzardi L, Bayer MJ: Emergency management of the poisoned patient. In Bayer M, Rumack BH, Wanke LA (eds): *Toxicologic Emergencies.* Bowie, MD, Robert J Brady, 1984.

TABLE 22.3.
Toxidromes[a]

Drug Involved	Clinical Manifestations
Anticholinergics (atropine, scopolamine, TCAs, phenothiazines, antihistamines, mushrooms)	Agitation, hallucinations, coma, extrapyramidal movements, mydriasis, flushed, warm dry skin, dry mouth, tachycardia, arrhythmias, hypotension, hypertension, decreased bowel sounds, urinary retention
Cholinergics (organophosphates and carbamate insecticides)	Salivation, lacrimation, urination, defecation, nausea and vomiting, sweating, meiosis, bronchorrhea, rales and wheezes, weakness, paralysis, confusion and coma, muscle fasciculations
Opiates	Slow respirations, bradycardia, hypotension, hypothermia, coma, meiosis, pulmonary edema, seizures
Sedative/Hypnotics	Coma, hypothermia, central nervous system depression, slow respirations, hypotension, tachycardia.
TCAs	Coma, convulsions, arrhythmias, anticholinergic manifestations
Salicylates	Vomiting, hyperpnea, fever, lethargy, coma
Phenothiazines	Hypotension, tachycardia, torsion of head and neck, oculogyric crisis, trismus, ataxia, anticholinergic manifestations
Sympathomimetics (amphetamines, phenylpropranolamine, ephedrine, caffeine, cocaine, aminophylline)	Tachycardia, arrhythmias, psychosis, hallucinations, delirium, nausea, vomiting, abdominal pain, piloerection
Alcohols, Glycols (methanol, ethylene glycol, also salicylates, paraldehyde, toluene)	Elevated anion gap metabolic acidosis

[a]From Mofenson NC, Greensher J: The unknown posion. *Pediatrics* 54:337, 1974.

TABLE 22.4. ──────────────────────────────
Routinely Available Laboratory Tests That May Suggest Poisoning

Test	Poison
Decreased hemoglobin saturation with normal or increased PO_2 (measured not calculated hemoglobin saturation)	Carbon monoxide, agents causing methemoglobinemia (nitrates, nitrites, benzocaine)
Elevated anion gap, metabolic acidosis	Methanol, ethanol, isopropyl alcohol, ethylene glycol, salicylates, isoniazid, paraldehyde, toluene, iron, phenformin, carbon monoxide, cyanide
Elevated osmolar gap	Ethanol, methanol, isopropyl alcohol, ethylene glycol
Hypoglycemia	Insulin, ethanol, isopropyl alcohol, isoniazid, acetaminophen, salicylates, oral hypoglycemic agents
Hyperglycemia	Salicylates, isoniazid, organophosphates, iron
Hypocalcemia	Ethylene glycol, methanol
Urinalysis	
Oxalic acid crystalluria	Ethylene glycol
Ketonuria	Isopropyl alcohol, ethanol, salicylates

ing removal of poisons for blood and tissues (Table 22.6) and a discussion of one of the more important modalities. Finally, a selected list of the more common important toxins and the choice of techniques used in their removal (Table 22.7) is included.

HASTENING THE ELIMINATION OF POISONS FROM BLOOD AND TISSUES

Forced Diuresis with or without Alteration of Urine pH

Forced diuresis is seldom used alone. It is usually combined with techniques that change urinary pH. Enhancing excretion by altering pH is based on the principle that efficient reabsorption across the renal tubular epithelium occurs only when the compound is unionized and relatively lipid soluble. The proportion of drug that exists in the ionized and unionized forms depends on the pK of the drug and the pH of the solution. A drug that is a weak acid or base will become ionized by gaining or donating a hydrogen ion. By altering the pH of the urine, the proportion of ionized or nonpolar drug can be enhanced, "trapping" this poorly resorbed compound in the tubular lumen, reducing reabsorption, and enhancing excretion. Since the pK of salicylate is 3, the ratio of the ionized to the unionized form is 1:1 at a pH of 3. At a pH of 7.4, the ratio is 25,000:1.

TABLE 22.5.
Specific Intoxications and Their Antidotes[a]

Poison	Antidote	Dosage
Acetaminophen	N-Acetylcysteine (Mucomyst)	140 mg/kg orally, initial dose, then 70 mg/kg every 4 hr for 17 doses (68 hr)
Anticholinergics	Physostigmine	*Adult:* 2.0 mg *Child:* 0.5 mg, i.v., i.m., s.c., repeat at 5-min intervals until desired effect is achieved, to maximum of 2 mg
β-Blocking agents	Glucagon	*Adult:* 3-mg bolus, followed by 5-mg/hr infusion *Child:* 0.05-mg/kg bolus, followed by 0.07-mg/kg infusion
	Isoproterenol, dopamine, epinephrine	Infusions: titrate to effect
Carbon monoxide	Oxygen	100% O_2; consider hyperbaric oxygen
Cyanide	Amyl nitrite, sodium nitrite	*Adult:* Amyl nitrite inhalation pending administration of i.v. sodium nitrite of 300 mg (3% solution), then sodium thiosulfate of 12.5 g (25% solution) *Child:* (For children of <25 kg, sodium nitrite and sodium thiosulfate doses are dependent on the hemoglobin concentration, since an overdose can cause fatal methemoglobinemia):
Ethylene glycol	Ethanol	Loading dose: *Adult:* 0.6 g/kg i.v. *Child:* 0.7 g/kg i.v. (Loading dose to achieve blood level of 100 mg/100 ml) Maintenance dose:

Hemoglobin (g/100 ml)	Initial dose of 3% Na nitrite (ml/kg i.v.)	then	Initial dose of 25% sodium thiosulfate (ml/kg i.v.)
8	0.22 (6.6 mg/kg)		1.10
10	0.27 (8.3 mg/kg)		1.35
12	0.33 (10 mg/kg)		1.65
14	0.39 (11.6 mg/kg)		1.95

		...fuse the sum of the loading dose and the first hour's maintenance dose over the first hour
		Infusions are adjusted to maintain blood levels at 100 mg/100 ml
Iron salts	Deferoxamine	Deferoxamine, 2 g/l in 1–2% sodium bicarbonate lavage
		Deferoxamine, 20–40 mg/kg i.m. or i.v. not to exceed 15 mg/kg/hr
		Repeat every 4–8 hr until urine color is normal or iron level is <100 µg/dl
Isoniazid	Pyridoxine (vitamin B₆)	When the dose of isoniazid is known, administer an equivalent amount of i.v. pyridoxine; if supplies are limited or the dose is unknown, administer 5 g; repeat dose if no response; cumulative dose is 20 g in children and 40 g in adults
Lead	Calcium disodium edetate (EDTA)	1500 mg/m²/24 hr i.m. in 6 divided doses
	British antilewisite (BAL)	500 mg/m²/24 hr i.m. in 6 divided doses
Methanol	Ethanol	For dosage, see under ethylene glycol
Methemoglobin-producing agents (nitrites, nitrates, phenacetin, phenazopyridine)	Methylene blue	1–2 mg/kg i.v. (0.1–0.2 ml/kg of a 1% solution over 5–10 min) (contraindicated in methemoglobinemia secondary to sodium nitrite administration for cyanide poisoning)
Narcotics	Naloxone	*Adult:* 0.4 mg i.v.; repeat at 10 times dose if no response and findings are consistent with narcotic overdose
		Child: 0.01 mg/kg i.v.
Organophosphate insecticides	Atropine	*Adult:* 2–5 mg i.v.
		Child: 0.05 mg/kg i.v.
		Repeat every 10–30 min to achieve adequate atropinization
	Pralidoxime	Only after atropine
		Adult: 1 g i.v.
		Child: 25 mg/kg i.v.
		Repeat after 1 hr if weakness and fasciculations persist
Phenothiazines (occulogyric crisis)	Diphenhydramine	0.5–1.0 mg/kg i.v. or i.m. (not to exceed 50 mg)

[a]From Henretig FM, Cupit GC, Temple AR: Toxicologic emergencies. In Ludwig S, Fleischer G (eds): *Textbook of Pediatric Emergency Medicine,* Philadelphia, WB Saunders, 1983.

TABLE 22.6. _____
Techniques of Hastening the Removal of Poisons from Blood and Tissues[a]

Forced diuresis
Urinary pH control ("ion trapping")
Hemodialysis, peritoneal dialysis
Hemoperfusion
Gastric suctioning
Activated charcoal ("gastrointestinal dialysis")
Exchange transfusion
Plasmapheresis
Drug antibodies

---

[a]From Pond SM: Diuresis, dialysis and hemoperfusion. Indications and benefits. *Emerg Clin North Am* 2:29, 1984.

Forced diuresis is accomplished by the administration of intravenous fluids at 2–5 times maintenance requirements, to establish a urine output of 2–5 ml/kg/hr. Bladder catheterization allows for the accurate measurement of urine output. Since some infants with salicylate intoxication may be considerably dehydrated, rapid rehydration may be necessary before diuresis can be accomplished. Diuretics such as mannitol and furosemide can be added to ensure high urine flow rates.

Alkalinization of the urine (pH of ≥ 7.0) is achieved by adding sodium bicarbonate in concentrations of 50–75 mEq/l to the intravenous fluids. Hypokalemia, whether pre-existent or induced by the bicarbonate administration, may make the patient relatively resistant to attempts at producing urinary alkalinization. Aggressive potassium supplementation will correct the situation.

Acid diuresis can increase the excretion of weak bases, but clinically this modality plays less of a role than alkalinization in the management of poisoned patients. Acidification of the urine to a pH of < 6.5 can be achieved by the oral or intravenous administration of ammonium chloride. Intravenous hydrochloric acid or oral ascorbic acid can also be used.

Dialysis

In general, drugs that are effectively dialyzed are poorly protein bound, are highly water soluble, and have a low volume of distribution. They should have a molecular structure and physical characteristics that enable rapid diffusion across the dialysis membranes. Methanol is an ideal candidate for removal by dialysis. It is a small molecular weight (32 daltons), poorly protein bound, highly water soluble compound that has a low volume of distribution ($V_D = 0.6$ l/kg). In addition, it is metabolized to toxic metabolities that are, themselves, dialyzable. In comparison, tricyclic antidepressants (TCAs), are poorly removed by dialysis. They are lipid soluble and >90% protein bound, with a large volume of distribution ($V_D = 20$ l/kg).

TABLE 22.7. _____
Choice of Techniques for Removal of Common Toxins in Which Eliminative
Therapy May Be Indicated[a]

Toxin	Levels Above Which Enhanced Elimination Techniques May Be Indicated (μg/ml)	Technique[b]
Amanita sp. (mushrooms)		HP
Amphetamines		D, HD, PD
Barbiturates		
Phenobarbital	100	HP, HD, D
Short and intermediate acting	50	HP
Carbon tetrachloride		HD, HP
Chloral hydrate (trichloroethanol)	50	HP, HD
Chloroquinone		D
Ethanol	300	HD
Ethchlorvynol	150	HP, HD
Ethylene glycol		HD
Glutethimide	40	HP
Isopropanol		HP, HD
Meprobamate	100	HP, HD
Methanol		HD
Methaqualone	40	HP, HD
Methotrexate		D
Methyprylon		HP
Paraquat		HP
Phencyclidine		D
Procainamide		HD
Salicylates	800	HD, PD, D
Theophylline	50	HP, HD

[a]From Wanke LA, Bennett WM: Enhancement of elimination: Diruesis, peritoneal dialysis, hemodialysis, and hemoperfusion. In Bayer MJ, Rumack BH,
Wanke LA (eds): *Toxicologic Emergencies.* Bopwie, MD, Robert J Brady, 1984.
[b]GD, gastrointestinal dialysis; D, diuresis; PD, peritoneal dialysis; HD, hemodialysis; HP, hemoperfusion. These are given in order of preference, when more
than a single technique is listed.

Hemoperfusion

Hemoperfusion is the process whereby compounds are cleared from the
blood as it comes into direct contact with an adsorbent material, contained in a cartridge, in an extracorporeal circuit.

The absolute indications for hemoperfusion remain unclear, though it
has been used with high serum levels of theophylline, paraquat, methypry-

lon, meprobamates, isopropanol, carbon tetrachloride, barbiturates, especially phenobarbital, and several other drugs.

In the past, the use of hemoperfusion in children was limited because of the large size of the available adsorption cartridges. However, infants weighing <5 kg have undergone successful hemoperfusion with use of the standard cartridges. Smaller cartidges with priming of volumes of 100 ml have recently become commercially available in the United States. Their use will facilitate hemoperfusion in small children.

The clinical use of hemoperfusion requires both the technical and the clinical expertise, as well as the equipment, needed to perform hemodialysis. Suitable vascular access via a double-lumen catheter placed in the subclavian or femoral vein must be obtained for establishing the extracorporeal circuit. Such a technique is suitable for children as small as 10 kg. The umbilical artery and vein can be used for vascular access in the newborn. For children beyond the newborn period but <10 kg, two separate venous sites must be cannulated because the double-lumen catheters are generally too large to be placed in these infants.

Activated Charcoal "Gastrointestinal Dialysis"

At present, activated charcoal "gastrointestinal dialysis" is the therapeutic modality recommended for phenobarbital, digoxin, and theophylline intoxication. Activated charcoal in a dose of 1 g/kg in a child, or 50–100 g in an adult, should be orally administered every 2–4 hours.

Plasmapheresis

Plasmapheresis, a process of plasma removal by continuous centrifugation, has been used in drug intoxications to facilite the removal of highly protein bound drugs. It has been successfully used in chromic acid and chromate poisoning but has largely been replaced, when indicated, by hemoperfusion.

Exchange Transfusion

Exchange transfusion has been used as a therapeutic modality in drug intoxications, especially in very small infants and in those intoxications complicated by intravascular hemolysis and methemoglobinemia. In addition to removing the intoxicating drug, fragmented and methemoglobin-containing cells are replaced by intact erythrocytes.

ORGANOPHOSPHATE AND CARBAMATE INSECTICIDE INTOXICATION

Pathophysiology

Acetylcholine is responsible for neurotransmission by occupying receptors at (a) certain sites within the central nervous system, (b) parasympathetic and sympathetic ganglia and the neuromuscular junction (nicotinic receptors), and (c) parasympathetic nerve endings to sweat glands (muscarinic receptors). After release from nerve endings and effecting action potentials at these synapses or the neuromuscular junction, acetylcholine is hydrolyzed to inactive choline and acetic acid by the enzyme, acetylcholinesterase.

The phosphate moiety of the organophosphate insecticide binds irreversibly to acetylcholinesterase to form a stable, inactive, phosphorylated enzyme complex. Acetylcholinesterase has an affinity for organosphosphate of approximately 106 times that of acetylcholine. Unhydrolyzed acetylcholine subsequently accumulates at the sites of acetylcholine synaptic transmission, stimulating neurotransmission. Because of the failure of acetylcholinesterase to hydrolyze the acetylcholine, the receptors become blocked and transmission ceases. Clinical manifestations are the result of the initial stimulation and subsequent paralysis of neurotransmission at the muscarinic and nicotinic receptor sites (Table 22.8).

Laboratory Tests

The specific diagnosis of organophosphate poisoning can be made by laboratory measurement of red cell acetylcholinesterase and serum pseu-

TABLE 22.8.
Clinical Manifestations of Organophosphate and Carbamate Poisoning[a]

Anatomic Site	Manifestation
Central nervous system effects	Headache, lethargy, restlessness, dizziness, confusion, coma, seizures, respiratory depression, convulsions
Nicotinic effects	
Skeletal muscle	Cramps, fasciculations, weakness, paralysis
Sympathetic ganglia	Tachycardia, hypertension, arrhythmias, pallor, mydriasis
Muscarinic effects	
Cardiac	Bradycardia, hypotension, heart block, arrhythmias
Respiratory	Bronchorrhea, wheezing, respiratory distress
Gastrointestinal	Cramps, vomiting, nausea, diarrhea, tenesmus, abdominal pain
Salivary glands	Excess salivation
Sweat glands	Sweating
Eyes	Meiosis, lacrimation, blurred vision
Bladder	Incontinence
Miscellaneous	Garlic odor, fever

[a]From Haddad LM: The organophosphate insecticides. In Haddad LM, Winchester JF (eds): *Clinical Management of Poisoning and Drug Overdose.* Philadelphia, WB Saunders, 1983.

doacetylcholinesterase. The levels of these enzymes reflect the degree of inactivation of synaptic acetylcholinesterase. Depressed red cell cholinesterase levels are more specific in the diagnosis of organophosphate poisoning, but this assay is generally a less readily available test. Low serum pseudocholinesterase levels are less specific, since they may also be present in patients with malnutrition, liver disease, preganancy, and various genetic deficiencies of the enzyme. Although clinical manifestations do not always parallel the degree of acetylcholinesterase activity, mild poisoning is usually associated with >20% activity, and severe intoxication is usually associated with <10% activity.

Treatment

Initial supportive care must be directed toward the maintenance of an adequate airway that can be easily compromised by muscular weakness, excessive secretions, emesis, and seizures (typical features of severe poisoning). Intubation and artificial ventilation must be instituted for respiratory failure.

Immediate decontamination is crucial. All clothing must be removed, and skin and hair should be thoroughly washed with soap and water. Either gastric lavage or emesis must be performed. Activated charcoal and cathartics are indicated.

Atropine and the oximes are the classic organophosphate poisoning antidotes. Atropine alone blocks the effects of acetylcholine in the central nervous system and at muscarinic receptors but has no effect on the neuromuscular junction. The recommended initial pediatric dose is 0.05 mg/kg intravenously (adult dose, 2 mg). Doses of 0.02–0.05 mg/kg must be repeated at 5–10 minute intervals until a therapeutic response is achieved as noted by signs of atropinization, judged chiefly by the decrease in oral and bronchial secretions, not by ocular findings, since, if meiosis is initially present in the poisoned patient, atropine will not necessarily produce mydriasis. Once adequate atropinization has been achieved, repeated doses should be given every 30–60 minutes because of the relatively short half-life of atropine. Some workers have suggested that control of clinical symptoms is best achieved by the use of a continuous infusion of atropine at 0.02–0.08 mg/kg/hr, depending on the degree and stage of intoxication. Enormous doses of atropine that may exceed 0.5 mg/kg/day may be required over the course of treatment.

Pralidoxime, an anticholinesterase reactivator, is administered intravenously over several minutes at a dose of 25 mg/kg to children or 1–2 g to adults. The dose may be repeated after 1 hour if weakness and fasciculations persist. In some severely poisoned patients, large amounts may be required for prolonged periods, and continuous infusions of up to 0.5 g/hr in adults have been effective. The introduction of highly fat soluble organophosphates has resulted in poisonings with a clinical course of several weeks duration. This has necessitated atropine and pralidoxime therapy for prolonged periods.

TRICYCLIC ANTIDEPRESSANT INTOXICATION

Pharmacology and Pharmacokinetics

The pharmacologic mechanism of toxicity of the TCAs is due to (a) central and peripheral anticholinergic actions, (b) a blockade of the amine pump, with a decrease in reuptake of norepinephrine at adrenergic nerve endings and subsequent enchanced catecholamine action in the central nervous system and peripheral tissues, and (c) a "quinidine-like" myocardial depressant effect. Different TCAs express these pharmacologic actions in varying degrees.

Clinical Manifestations and Pathophysiology

TCA toxicity is characterized by central nervous system disturbances, peripheral anticholinergic manifestations, and cardiovascular effects of hypotension and arrhythmias.

The central nervous system changes are characterized by a clinical spectrum varying from drowsiness, lethargy, confusion, and agitation in milder cases to delirium, respiratory depression, and coma in more severely overdosed patients. Twitching, myoclonic jerks, pyramidal tract signs, and choreoathetosis are not infrequently seen.

Respiratory depression with hypoventilation and respiratory acidosis may be a feature of severe intoxication. The peripheral anticholinergic effects observed in TCA intoxication include: dry mucous membranes; flushed, warm skin without sweating; mydriasis; blurred vision; urinary retention; decreased bowel sounds; and constipation.

The three pharmacologic effects of TCAs on the heart include: (a) anticholinergic actions, (b) blockage of norepinephrine reuptake at the adrenergic synapse, and (c) "qunidine-like" myocardial depressant effects.

Laboratory Tests

Apart from the demonstration of TCA in blood or urine, there is no specific laboratory test of TCA poisoning. The serum levels can, however, provide some prognostic information. Several investigators have shown that in both adults and children a serum TCA concentration of >1000 ng/ml is indicative of severe intoxication and correlates well with a QRS interval of >100 msec, as well as with the presence of other signs of severe poisoning.

Treatment

After the adequacy of the airway, ventilation, blood pressure, and peripheral perfusion are ensured, gastric decontamination must be initiated with either syrup of ipecac or lavage. Since the anticholinergic actions of the TCA may dramatically delay gastric emptying, attempts at gastric decontamination, even 24 hours after ingestion, may yield unabsorbed drug and should be performed.

Activated charcoal administration plays a particularly important role in the therapy of TCA poisoning, initially by binding the TCA not removed by the gastric decontamination. Such repeated doses should be given every 4 hours. Since 5–15% of an ingested dose may be excreted by the stomach in the gastric juices, some authorities have suggested the use of continuous nasogastric suctioning to prevent reabsorption of this fraction of drug.

Management of Central Nervous System Toxicity

Physostigmine is a short-acting, nonspecific cholinesterase inhibitor that, because of its structure, can cross the blood-brain barrier to exert a central nervous system, as well as a peripheral, cholinergic affect. It has been used by some toxicologists to reverse TCA-induced neurologic abnormalities, but because of its short half-life, frequent doses or a continuous infusion is required.

Some suggested indications for the use of physostigmine include severe agitation, with or without myoclonic and choreathetoid movements, seizures, and hypotension, but only after more conservative therapy, such as diazepam, airway management and controlled ventilation for seizures and volume replacement for hypotension, has failed. Physostigmine must be administered over several minutes at a dose of 1–2 mg to adults and 0.5 mg to children.

Management of Cardiovascular Toxicity

Arrhythmias

Sinus tachycardia is a universal occurrence in any patient with TCA poisoning. In the child with a healthy heart, this requires no specific therapy.

The most frequently occurring ventricular arrhythmias are premature ventricular beats, bigeminy, and ventricular tachycardia. Alkalinization is the treatment of choice for ventricular arrhythmias and intraventricular conduction delay. Supraventricular tachycardia may also be responsive to this therapeutic modality. Alkalinization may be accomplished by either sodium bicarbonate administration (2–3 mEq/kg), hyperventilation, or both, to achieve a pH of 7.45–7.55. The mechanism of action alkalinization as an antiarrhythmic is not precisely known.

Other more conventional antiarrhythmics, such as lidocane and Dilantin, may be effective in the management of TCA-induced ventricular arrhythmias, should alkalinization fail. Propranolol and physostigmine have also been used for the treatment for these arrhythmias, but their side effects relegate them to second-line drugs.

Hypotension

Hypotension in TCA intoxication is due to the coexistence of relative hypovolemia with decreased filling pressures, decreased peripheral resistance, depressed myocardial contractility, and possibly arrhythmias. Initial management should consist of the Trendelenburg position and volume infusion, if necessary, guided by central venous pressure or Swan-Ganz catheter monitoring. Vasoactive agents are warranted for persistence of

severe hypotension in spite of volume replacement. Directly acting α-ago-
nists, such as norepinephrine or phenylephrine, are more effective than
the indirectly acting agents, such as dopamine, because by preventing
neuronal reuptake of catecholamines, TCAs result in norephineprine-de-
pleted sympathetic neurons unable to respond to indirectly acting agents.

OPIOID INTOXICATION

Opioid intoxication in children occurs under several circumstances. It is
frequently the result of the accidental or suicidal ingestion of potent opioids,
such as methadone, propoxyphene, or pentazocine, or by the large overdose of cough mixtures, pain medications, and antidiarrheal agents.

Pharmacology and Pathophysiology

Results of extensive research over the past 20 years have suggested that
the action of the exogenously administered opioids is mediated by their
interaction with three different stereospecific, saturable receptors in the
central nervous system—the μ, κ, σ receptors. Different opioids bind with
different affinities to these receptors to exhibit variable agonistic or antagonistic actions (Table 22.9). On the basis of their variable interactions with
these receptors, the exogenous opioids may be classified as agonists (e.g.,
morphine), antagonists (e.g., naloxone), or mixed agonist-antagonist (e.g.,
nalorphine, cyclazocine, and levallorphan) for particular receptors (Table
22.9). An opioid may, therefore, act as an agonist at one receptor but as
an antagonist at another—an example of receptor dualism.

Clinical Manifestations

In general, the clinical manifestations of opioid drug poisoning in children are similar, irrespective of the drug ingested. The differences are due
mostly to the time course of toxicity. The triad of respiratory depression,
miosis, and impaired consciousness is very typical of opioid intoxication.

Although miosis is classic, mydriasis with opioid intoxication can occur
with severe hypoxia and may also be seen with the injestion of Lomotil, a
fixed combination preparation of the opioid diphenoxylate and atropine.
The clinical manifestations of intoxication with this compound are the results of either the sequential or combined manifestations of anticholinergic poisoning (flushing, fever, lethargy, tachycardia, ileus, and urinary
retention) and those of narcotic intoxication. Meperidine produces miosis
less consistently than the other opioids because of a slight atropine-like
action.

Cardiovascular collapse in opioid intoxication is uncommon and is usually secondary to severe hypoxia. Hypotension and bradycardia are not uncommon, however, with intravenous heroin abuse.

The pulmonary edema associated with opioid intoxication is noncardiac
in origin and reflects increased pulmonary capillar permeability. This is
evidenced by normal or low pulmonary capillary wedge pressures and by a

TABLE 22.9.
Central Nervous System Opioid Receptor System[a]

Receptor	Agonist	Antagonist	Postulated Clinical Effects
μ	Morphine	Pentazocine	Analgesia
	Codeine	Cyclazocine	Euphoria
	Heroin	Nalorphine	Respiratory depression
	Dihydromorphinone	Naloxone	Miosis
	Oxymorphine	Naltrexone	
	Oxycodeine		
	Methadone		
	Meperidine		
κ	Pentazocine	Naloxone	Analgesia
	Nalorphine	Naltrexone	Sedation
	Cyclazocine		Miosis
	Morphine-like analgesics		
	Levallorphan		
σ	Pentazocine	Naloxone	Dysphoria
	Cyclazocine	Naltrexone	Delusions
	Nalorphine		Hallucinations
	Levallorphan		

[a] From Bradberry JC, Raebel MA: Continuous infusion of naloxone in the treatment of narcotic overdose. *Drug Intell Clin Pharm* 15:945, 1981.

protein concentration in the edema fluid that approximates that of serum. The mechanism whereby the opioids produce damage of the alveolar-capillary-membrane is unclear but is probably multifactorial in nature.

Seizures are occasionally part of the clinical picture of opioid intoxication. They are, however, particularly associated with propoxyphene overdose.

Rhabdomyolysis secondary to deep coma and pressure necrosis of muscle occasionally complicates severe narcotic intoxication and may result in renal failure.

Laboratory Tests

The qualitative detention of opioids or their metabolites in urine is available in most clinical laboratories, to confirm the clinical diagnosis of opioid intoxication. Quantitative assays are technically difficult and play no role in the diagnosis or management of those intoxications. The laboratory can play a vital role in the determination of coingestants, or drugs such as acetaminophen, that are present in fixed combinations with some opioids, such as propoxyphene or codeine.

Treatment

The initial use of naloxone is both diagnostic and therapeutic. It has always been considered that a response to naloxone in a comatose patient with respiratory depression and miosis confirms the diagnosis of opioid intoxication. However, recent reports in the literature have suggested that the specificity of naloxone for opioid receptors might be less than previously considered. Naloxone has been shown to reverse the central nervous system depression caused by ethanol, clonidine, and diazepam intoxication. Naloxone should be given intravenously for its most rapid effect but may be administered intramuscularly or even intratracheally if intravenous access is unavailable. Since the displacement by naloxone of the opioid from its central nervous system receptor is governed by the law of mass action, the dose of naloxone required for antagonism is a function of the concentration of both the opioid and naloxone, as well as the affinity of the receptors involved, for these agents. Initially, the recommended dose of naloxone was 0.4 mg/kg in adults and 0.01 mg/kg in children. The literature, however, is now replete with many case reports in which patients have required 10 times or greater the recommended dose of naloxone to reverse the actions of the intoxicating opioids. This is particularly so of opioids with high affinities for κ and σ receptors, e.g., methadone and pentazocine. If there is no response to the usual dose within 2–3 minutes, 10 times the original dose, i.e., 4.0 mg/kg for adults and 0.1 mg/kg for children, should be given. Narcotic overdose should be excluded only after there has been no clinical response to 10 times the original dose. Since the duration of action of most narcotics that are responsible for intoxication is significantly longer than that of naloxone (half-life of several hours versus half-life of 1 hour), additional doses of naloxone may be necessary to prevent the recurrence of central nervous system depression. These repeated doses may be necessary for more than 24 hours, particularly after intoxication with very long-acting opioids, such as methadone. To maintain adequate reversal by maintaining high brain levels of naloxone and to obviate the need for frequent, intermittent doses, several reports have proposed and have demonstrated the efficacy of a continuous naloxone infusion. After the initial intravenous bolus of naloxone, continuous naloxone infusion with an initial starting dose of approximately 5 μg/kg/hr is begun. The dose must be titrated according to the patient's clinical response. Doses as low as 2.5 μg/kg/hr and as high as 33 μg/kg/hr have been noted in the literature.

THEOPHYLLINE INTOXICATION

The widespread availability of this drug and its narrow therapeutic index have made theophylline intoxication a common pediatric problem that occurs in two distinct clinical settings. Iatrogenic, subacute, or chronic intoxication usually results from either a therapeutic dosage error or a reduction in theophylline clearance. Acute, massive intoxication occurs as a result of a suicidal ingestion in older children and adolescents or from an accidental ingestion in young children.

Pathophysiology

The biochemical pathogenesis of theophylline toxicity is unclear, but theophylline toxicity may be considered as an example of "hyperadrenergic syndrome." Very high levels of epinephrine and norepinephrine have been measured in intoxicated patients and in animal models of theophylline intoxication.

Clinical Manifestations

Theophylline toxicity is characterized by multisystem manifestations that may include nausea, vomiting, tachyarrhythmias, cardiovascular collapse, agitation, tremors, seizures, lethargy, and coma.

The central nervous system manifestations include agitation, hypernea, tremor, hyperreflexia, confusion, disturbed behavior, hallucinations, and seizures, as well as signs of central nervous system depression—lethargy, obtundation, and coma. In children, seizures generally occur with theophylline levels of >60 µg/ml, although seizures may develop with levels as low as 25 µg/ml in adults. Clearly, the serum theophylline concentration alone is not the only factor determining the likelihood of seizures.

The metabolic abnormalities that occur with theophylline intoxication have recently been emphasized. These disturbances include hypokalemia, hypophosphatemia, hyperglycemia, leukocytosis, metabolic acidosis, and respiratory alkalosis.

Hypokalemia is the most significant of these abnormalities because of its potential arrhythmogenic effect. Several factors may play a role in the production of this disturbance. Gastrointestinal loss by emesis and diarrhea and renal loss are probably insignificant. A shift of potassium from the extracellular to the intracellular compartment is the most likely explanation for the hypokalemia.

Hyperglycemia is also a consistent finding in severe theophylline intoxication. Suggested pathophysiologic mechanisms include the stimulatory effects of elevated concentrations of catecholamine and adenosine $3':5'$-cyclic phosphate on hepatic glucose production by enhancing gluconeogenesis.

The most consistent cardiovascular manifestation of theophylline intoxication is supraventricular tachycardia. With more serious intoxication, ventricular arrhythmias including ventricular ectopic beats, bigeminy, and ventricular tachycardia, as well as hypotension and refractory cardiovascular collapse, can develop. Theophylline has demonstrable cardiovascular effects at therapeutic levels that include an increase in chronotropy and inotropy.

Treatment

The therapy of theophylline toxicity is largely supportive. Priority, as in all cases of intoxication, must initially be directed toward the maintenance of an adequate airway, effective ventilation, and stable circulation. Gastric decontamination must then proceed with haste. In awake patients, ipecac-induced emesis must be initiated. Gastric lavage, after endotracheal tube placement, is the alternative in the obtunded patient.

There has been a move among toxicologists to utilize techniques to enhance the elimination of theophylline, because of the reduced endogenous clearance of theophylline in the intoxicated patient. Such techniques include repeated oral administration of activated charcoal, exchange transfusion, dialysis, and charcoal or resin hemoperfusion.

Several studies have demonstrated the efficacy of the repeated oral administration of activated charcoal in decreasing the half-life ($t_{1/2}$) and in increasing the clearance of theophylline both in normal subjects given either oral or intravenous theophylline and in patients with theophylline toxicity.

Because it is less invasive and safer than other techniques that enhance theophylline elimination, oral activated charcoal therapy should be started as the initial therapy of theophylline toxicity.

Exchange transfusion has been attempted in pediatric patients with theophylline toxicity, but it is not effective. Hemodialysis does enhance theophylline clearance, but it is not as effective as hemoperfusion.

Resin and charcoal hemoperfusion has been emphasized in the adult literature as a therapeutic modality in the management of theophylline intoxication. There is, however, substantially less experience with this technique in intoxicated children. Although there are many data to attest to the efficacy of hemoperfusion in dramatically enhancing theophylline clearance and rapidly lowering serum levels, the benefits of rapid drug removal remain speculative, especially in children.

Although aminophylline-induced seizures in adults are difficult to control, those that develop in intoxicated children generally respond well to the administration of diazepam alone or its combination with phenytoin or phenobarbital.

Of the metabolic disturbance, hypokalemia should be aggressively treated because of its potential role in aggravating cardiac arrhythmias. Insulin is not indicated for hyperglycemia because glucose levels will return to normal as intoxication lessens. Sodium bicarbonate should be administered to partially correct a severe metabolic acidosis.

The specific therapy of supraventricular tachycardias is usually not indicated in children. Little information is available on the specific management of theophylline-induced ventricular arrhythmias, particular in children. Lidocaine and procainamide may be used. Based on an understanding of the pathophysiology of the intoxicated state, β-adrenergic blocking agents would appear to be the most logical agents to use, but they are contraindicated in asthmatic patients—frequently those with aminophylline toxicity.

ACETAMINOPHEN INTOXICATION

The widespread availability of acetaminophen in over-the-counter preparations has resulted in a dramatic increase in accidental and suicidal intoxications over the past 10 years. It is a safe drug when used in recommended doses, but striking hepatic dysfunction can develop with an acute ingestion of >7.5 g in adults or 140 mg/kg in children.

Pharmacology and Pathophysiology

Acetaminophen is rapidly absorbed after a therapeutic dose and peak levels are achieved within 1–2 hours. It is rapidly taken up and concentrated by the liver, the primary site of metabolism. Here, >90% of acetaminophen is conjugated with sulfate and glucuronate, to form inactive, nontoxic polar compounds that are excreted by the kidney. Under therapeutic circumstances, <2% of acetaminophen is excreted unchanged in the urine, and approximately 4% is conjugated with glutathione by the cytochrome P-450-dependent mixed-function oxidase enzyme system to form renally excreted mercapturic acid and cysteine conjugates. This mercapturic acid conjugate is considered the toxic intermediate of acetaminophen metabolism. Hepatic toxicity is caused by these intermediates that accumulate in the face of gluthathione depletion, to produce cellular necrosis.

Clinical Manifestations

The clinical course of significant acetaminophen intoxication in adolescents and adults can be divided into four stages.

Stage 1: The first 12–24 hours are remarkable for nausea, anorexia, and vomiting. Some patients may, however, remain entirely asymptomatic. Central nervous system, respiratory, and cardiac manifestations are not features during this early phase, and their presence should alert one to the possible ingestion of additional drugs.

Stage 2: Stage 2 is marked clinically by the resolution of the early gastrointestinal symptoms, but the clinician should not be reassured, since the resolution of these symptoms is of no prognostic importance. Most patients will become asymptomatic for a period even if severe liver dysfunction subsequently appears. Biochemical evidence of hepatic dysfunction with elevation of transaminases, bilirubin, and prothrombin time will begin to appear approximately 36 hours after ingestion.

Stage 3: Liver function abnormalities reach their peak on the third or fourth day. This is associated with a recrudescence of nausea, vomiting, and anorexia—symptoms of hepatitis. The extraordinary high levels of transaminases that may exceed 10,000 IU/ml do not necessarily herald liver failure. Fulminant liver failure, with jaundice, encephalopathy, and bleeding, is an infrequent occurrence and does not inevitably complicate untreated acetaminophen poisoning. Other known complications of severe intoxication include renal failure, pancreatitis, and myocardial injury.

Stage 4: Stage 4 is the recovery stage and lasts approximately 7–8 days. Chronic hepatitis is not a feature of acetaminophen intoxication, and liver function tests and the liver biopsy and histology of patients who survive return to normal.

The clinical manifestations and the course of acetaminophen intoxication in infants and young children are somewhat different from that described above. With rare exceptions, children who have ingested acetaminophen in doses well in excess of the toxic range for adults and adolescents appear strikingly resistent to its toxic effects. Overwhelming liver failure is extremely rare. The precise mechanisms responsible for the young child's tolerance to acetaminophen intoxication are not precisely known.

Prediction of Toxicity

As a rough guide, an ingestion of 150 mg/kg in a child and 7.5 g in an adult should be considered potentially toxic. Liver damage is very uncommon with ingestions of <125 mg/kg, but severe damage will occur in about 50% of adults with intoxications of 250 mg/kg and in almost 100% of those with a 350-mg/kg ingestion.

Various studies have resulted in the formulation of a nomogram (Fig. 22.1) that defines, with good correlation, the risk of hepatic damage in with good correlation, the risk of hepatic damage in terms of serum levels and duration of time since ingestion. Clinically significant liver damage is generally defined as an SGOT (aspartate aminotransferase) level of >1000 IU/l. The nomogram that begins at 4 hours postingestion and ends at 24 hours applies only to acute intoxication. Values obtained before 4 hours do not yet reflect peak serum levels. After 24 hours, hepatocellular damage has already occurred.

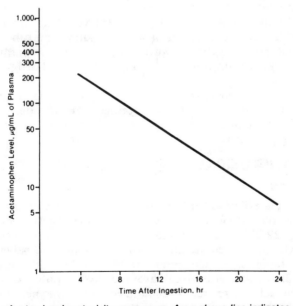

FIGURE 22.1. Acetaminophen toxicity nomogram. *Area above line* indicates probable hepatotoxic reaction. *Area below line* indicates no hepatotoxic reaction. (From Rumack BH, Peterson RC, Koch GC, et al: Acetaminophen overdose. *Arch Intern Med* 141:380, 1981.)

Treatment

The initial state of treatment should consist of emesis or lavage and ca-thartics. If other drugs have been ingested in addition, activated charcoal should be administered as well.

N-Acetylcysteine is the only antidotal agent available in the United States for the treatment of acetaminophen poisoning and, when administered for < 16 hours and even up to 24 hours after ingestion, has the profound effect of lowering the morbidity and mortality. Although both intravenous and oral preparations of the drug are efficacious, there is dispute as to the preferred route of administration. The oral form is the therapy of choice in the United States.

The precise mode of action of N-acetylcysteine is unclear, but after being taken up by the liver cells, it is metabolized to cysteine, a precursor of glutathione that binds the reactive toxic intermediate of acetaminophen metabolism.

If on the basis of the 4-hour postingestion level plotted on the nomogram the patient appears at risk for hepatic toxicity, therapy with N-acetylcys-teine should begin with a loading dose of 140 mg/kg. The commercially available 20% solution (Mucomyst) is unpalatable and must be mixed with 3 parts of soda or grapefruit juice to make a drinkable 5% solution that reduces vomiting to a minimum. A maintenance dose of 70 mg/kg should follow every 4 hours for 17 doses. A dose should be repeated if vomiting occurs within 1 hour of administration. If activated charcoal has been pre-viously administered, it should be removed by nasogastric lavage prior to N-acetylcysteine administration. If persistent vomiting prevents oral ad-ministration, the drug can still be given via a duodenal tube, and consid-eration may be given to the use of the intravenous preparation. This is available in Great Britain but is still an investigational drug in the United States.

If acetaminophen blood levels are not readily available on an emergency basis, a blood specimen should be obtained, and the decision to begin therapy should be made on the basis of a suggestive history. Treatment can then be stopped if the reported level is nontoxic.

SALICYLATE INTOXICATION

Pharmacology

Salicylic acid is excreted from the body by the kidney after conversion by several hepatic biotransformation pathways to five inactive conjugated me-tabolites (Fig. 22.2). With low therapeutic doses of aspirin, approximately 70% of salicylic acid is conjugated with glycine to yield salicyluric acid— the major metabolite. Smaller amounts of salicylic acid are converted to salicyl phenolic or salicyl acyl glucuronide, hydroxylated to gentisic acid and gentisuric acid, or excreted unchanged as salicylic acid by glomerular filtration and tubular secretion. Except in renal failure, the metabolites of salicylic acid are excreted as rapidly as they are formed and are of no toxi-cologic importance.

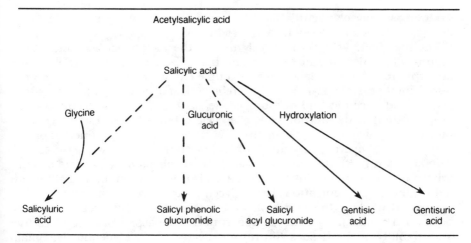

FIGURE 22.2. Metabolism of acetylsalicylic acid. – – – –, zero-order kinetics at toxic levels; — —, first-order kinetics at toxic levels.

The metabolic pathways for the synthesis of the two quantitatively most important metabolites—salicyluric and salicyl phenolic glucuronide—are, however, saturable and obey zero-order kinetics at high therapeutic and toxic plasma levels, even though first-order kinetics are followed at therapeutic levels. The other metabolic pathways obey first-order kinetics.

Clinical Manifestations and Pathophysiology

Salicylate poisoning is characterized by a wide-range of clinical symptoms and signs that characteristically include tinnitus in older children and adults, fever, sweating, tachycardia, hyperventilation, nausea, vomiting, dehydration, and central nervous system signs of lethargy, coma, and even seizures.

Fever is a common feature of salicylate intoxication in children. It is primarily due to the potent metabolic stimulant effect of salicylates that uncouples oxidative phosphorylation in a manner similar to that of 2,4-dinitrophenol, depleting the tissues of intracellular high-energy phosphates. This enhances total body oxygen consumption, carbon dioxide production, basal metabolic rate, and heat production—biochemical events that are clinically manifest by fever, flushed skin, sweating, and signs of a hyperdynamic circulation. Dehydration, so frequent a finding in salicylate intoxication, reduces physiologic sweating, further aggravating the pyrexia.

Acid-base disturbances that consist of either respiratory alkalosis, metabolic acidosis, or a mixed acid-base disturbance of metabolic acidosis and respiratory alkalosis frequently accompany salicylate intoxication in both children and adults. This is caused by a combination of three processes:

(a) increased alveolar ventilation, (b) increased carbon dioxide production, and (c) increased endogenous acid production.

The metabolic acidosis is largely due to the metabolic disruption that occurs with salicylate intoxication and that affects primarily carbohydrate and lipid metabolism. Salicylates uncouple oxidative phosphorylation and also inhibit several enzymes of the Krebs cycle, particularly α-ketodehydrogenase and succinic acid dehydrogenase, with subsequent accumulation of pyruvate, lactate, and other Krebs cycle intermediates. Enhanced metabolism, in turn, stimulates lipolysis with the increased production of ketone bodies, β-hydroxybutyrate, and acetoacetate.

In addition to its influence on acid-base metabolism, the effects of salicylates on carbohydrate metabolism are also reflected in abnormalities of blood glucose concentration. Hyperglycemia and glycosuria are common, particularly early in the course of acute intoxication. This possibly reflects both an increase in the rate of absorption of glucose from the intestine and inability of the tissues to utilize delivered glucose adequately. Small children, particularly those with chronic salicylate intoxication, as well as those late in the course of acute intoxication, may develop life-threatening hypoglycemia.

Disturbances of water and electrolyte metabolism frequently accompany salicylate intoxication. Dehydration is an almost universal feature of severe salicylate intoxication and is multifactorial in its etiology. Hyponatremia may occasionally be associated with the syndrome of inappropriate release of antidiuretic hormone. Potassium metabolism is also frequently disturbed. Total body potassium is depleted by the obligatory urine loss associated with the organic aciduria. Hypocalcemia can be precipitated by either respiratory or iatrogenic metabolic alkalosis induced by forced alkalinization.

Central nervous system toxicity is manifest clinically in moderate and severe toxicity by restlessness and lethargy that progress to coma and even seizures. These findings of severe toxicity are more frequently observed in young children in whom a severe metabolic acidosis is usually present.

Seizures occasionally complicate salicylate intoxication and may be caused by high fever, hypernatremia, cerebral edema, hypocalcemia, or decreased cerebral and cerebrospinal fluid glucose concentrations, even in the face of normal blood levels.

The pathogenesis of cerebral edema in salicylate intoxication is unclear but is probably multifactorial in origin. Occasionally, it may be attributed to rapidly developing hyponatremia with the syndrome of inappropriate antidiuretic hormone secretion. The entry of salicylate into the brain under circumstances of severe metabolic acidosis and the possibility of low central nervous system concentrations of glucose that result from brain glucose utilization in excess of supply have been implicated in the developmental of cerebral edema.

The hemorrhagic complications associated with salicylate intoxication are uncommon in acute intoxication and are usually associated only with severe, chronic poisoning. Decreased platelet adhesiveness and hypopro-thrombinemia contribute to the coagulopathy.

Pulmonary edema is an uncommon complication associated with salicy-late intoxication in children, developing more frequently in severely intox-icated adults with concurrent medical problems during the course of chronic rather than acute intoxication. In some patients, pulmonary edema may occasionally result from overhydration during forced diuresis, particularly in the presence of renal failure or the syndrome of inappropriate antidi-uretic hormone secretion. Other patients have developed pulmonary edema prior to forced diuresis and with evidence of volume contraction. The nor-mal or low filling pressures suggest that the edema is noncardiogenic in origin and is due to alveolar capillary leakage.

Assessment of the Severity of Intoxication

The amount of drug ingested in a single acute ingestion can be used to predict the subsequent degree of toxicity (Table 22.10). These guidelines do not apply to chronic salicylate intoxication. It has, however, been sug-gested that chronic toxicity is likely when salicylate at > 100 mg/kg/day has been administered for 2 or more days.

In studies performed in the 1960s, the severity of acute intoxication was shown to correlate poorly with the blood salicylate level at the time of di-agnosis. Although symptoms of intoxication were uncommon at concen-trations of <30 ng/dl, there was much overlap in serum concentrations between mildly and fatally intoxicated children. Nevertheless, there is a nomogram (Fig. 22.3) to be used for predicting the severity of intoxication after a single acute ingestion, via salicylate levels obtained 6 hours or longer after ingestion.

Although disturbances in acid-base status do not necessarily correlate with the level of serum salicylates, the severity of acidosis is considered by some to reflect the severity of poisoning, since the degree of acidosis largely

---

TABLE 22.10.
Assessment of the Severity of Acute Salicylate Intoxication Based on the Estimated Dose Ingested[a]

Ingested Dose (mg/kg)	Estimate Severity
<150	No toxic reaction expected
150–300	Mild-moderate toxic reaction
300–500	Severe toxic reaction
>500	Potentially lethal toxic reaction

[a]From Temple AR: Acute and chronic effects of aspirin toxicity and their treat-ment. *Arch Intern Med* 141:364, 1981.

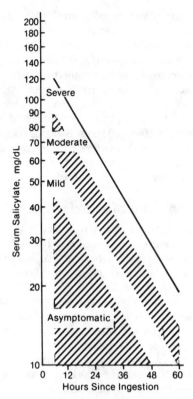

FIGURE 22.3.   The Done nomogram for estimating the severity of poisoning via serum salicy-late levels. (From Temple AR: Acute and chronic effects of aspirin toxicity and their treatment. *Arch Intern Med* 141:364, 1981, ©1981, American Medical Association.)

determines the amount of salicylate that enters the brain and other target organs.

The clinical findings, in both acute and chronic intoxication, reflect the severity of intoxication. Mild intoxication is characterized by mild hypernea, some lethargy, vomiting, and tinnitus. Hyperpnea and prominent neurologic disturbances with depressed consciousness but without coma or convulsions suggest moderate poisoning. Severe intoxication is marked by severe hyperpnea, hyperthermia, coma, and possibly convulsions.

Treatment

As with all intoxications, initial therapy is directed toward ensuring ventilation, oxygenation, and cardiovascular stability.

Prevention of further absorption can be accomplished by ipecac-induced emesis or gastric lavage, followed by activated charcoal and saline cathartic administration. Since salicylates delay gastric emptying time, emesis or lavage should be initiated even 12–24 hours after ingestion to remove residual pill fragments.

Severe dehydration frequently accompanies severe intoxication, and rapid fluid replacement with large volumes of an isotonic solution such as Ringer's lactate may be necessary to restore the circulating blood volume, correct hypotension, improve peripheral perfusion, and restore urine flow. Subsequent fluid replacement will depend upon the degree of dehydration. Saline (0.45%) with 35–70 mEq sodium bicarbonate per liter is a suitable replacement solution for a dehydrated acidotic child. Dextrose should be added to the solution as needed.

The therapy of acidosis in salicylate intoxication is of critical importance. The role of acidosis in enhancing the passage of salicylates from the extracellular space into the cells where they disrupt mitochondrial function and intermediary metabolism has been discussed previously. Sodium bicarbonate is the alkalinizing agent of choice. Since it is almost solely an alkalinizer of the extracellular space, it increases the intracellular-to-extracellular gradient of diffusible, nonionized drug, enhancing the trapping of salicylate in the extracellular plasma.

Acidosis may be treated by repeated intravenous boluses of sodium bicarbonate or by adding the drug to the rehydrating fluid in concentrations of 30–75 mEq/l. Dosage is guided by repeated blood gas determinations. Alkalinizing therapy is not without hazards, however. Sodium bicarbonate administration may aggravate hypernatremia and hypokalemia. It may also precipitate hypokalemia and subsequent seizures. The increased sodium administration may also aggravate pulmonary edema.

Close monitoring of the concentration of serum salicylates, glucose, calcium, electrolytes, and determinations of acid-base status are mandatory.

Several techniques have been employed to enhance the elimination of salicylates from the intoxicated patient. Of these, forced alkaline diuresis and dialysis are most used. Although charcoal hemoperfusion is very efficient in removing salicylates, it does not allow for the correction of electrolyte disturbances, acidosis, or fluid overload. Alkaline diuresis should be initiated in the moderately and severely intoxicated patient. The rationale for instituting forced diuresis with alkalinization is as follows. In the intoxicated state the hepatic pathways for metabolism become saturated and are unable to detoxify the additional load of substrate. The kidneys then become the prime organ of salicylate excretion. By enhancing diuresis, the concentration of salicylate in the distal tubular lumen is decreased, reducing the urine-tubular cell concentration gradient for reabsorption. In addition, since salicylates are weak acids, with a pK_a of 3.5, they become more ionized and less absorbable from the tubular lumen in an alkaline urine.

In a critical patient, hemodialysis has the advantage of being able to correct electrolyte disturbances, severe acidosis, and fluid overload. Peritoneal dialysis is much less effective than hemodialysis; it can, however, be rapidly instituted in the critically ill child while arrangements are being made to set up for hemodialysis. Indications for dialysis are not strictly defined. It should be reserved for the severely ill patient with renal failure, severe central nervous system manifestations, pulmonary edema, or severe acidosis unresponsive to conventional therapy, as well as for patients with very high salicylate levels, e.g., projected at the salicylate level time of ingestion (S_0) of >160 mg/dl or a 6-hour level of >130 mg/dl.

IRON INTOXICATION

The severity of iron intoxication is directly related to the amount of elemental iron that has been ingested. As estimation of this may provide a rough guide to the potential severity of the intoxication. These estimations are, however, notoriously unreliable. When the ingested dose is being calculated, it must be realized that the amount of contained elemental iron will depend on the particular iron compound ingested. The iron content of the ferrous gluconate, sulfate, and fumarate salts is 12, 20, and 33%, respectively. It is generally considered that ingestions of elemental iron of <20 mg/kg will be insignificant. Moderate to serious toxicity is likely after ingestion of 20–60 mg/kg. An ingestion of >200 mg/kg is potentially lethal unless the patient is rapidly and appropriately treated.

Pathophysiology

The vomiting, diarrhea, and abdominal pain that occasionally progress to lethal hemorrhagic gastroenteritis are attributed to the direct corrosive and toxic effects of the ingested iron salts on the mucosal surfaces of the gastrointestinal tract. Acute, focal gut necrosis that complicates vascular thrombosis may lead to perforation and peritonitis.

The pathogenesis of shock and cardiovascular depression is unclear. There are scant hemodynamic data on humans with iron intoxication and only a limited number of animal studies. It has been suggested that the high concentration of circulating iron or ferritin produces venous pooling.

Several factors account for the metabolic acidosis associated with severe iron poisoning. Shock and hypotension result in reduced tissue perfusion, anaerobic metabolism, and lactic acidosis.

A coagulopathy is the hallmark of severe iron poisoning in humans and laboratory animals. It is multifactorial in this etiology with disseminated intravascular coagulation, depressed synthesis of hepatic coagulation factors, and iron-induced alteration of factors of both intrinsic and extrinsic coagulation cascades playing a role. The coagulopathy is characterized by prolongation of the prothrombin, thrombin, and partial thromboplastin times.

Clinical Manifestations

The clinical manifestations of iron intoxication have been divided into four phases. The initial phase, attributed primarily to the direct effects of iron on the stomach and ileum, is characterized by nausea, vomiting, diarrhea, and abdominal pain. Severe iron poisoning does not develop in the absence of these gastrointestinal symptoms. With severe intoxication, these manifestations may progress to a severe hemorrhagic gastroenteritis with hematemesis and melena. Fever and leukocytosis may also reflect mucosal damage when intoxication is severe. In severe poisoning, shock and encephalopathy may develop during this very early stage. Approximately 25% of deaths from iron poisoning occur during this early phase.

The second phase, one of temporary recovery after initial successful resuscitative measures, occurs between 6 and 12 hours after ingestion. It is one of deceptive quiescence, lasting from 6 hours to several days. It is characterized by amelioration of the gastrointestinal and neurologic symptoms and with intensive appropriate therapy, even the restoration of hemodynamic stability. Some patients will, in fact, completely recover from this point. For others, this improvement is short-lived. They progress to the third phase, with recrudescence of both the gastrointestinal symptoms, the metabolic acidosis, the shock, and the central nervous system depression with lethargy and coma. The liver dysfunction is characterized by jaundice, elevated bilirubin and serum transaminases, profound hypoglycemia, and coagulopathy. Renal failure may also develop. Some patients will progress to this phase of severe multisystem failure without experiencing the quiescent second phase.

The fourth phase of iron intoxication is occasionally experienced 4–6 weeks after ingestion by those who have survived severe iron poisoning. It is characterized by pyloric, gastric, or intestinal stenosis, the result of the healing and scarring of the gastrointestinal tract lesions.

Prediction of Toxicity

The serum iron concentration and particularly the extent by which it exceeds the iron-binding capacity, has repeatedly been shown to correlate with the severity of iron intoxication (Table 22.10). Serum iron levels peak between 2 and 4 hours after a large ingestion. This is the optimal time to obtain a serum iron level. After 6 hours, the serum iron has been rapidly cleared from the serum, especially by the liver. A level drawn after this may be normal even in the face of a potentially lethal ingestion. When iron levels exceed the iron-binding capacity, free, toxic iron will circulate. With levels of <100 μg/dl, toxicity is unlikely. Levels that range between 100 and 300 μg/dl usually produce only mild symptoms. Moderate toxicity can be expected with levels between 300 and 500 μg/dl.

Although serum iron levels are fairly predictive of the severity of iron poisoning, they are not always available on an emergency basis. In addition, since there have been cases of serious iron poisoning with serum levels of <300 μg/dl, normal serum iron levels do not rule out potentially serious intoxication.

Studies have, however, demonstrated that certain clinical findings as well as simple laboratory tests are also useful in selecting those patients who are more likely to have a serum iron level of >300 μg/dl and significant toxicity. Vomiting and diarrhea that develop in the 6 hours after ingestion, hyperglycemia (a blood glucose concentration of >150 mg/dl), leukocytosis (a white cell count of >15,000 cells/mm^3), and an abdominal radiograph that demonstrates the presence of radiopaque material are each highly predictive of and specific for a serum iron level of >300 $\mu g/dl$.

Treatment

The prompt gastric emptying by ipecac-induced emesis is the initial step in gastric decontamination in the alert patient with an intact gag reflex. Gastric lavage via a large-bore orogastric hose must be performed after airway protection is ensured, if there is any question about the ability of the patient to protect the airway. Lavage reduces the contact of residual iron particles with the gastrointestinal mucosa and decreases the absorption of the remaining iron by precipitating insoluble iron compounds. Sodium bicarbonate of 1–1.5%, the solution of choice, precipitates iron as relatively insoluble ferrous bicarbonate and hydrous iron oxide. Disodium phosphate lavage solutions that convert iron to ferrous phosphate have been used as lavage solutions but have fallen into disfavor because of severe hyperphosphatemia, hypocalcemia, tetany, and hypernatremic dehydration that have occasionally followed their use. If, in spite of vigorous gastric lavage, abdominal radiographs continue to demonstrate the presence of gastric iron-containing aggregates, consideration must be given to the removal of the drug mass by gastrotomy.

Specific Chelation Therapy

Deferoxamine, an avid iron-binding ligand, is a safe and effective chelating agent for the therapy of iron intoxication. It may be administered by either enteral or parenteral routes. The mechanism of action is unclear and remains controversial. Parenteral deferoxamine chelates free iron, as well as iron in storage as ferritin and hemosiderin, to form water-soluble, renally excreted feroxamine.

In mild to moderate intoxication, deferoxamine therapy should be instituted in a dose of 40 mg/kg up to a maximum of 1 g, administered intramuscularly or, in more severe cases, as an intravenous infusion. Deferoxamine should not be administered in excess of 15 mg/kg/hr, to prevent tachycardia and hypotension. Repeated doses of deferoxamine should be administered every 4–6 hours until the urine no longer exhibits a vin rosé color or until the serum iron is <100 $\mu g/dl$. No more than 6 g of deferoxamine should be given in a 24-hour period.

If the pathophysiologic events of iron poisoning involve the iron-induced generation of free radicals and subsequent membrane peroxidation, then therapy with either free radical scavengers or antioxidants might be effective. At the present time, however, there are insufficient data to recommend the use of any such agent for the treatment of iron poisoning.

PHENCYCLIDINE INTOXICATION

Phencyclidine (PCP) intoxication of pediatric patients occurs under two circumstances. Whereas adolescents become intoxicated by purposefully experiencing the mood-altering properties of PCP, infants and young children are exposed by accidental ingestion of PCP, by passive inhalation of ambient, PCP-tainted cigarette smoke, or, occasionally, by intentionally being administered PCP—a form of child abuse.

Pharmacology and Toxicology

The mechanisms of action of PCP have undergone intensive investigation, but the pathophysiology of the intoxication is still unclear. The prominent sympathomimetic effects of PCP intoxication have been attributed to both α-agonistic and anticholinergic actions. The neurologic and psychomimetic manifestations have been variously associated with anticholinergic and dopaminergic antagonistic actions.

Clinical Manifestations

PCP of < 10 mg generally produces low-dose intoxication. These patients usually present with the psychiatric, behavioral, and other neurologic and cardiovascular manifestations of PCP intoxication. Patients with high-dose intoxication caused by > 10 mg of PCP are usually comatose with the more marked neurologic findings noted below.

The hemodynamic findings of PCP intoxication are characteristically those of mild systolic and diastolic hypertension.

Ventilation is well maintained in most low- and moderate-dose PCP-intoxicated patients, a feature that promoted its early use as an anesthetic agent. Hypoventilation and apnea may develop with massive overdoses.

The central nervous system manifestations of PCP intoxication are profound and best known. Nystagmus, which may be either vertical, horizontal, or rotary, is usually present. The pupils are typically midsize or miotic and reactive. Dilated pupils are an infrequent finding. The characteristic motor disturbances of PCP intoxication include hyperactive reflexes, muscle rigidity, catalepsy, opisthotonus, localized dystonic reactions, purposeless facial grimacing, myoclonus, athetosis, and ataxia. Seizures are not infrequently a complication in large overdoses.

Rhabdomyolysis with myoglobinuria and even acute renal failure may complicate the muscle contractions associated with the dystonic motor activity. This can occur with isometric muscle contraction even in the absence of convulsions.

Coma is a feature of moderate- or high-dose intoxication. It may last for hours or, in the most severe intoxications, for many days. Patients may be completely unresponsive but remain with open eyes.

Deaths due to PCP intoxication are usually the result of accidents associated with behavioral disturbances. Occasionally, fatalities are caused by uncontrolled seizures, intracranial bleeding, and respiratory depression. Patients with moderate or severe PCP intoxication may clinically resemble cases of sedative-hypnotic overdose. Hypertension, hyperreflexia, abnormal posturing, and the absence of significant respiratory depression will support the diagnosis of PCP intoxication.

Laboratory Findings

Several chromatographic and enzyme immunoassay techniques of varying sensitivities are available for the detection of PCP in urine, blood, and other body fluids. Quantitative determinations are not of particular importance, since there is no constant relationship between the serum or urine levels of PCP and the severity of intoxication.

Treatment

Since most adolescents and adults are intoxicated by snorting or smoking PCP, inducing emesis and the routine administration of activated charcoal and cathartics are not indicated unless exposure is by ingestion. In the comatose patient where the mode of exposure is unknown, gastric lavage through an orogastric hose and the administration of intragastric activated charcoal and a cathartic should be performed after airway protection is ensured.

General supportive care is the key to successful treatment in the PCP-intoxicated patient. The mildly intoxicated patient should be observed in a quiet, darkened environment. Patients must be continuously observed and prevented from injuring themselves. The technique of "talking down" patients, sometimes successfully used for the management of the agitated patient intoxicated with other hallucinogens, is frequently unsuccessful with the PCP-intoxicated patient. Seizures are usually easily controlled with intravenous diazepam. Severe hypertension is uncommon, but hydralazine, diazoxide, nitroprusside, and propranolol may be used. Rhabdomyolysis with myoglobinuria should be managed with intravenous fluids and a diuretic such as mannitol or furosemide to ensure a diuresis. Urinary alkalinization, the usual therapy for rhabdomyolysis in other clinical circumstances, is contraindicated in the setting of PCP intoxication, because of its action in enhancing the renal absorption of this drug.

Techniques to enhance the elimination of PCP from intoxicated patients have been proposed, but since their efficacy remains unproven, their use should probably be reserved only for severely intoxicated cases. Since PCP has a pK of 8.5 urinary acidification will dramatically increase the renal excretion of the drug by the mechanism of ion trapping. Acidification can be accomplished by the administration of ascorbic acid or ammonium chloride.

CHAPTER 23

Disseminated Intravascular
Coagulation and Hemophilia

DISSEMINATED INTRAVASCULAR COAGULATION

Critically ill children in the intensive care unit may develop the cata-strophic thrombotic and proteolytic syndrome of disseminated intravas-cular coagulation (DIC) as a final common pathway complicating their un-derlying illness. The pathophysiology of the syndrome is discussed, with the focus placed on acute, hemorrhagic, sepsis-induced DIC, the most common manifestation of the syndrome in children, rather than on the thrombotic, chronic DIC more commonly seen in adults. Then an ap-proach to management, emphasizing control of the etiologic disorder but also describing some of the newer antithrombin agents, is outlined.

Thrombin Generation

Thrombin stands at the center of the coagulation mechanism (Fig. 23.1). It is generated from prothrombin by a dual cleavage effected by the pro-thrombinase complex consisting of activated factor X (Xa), activated factor V (Va), and calcium (Ca^{2+}) assembled on the platelet phospholipid mem-brane. In turn, the prothrombinate complex components are activated by factors XII, XI, IX, VIII, and VII as described previously (see the section on general principles of coagulation, briefly outlined in Fig. 23.2).

Once activated, thrombin has manifold effects. It cleaves fibrinopeptides A and B from fibrinogen, leaving fibrin monomer. Fibrin monomers then spontaneously polymerize into large fibers. These fibers are cross-linked by activated factor XIII (XIIIa), which may also further the binding of fibrin to fibronectin and thence to collagen, anchoring the clot to connective tissue. Factor XIII itself is activated by thrombin, so that thrombin catalyzes both the formation and the stabilization of the fibrin clot.

Furthermore, thrombin positively reinforces its own formation by acti-vating factors V and VIII and by stimulating platelet aggregation, mem-brane inversion, and secretion. However, the activation of V, VIII, and platelets by thrombin results in their subsequent degradation. In patho-

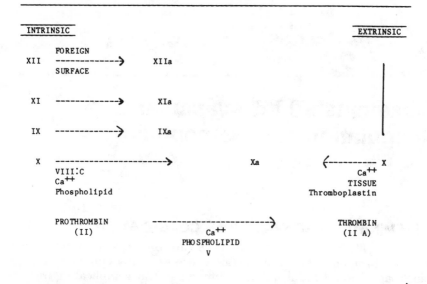

FIGURE 23.1. During clot formation, intrinsic and extrinsic pathways activate factor X (phase I) prior to the formation of thrombin (phase II). (From Rodman G Jr: *Bleeding and Clotting Disorders in the Critically Ill* (a video). Miami, University of Miami, 1980.)

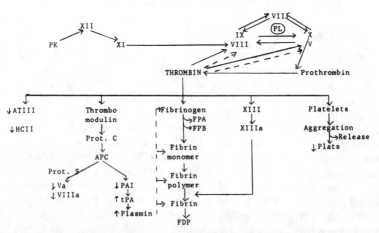

FIGURE 23.2. The role of thrombin in DIC. *Symbols and abbreviations:* ↑, increased; ↓, decreased; →, increases activity; – – →, decreases activity; *PK*, prekallikrein, *ATIII*, antithrombin III; *HCII*, heparin cofactor II; *Prot. C*, protein C; *APC*, activated protein C; *Prot. S*, protein S; *PAI*, plasminogen activator inhibitor; *tPA*, tissue plasminogen activator; *FPA*, fibrinopeptide A; *FPB*, fibrinopeptide B; *FDP*, fibrin degradation products; and *PL*, platelet. (From Corrigan JJ: Disseminated intravascular coagulopathy. *Pediatr Rev* 1:37, 1979.)

logic overactivation of thrombin, therefore, these components (platelets, V, VIII) will be consumed and will contribute to hemostatic failure.

Thrombin is inactivated by both antithrombin III (ATIII) and heparin. Heparin-like molecules are present on the endothelial cell surface and are important in localizing the thrombotic process. ATIII binding to the endothelial surface may be antagonized by platelet factor 4, which competes for its binding site. The platelet also releases an endoglucuronidase that degrades heparin. And the endothelial cell itself may be modulated into a prothrombotic state by pathologic stimuli.

Fibrinolysis

The widespread activation of thrombosis in DIC is countered by secondary fibrinolysis. Thrombin results in the generation of the serine protease plasmin. Plasmin is a proteolytic enzyme with many substrates. It hydrolyzes fibrinogen and fibrin with equal affinity. Fibrin degradation products (FDP) themselves add to the hemostatic failure in DIC.

Plasmin also hydrolyzes V, VIII, IX, and XI. In a feedback loop that may be of particular importance in sepsis-induced DIC, plasmin degrades activated factor XII (XIIa). XIIa fragments, as well as XIIa, catalyze the conversion or prekallikrein into kallikrein on a negatively charged surface that may normally be the activated plated membrane and, in many disorders leading to DIC, may be the denuded collagen basement membrane.

In fulminant DIC there is both an activation and an escape from inhibitory control of the thrombotic and compensatory fibrinolytic (and proteolytic) systems, resulting in hemostatic failure. Platelets, fibrinogen, prothrombin, and factors V, VIII, IX, and XI are consumed to a variable degree. Prekallikrein and protein C will also be activated and then degraded. Coexistent kinin generation results in vasodilation, hypotension, and increased vascular permeability.

Clinical Syndromes (Table 23.1)

Sepsis

Any sepsis syndrome may lead to DIC, and a wide variety of organisms have been implicated. Most characteristic, however, are Gram-negative infections associated with endotoxin release. Endotoxin can directly injure the vessel wall, exposing the subendothelium. The exposed subendothelial surface can initiate contact activation, allowing assembly of factor XII and the associated kallikrein–high-molecular-weight kininogen complex. Pathologically, endotoxin can directly activate factor XII, thus beginning the reciprocal cleavage into active products. Kallikrein can then liberate bradykinin from kininogen. In addition, endotoxin directly binds to a specific platelet receptor, causing the release reaction and furthering both pathologic thrombosis and subsequent platelet exhaustion. Endotoxin also stimulates the synthesis of tissue factor activity by monocytes, which can then activate X in the presence of VIIa. Lymphocytes may amplify this syn-

TABLE 23.1.
Causes of DIC

1. Infection
   A. Gram negative
      a. Endotoxin
         i. Kallikrein—Kinins (e.g., bradykinin) (↓ blood pressure)
         ii. Activates factor XII, platelets
         iii. Endothelial damage
         iv. Activates factor VII (monocyte tissue factor production)
   B. General mechanisms
      a. Direct endothelial damage
      b. Antigen-antibody complexes
         i. Platelet activation
      c. Direct platelet activation
      d. Venous/vascular stasis
2. Tumor
   A. Leukemia
      a. Acute promyelocytic leukemia
         i. Factor VII-like activity
   B. Solid tumors
      a. X-activating activity (especially in mucinous adenocarcinoma)
      b. Endothelial injury and prothrombinase assembly
3. Severe head injury
   A. Tissue thromboplastin activity
4. Obstetric
   A. Abruption
   B. Retained dead fetus
5. Neonatal
   A. Necrotizing enterocolitis
   B. Respiratory distress syndrome
6. Hemolytic-uremic syndrome
7. Giant hemangioma
8. Miscellaneous
   A. Shock (anaphylaxis, heat stroke, etc.)
   B. Snakebite
   C. Transfusion reactions

thesis. The endothelial cell itself may also modulate into a prothrombotic state under the influence of endotoxin.

Both Gram-negative bacteria and other infectious organisms can induce DIC through other mechanisms. These include direct endothelial damage worsened by generalized vascular stasis in shock states or by locally decreased flow in organs injured by the accumulation of organisms and inflammatory cells. The leukocytes may further cause damage by releasing mediators, including proteolytic granular enzymes, superoxides, and sulfated mucopolysaccharides, that nonenzymatically precipitate fibrin monomer. Antigen-antibody complexes may form, resulting in platelet injury.

Sometimes, the attachment of the organism is followed by specific anti-body binding and platelet destruction. Nonspecific lymphocyte stimulation may result in autoantibody production. Although these mechanisms may further the thrombocytopenia in DIC, they may also result in an isolated decrease in the platelet count.

Overall, sepsis-related DIC is a fulminant process whose predominant clinical manifestation is hemorrhage. Nonetheless, it is important to re-member that widespread microthrombosis leading possibly to organ is-chemia is an ongoing process. This is dramatically evident in purpura ful-minans. Intravascular occlusion of the terminal arterioles in the skin gives rise to sharply demarcated areas of hemorrhagic necrosis, which may co-alesce if larger vessels are subsequently occluded. Digit or even limb gan-grene may supervene. Renal damage varying from glomerular injury to cor-tical necrosis may also occur, and a confusional state, convulsions, or coma may be furthered by microvascular occlusion in what may be an underper-fused brain. Pulmonary injury and gastrointestinal ulceration may also re-sult from clots in small vessels.

Associated with Tumor

In adults, DIC associated with cancer is most often a chronic, low-grade, primarily thrombotic process seen most frequently in patients with muci-nous adenocarcinomas. Pancreatic carcinoma leading to migratory throm-bophlebitis is the classic example. The mucin may have X-activating activ-ity. Some malignant cells can also assemble the prothrmbinase complex on their surface. The necessary coagulation factors may have easy access to the malignant cell due to endothelial damage induced by the tumor, allowing extravasation of plasma proteins into the vicinity of the malig-nant cell.

In acute promyelocytic leukemia (APL), the abnormal granules have tis-sue factor activity. The cells may also have fibrinolytic capacity. Hemor-rhage is a frequent presenting manifestation of APL and may worsen with the initiation of therapy, when the disrupted cells release their abnormal granules. Any widespread malignancy may cause enough endothelial in-jury to induce a low-grade state of DIC, although this is rarely of hemo-static significance.

Severe Head Injury

Brain tissue is known to be a potent thromboplastin. In fact, it is the thromboplastic used in the laboratory evaluation of the classic extrinsic pathway determined by prothrombin time (PT). Severe brain injury may, therefore, release thromboplastic substances into the circulation where they initiate coagulation. Studies of brain-injured patients who died within 24 hours of admission demonstrated histopathologic evidence of DIC in a vast majority of these patients, when careful search for this evidence was made. Large thrombi were found most frequently in the brain and spinal cord, liver, lungs, kidneys, and pancreas, while microthrombi were found most frequently in the liver, pituitary, pancreas, thymus, brain and spinal cord, large intestine, kidneys and lungs. Concomitant hypotension, respiratory impairment, or both were common.

Other studies have found that the severity of injury correlates with the presence of DIC defined by abnormalities in three of the following five: tests for PT, activated partial thromboplastin time (aPTT), and FDP, platelet count, and fibrinogen level. Moreover, the prognosis is worse for those with DIC even within the same clinical and radiologic category of severity, reflecting either underestimation of the extent of injury or the worsening of that injury by microthrombus formation.

Neonatal Illness

Birth depression (defined as a 1-minute Apgar score of <3 and a 5-minute Apgar of <7) and sepsis are the most common etiologies of DIC in the newborn. Necrotizing enterocolitis, a syndrome of intestinal mucosal injury most closely related to infection but also related to ischemic bowel injury, which disproportionately affects the small premature infant, may also lead to either thrombocytopenia or DIC. The release of thromboplastic material from the injured bowel may well be etiologic. Certainly, in those cases associated with infection, sepsis-associated thrombocytopenia or DIC may supervene. The respiratory distress syndrome may occasionally be complicated by DIC. Obstetrical problems such as toxemia and third-trimester bleeding figure prominently in neonatal as well as maternal DIC. As always, the small premature (<1500 g at 32 weeks gestation) is at increased risk.

Hemolytic-Uremic Syndrome

Hemolytic-uremic syndrome (HUS) is a triad of uremia, microangiopathic hemolytic anemia, and thrombocytopenia, which most frequently affects children following gastroenteritis. Verotoxin-producing *Escherichia coli* may be the causative organism in many of these enteritis-associated cases, and neuramidase-producing organisms have also been implicated. Other etiologies of the syndrome include shigellosis, familial prostacyclin deficiency, and inherited C2 deficiency. Thrombocytopenia is usually more prominent than DIC, and thrombosis, particularly in the renal microvasculature and perhaps in the brain also, is more important than hemorrhage. The verotoxin, in particular, may act by inducing a plasma factor that causes platelet aggregation by use of glycoproteins IIB and IIIA. Microvascular occlusion in cerebral vessels is particularly pronounced in thrombotic thrombocytopenic purpura, a closely related if not identical syndrome in adults.

Miscellaneous

Any shock state can result in sufficient tissue injury to activate the coagulation mechanism in a widespread fashion. Antibody-mediated hemolytic transfusion reactions can induce DIC. Red cell stroma or hemoglobin alone is not sufficient; antibody also must be bound to the red cell surface. Diseases as disparate as juvenile rheumatoid arthritis and snake bites have had classically defined DIC.

Laboratory Abnormalities

The laboratory abnormalities characteristic of DIC (Table 23.2) reflect the combination of excess thrombosis and fibrinolysis. The least specific is the blood smear, which will show fragmented red cells (schistocytes damaged presumably by passage through small vessels occluded by fibrin. The absence of schistocytes does not rule out DIC, and their presence may be prominent in disorders such as HUS, which have a lesser activation of the coagulation mechanism as a whole.

In acute DIC, the platelet count is frequently decreased. Mean values approximate 50,000/μl, and nearly all are below 150,000/μl. Fibrinogen is less often decreased, perhaps because it is an acute phase reactant that rises in both infection and malignancy, two common underlying conditions predisposing to DIC.

The common screening tests aPTT and PT are abnormal in about two-thirds of patients. FDP are detectable in three-quarters, and fibrin monomer (determined by ethanol and/or protamine gelation) is present in roughly the same number.

In general, a decreased platelet count with a prolonged PT or aPTT and

TABLE 23.2.
Laboratory Tests in DIC, Liver Disease, and Primary Fibrinolysis[a]

Test	DIC	Liver Disease	Primary Fibrinolysis
Blood smear	Fragmented red blood cells; ↓ platelets	Targets; occ. ↓ platelets	
Platelet count	<150,000; may be <50,000	Variable; rarely <50,000	nl
aPTT (intrinsic)	Prolonged	Prolonged	Prolonged
PT (extrinsic)	Prolonged	Prolonged	Prolonged
Fibrinogen	<150 mg/dl	<150 mg/dl only if very severe disease or fibrinolysis	<150 mg/dl
FDP	>40 μg/ml	Usually <40 μg/ml	>40 μg/ml
B-β-related peptides	+	+	+
Fibrinopeptide A	+	?−	−
D dimer	+	?−	−
VIII:C/VIII:CAg or VIII:C/VIII:Ag	↓	?	Probably ↓
ATIII	↓	↓	? nl
Prekallikrein	↓	↓	

[a]Symbols and abbreviations: +, present; −, absent; ,?, uncertain; ↑, increased; ↓, decreased; VIII:C, VIII coagulant activity; VIII:CAg, VIII coagulant antigen; VIII:Ag, VIII-related antigen; and nl, normal.

an elevated titer of FDP in the appropriate clinical setting is sufficient for the diagnosis of DIC. The fibrinogen level may be normal, and the smear may not show red cell abnormalities.

More specialized testing may confirm the overactivation of thrombin or secondary fibrinolysis in doubtful cases, may be used to study the underlying pathophysiology and so perhaps determine treatment, or may give prognostic information. The thrombin time measures the time taken for a specified amount of thrombin to convert fibrinogen to fibrin. It is prolonged in hypofibrinogenemia or dysfibrinogenemia, either inherited or acquired. FDP interfere with fibrin formation and so lengthen the thrombin time. Heparin will also prolong the thrombin time, owing to its antithrombin effect. Measurement of the thrombin time is rapidly performed and so may be helpful in evaluation of the final stages of clot formation in DIC.

When thrombin acts on fibrinogen, it first cleaves a 16-amino acid peptide, fibrinopeptide A, from the A-α chain. Plasma does not effect this cleavage, so the presence of fibrinopeptide A is specific to the action of thrombin. Unfortunately, the radioimmunoassay is time consuming and may be positive even in localized clot formation, not just in DIC. When thrombin forms fibrin from fibrinogen, the fibrin monomers are cross-linked by activated factor XIII through the formation of α-α bonds (D-D dimers). Plasmin degradation leaves these bonds intact. Therefore, detection of an elevated titer of cross-linked FDP is specific for the combined action of thrombin and plasmin. A new monoclonal antibody-based latex bead aggregation assay is commercially available and may be a useful adjunct to diagnosis. Plasmin degradation of fibrin or fibrinogen will lead to the formation of peptides from the B-β chain containing amino acids 15–42. These are measurable by radioimmunoassay and provide a sensitive measure of fibrinolytic activity. Although a lengthy review of all laboratory tests is not possible in a short synopsis of the subject, Table 23.2 does include a list of all tests likely to be relevant at the time of publication.

Differential Diagnosis
Primary Fibrinolysis (Tables 23.2 and 23.3)

Primary fibrinolysis is rare in pediatrics, being most common in adults undergoing pelvic surgery, especially surgery involving the prostate gland. Generally, primary activation of plasmin will leave platelet numbers intact. Platelet secretory products such as β-thromboglobulin will not be elevated, nor will those fibrin fragments that require the initial action of thrombin

TABLE 23.3. ————————————————————————————
Conditions with Increased Fibrinolytic Activity

1. Giant hemangioma
2. Postbypass
   a. Platelet activation
   b. Factor XII activation

(fibrinopeptide A, D-D dimers). Two situations deserve mention. The cardiopulmonary bypass pump may lead to primary fibrinolysis, perhaps by contact activation due to the rapid flow of blood. This may complicate the thrombocytopenia with dysfunctional residual platelets usually found after extracorporeal circulation. Second, in the consumption coagulopathy occurring within a giant hemangioma (Kasabach-Merritt syndrome), fibrinolysis induced by the abnormal endothelium may play a role, although thrombopenia is also commonly prominent.

Liver Disease (Tables 23.2 and 23.3)

Severe liver failure profoundly affects the coagulation mechanism, the fibrinolytic system, and their inhibiting proteins. The liver synthesizes fibrinogen and the vitamin K-dependent factors II (prothrombin), VII, IX, X, protein C, and protein S, as well as factors V, XI, XII, and XIII. In addition, an abnormal fibrinogen with excess sialic acid content may be synthesized in patients with a variety of hepatic disorders, particularly chronic active hepatitis, cirrhosis, and acute liver failure. This acquired abnormality impairs fibrin polymerization, giving abnormally long thrombin and reptilase times. The thrombin time is correctable by the addition of excess calcium chloride, since calcium ions accelerate fibrin polymerization. Plasminogen, antithrombin III, and prekallikrein are also synthesized in the liver. Their levels decrease in liver failure. Prekallikrein, in particular, has been suggested as a marker of hepatic protein synthetic failure. Congestive splenomegaly may develop in liver failure, leading to platelet sequestration in the spleen and to thrombocytopenia.

The damaged liver may poorly clear plasminogen activators and may synthesize decreased amounts of α_2-antiplasmin. Accelerated fibrinolysis may, therefore, contribute to the hemostatic defect in liver failure and may be more frequent than DIC in the absence of complicating infection. The distinction between these two conditions may be difficult. Relative preservation of platelet numbers, with negative assays for fibrinopeptide A and the D dimer, low levels of FDP, and shortened clot lysis times, would support a diagnosis of fibrinolysis rather than DIC.

Therapy (Table 23.4)

The mainstay of therapy in DIC is treatment of the underlying disease. The most clear-cut example of the efficacy of such therapy is in obstetrical disorders, in which evacuation of the uterine contents removes the thrombotic stimulus and allows for rapid normalization of hemostasis.

Elimination of the thrombotic initiators is more difficult in sepsis or in other shock states in which there may be diffuse vascular damage. Antithrombin therapy has, therefore, been suggested as an adjunct to treatment of the underlying disorders. This has classically been heparinization. Unfortunately, the main side effect of heparin is hemorrhage, so that heparin has been a controversial medication for use in DIC. Some respected authorities still advocate its cautious use, although some retrospective reviews suggest no benefit in either the neonate or the adult. A recent con-

TABLE 23.4.
Therapy in DIC

1. Interrupt the process
   a. Treat the underlying disease
2. Replacement
   a. Platelets: 1 unit/5 kg body weight
   b. Plasma: 10–15 ml kg body weight
   c. Cryoprecipitate (fibrinogen source): 1 bag/5 kg body weight
3. Pharmacologic intervention
   a. Heparin
      i. APL
      ii. Purpura fulminans
   b. Investigational
      i. ATIII
      ii. Synthetic antithrombins
      iii. Heparin fragments
4. Exchange transfusion

trolled trial in the adult showed no benefit to heparinization and, in fact, demonstrated increased bleeding in those with hemorrhage shock who had been treated with heparin.

Nonetheless, there are at least two specific indications for heparin therapy. In purpura fulminans, fibrin deposition in small vessels is of major pathologic significance, and heparin therapy may improve outcome. Heparin may also normalize coagulation in acute promyelocytic leukemia by interfering with the action of the tissue factor-like activity in the granules.

Recently, antithrombin III concentrates have become available in Europe. Preliminary experience suggests efficacy, and earlier correction of coagulation abnormalities in patients with low levels of ATIII who receive substitution therapy. No difference in survival was found, however, emphasizing the crucial role of the underlying disorder in determining outcome. Other investigational antithrombin agents that show promise include a synthetic thrombin inhibitor and perhaps some of the newer heparin fragments and derivatives.

In the neonate, exchange transfusion has been advocated. However, a controlled trial in a small number of patients showed no benefit when compared with either supportive care alone or supportive care plus transfusion therapy. Supportive care is also crucial to the outcome of the HUS, consisting mainly of management of the renal failure. Plasma infusion has an uncertain role, except in patients with hereditary prostacyclin deficiency. In patients with giant hemangioma (Kasabach-Merritt syndrome), evidence of fibrinolysis has prompted the use of fibrinolytic inhibitors, with resultant improvement in outcome. Fibrinolytic inhibitors have also been suggested in liver disease when excess fibrinolysis is demonstrable. Replacement therapy is also important in liver disease. Platelets may be rapidly sequestered, unfortunately. Prothrombin concentrates containing factors II, VII, IX, and X have been used also, although the damaged liver may poorly clear the activated clotting factors they contain, leading to the risk of thrombosis. Fresh frozen plasma (FFP) can be used, although the volume required may be a problem.

In general, replacement is probably indicated in patients with DIC and significant hemorrhage, despite the risk of "feeding the fire," along with vigorous treatment of the etiologic disorder. FFP in a dose of 10–15 ml/kg supplies all factors in limited concentration. One unit of platelets per 5 kg of body weight is estimated to raise the platelet count 50,000/μl. One unit of cryoprecipitate per 5 kg of body weight will raise the fibrinogen concentration about 75 mg/dl. This replacement should also be undertaken in victims of snake bite, along with the administration of specific antivenom.

Summary

DIC is a syndrome that results from a pathologic activation of thrombin with secondary fibrinolysis. The contact system (factor XII) with subsequent kinin generation is importantly involved in furthering the pathophysiologic process, especially in sepsis-associated DIC. The diagnosis is confirmed by a constellation of laboratory abnormalities, most prominently thrombocytopenia, a prolonged PT and aPTT, a decreased fibrinogen level, and the pressure of FDP in the appropriate clinical setting. The VIII:C/VIII:CAg or VIII:C/VIII:Ag ratio will decline, and inhibitors of thrombosis of fibrinolysis such as antithrombin III, α_2-antiplasmin, α_2-macroglobulin, and heparin cofactor II will be consumed.

Treatment of the underlying disorder is the agreed-upon mainstay of therapy. Replacement therapy in hemorrhagic states has been more controversial, as has antithrombotic intervention with heparin. A defined role for heparin is limited to its use in acute promyelocytic leukemia and purpura fulminans. More specific antithrombin treatment is becoming available in the form of heparin fragments, antithrombin III concentrates, and synthetic antithrombins and may improve outcome if the etiologic disorder can be effectively controlled.

HEMOPHILIA IN THE INTENSIVE CARE UNIT

The most common severe inherited bleeding disorders are the hemophilias. Hemophilia A, or classical hemophilia, is a deficiency of functional factor VIII:C, the coagulant portion of the factor VIII molecule. The VIII:C may be functionally absent but immunologically present (low VIII:C, higher VIII:CAg), implying production of an aberrant molecule. Alternatively, no molecule may be synthesized, with consequent low values of both VIII:C and VIII:CAg. The factor VIII-related antigen, VIII:Ag, and the platelet-aggregating activity of its multimer, the Rcof, will be normal. Similarly, in Christmas disease or hemophilia B, factor IX activity will be decreased. Cross-reacting material representing a functionally deficient IX may be present.

Both disorders are X-linked, so that the severe expression is limited to the hemizygous male. Occasionally, heterozygous females will inactivate enough of the normal X chromosome in precursor cells to have a level lower than the predicted 50%, although often that level is not <20%. Bleeding manifestations vary with the factor level, with severely affected patients having levels usually of <1% and patients with moderately severe defects having levels of between 1 and 5%. Moderately affected patients have VIII:C values between 5 and 15%, and mildly affected patients have values between 15 and 25%. Patients with values of >25% rarely bleed excessively, except with major traumatic or surgical stress. The overall incidence of both hemophilias is variably quoted as 1:10,000 males or 1:10,000 population, with VIII:C deficiency being about 4 times as common as IX deficiency.

Most bleeding episodes involve the muscles and joints and, more rarely, mucosal surfaces, perhaps because muscles and joints are relatively deficient in tissue factor activity and so require the augmentation pathway of VIII:C and IX for factor X activation. These bleeds rarely require intensive care and so are not further discussed.

Bleeding in the hemophiliac may be life-threatening either because of quantitative loss or because of location. Volume loss and the oxygen-carrying capacity (red cells) should be replaced in accordance with the general principles of patient management in these situations. In addition, factor replacement therapy is required. If the bleeding disorder is not yet specifically diagnosed but has been suspected because of excessive bleeding in relation to the extent of injury, a screening PT and aPTT should be performed. In VIII:C and IX deficiency, the PT is normal but the aPTT is prolonged, usually at least 60 seconds in patients with severe deficiencies. FFP contains both factors and should be administered in a dose of at least 15 ml/kg in a patient with excessive bleeding, a normal PT, and a prolonged aPTT. An emergency factor assay can usually be performed within 1 hour and can give an idea as to which factor is deficient. The level following a bleed may be lower than the patient's usual level, due to consumption of limited stores. Once a determination as to which factor is deficient has been made, more definitive replacement therapy can be given. One unit of VIII:C activity per kilogram will raise the VIII:C level about 2%. FFP contains 1 unit/ml, so that a large volume is required for adequate replacement. Cryoprecipitate contains 60–80 units of VIII:C activity per bag, and each bag is usually about 10 ml in volume. The lyophilized VIII:C concentrates vary by batch. As an example, a vial of a current batch contains about 280 units/bottle, requiring 10 ml of normal saline for reconstitution prior to administration. The concentrates are now heat treated, inactivating the HTLV-III, the putative agent causing acquired immune deficiency syndrome. Heat treatment does not, however, destroy the hepatitis viruses. For major bleeding, correction to at least 70% and perhaps to 100% activity (50 units/kg) is recommended. In factor IX-deficient patients, 1 unit of factor IX per kilogram will raise the activity only slightly more than 1%. Replacement to >80% would, therefore, require the administration of 80 units of lyophilized IX concentrates per kilogram, which are heat treated, as are the VIII:C concentrates. Blood precautions should be observed both when the concentrate is drawn up and when the venipuncture is performed. The concentrate may be administered either through a filtered needle or through a filtered Soluset.

Bleeding may also be life-threatening due to location. The central nervous system and the airway are the two most common potentially lethal areas of bleeding, as in the hemophiliac. The risk of intracranial bleeding is estimated in hemophiliacs as being between 2.0 and 3.5%/yr. After all but the most minor head trauma, replacement therapy to levels of 100% activity should be given. In patients with mild to moderate classical hemophilia who have suffered a relatively minor injury, DDAVP, a vasopressin analog, may be administered in a dose of 10 $\mu g/m^2$ (maximum, 24 μg), diluted to a final concentration of 0.5 $\mu g/ml$ to normal saline, given intravenously over 20 minutes, since it raises the VIII:C levels twofold to threefold, probably by release from endogenous stores. However, if brain swelling is suspected, DDAVP should not be used, since it may result in water retention, although water intoxication has not been reported at this dose. The most frequent side effects are facial flushing (possibly from prostacyclin release) and mild light-headedness. Hypotension during the first hour (also presumably from prostacyclin release) may be seen, although it is rarely severe. Headache and backache occur less commonly. A computed axial tomography scan of the brain should be performed to rule out intracranial bleeding. However, a negative result should not be overly reassuring, since the bleeding may be delayed. Therefore, a repeat computed axial tomography scan should be done if the patient clinically deteriorates.

Airway bleeding may follow local trauma, including prolonged dental work. Again, replacement to levels of 100% activity should be given.

Ten to fifteen percent of patients with VIII:C deficiency develop anti-VIII:C antibodies or inhibitors. Management of these patients remains a clinical challenge. In patients with low-titer inhibitors (<5 Bethesda units), the antibody may be overwhelmed with large doses of VIII:C, followed by a continuous VIII:C infusion. This will cause an anamnestic antibody rise in 4–5 days and so is reserved for life-threatening situations. In patients with higher titer inhibitors, IX concentrates or activated IX concentrates are given. Factor VIII:C bypassing activity is present in IX concentrates, perhaps reflecting activated factor X (Xa) activity. Activated complexes, which presumably contain more of this activity, are commercially available although expensive (e.g., FEIBA, Autoplex). They are titered for IX levels, not for bypassing activity levels, so the dose recommended for bleeding, 80 units/kg, is an empirical one. The Xa may cause a low-grade state of DIC through widespread thrombin activation, so that fibrinolytic inhibitors such as tranexamic acid or ϵ-aminocaproic acid (Amicar) must be avoided when IX complexes are given.

CHAPTER 24

Burns, Inhalational Injury, and Electrical Injury

PATHOPHYSIOLOGY OF THERMAL INJURY

The initial thermal injury to tissue results in areas of coagulation necrosis and cell death. In damaged tissues, an increase in capillary permeability occurs, ultimately resulting in edema formation. Large endothelial gaps that persist for several days have been demonstrated by electron microscopy. Other factors contributing to edema formation include hypoproteinemia and increased osmotic pressure in burned tissue.

Cardiovascular (Fig. 24.1)

Profound alterations in the cardiovascular system occur in association with thermal injury. Cardiac output is initially decreased largely due to decreased circulating blood volume and an increase in systemic vascular resistance. Cardiac output usually returns to normal before complete restoration of intravascular volume. Central venous pressure and pulmonary capillary wedge pressure are usually low normal and may remain so after adequate resuscitation.

Hypertension is a common phenomenon following thermal injury in pediatric patients. Hypertensive encephalopathy has been reported and is characterized by any one of the following: (a) convulsions, (b) marked irritability, (c) extreme lethargy, or (d) disorientation.

Pulmonary

Pulmonary dysfunction associated with thermal injury may be secondary to inhalational injury, aspiration, sepsis, congestive heart failure, shock, or associated trauma. Significant pulmonary disease is well described in thermal injury without associated inhalational injury. Experimental evidence reveals an initial increase in pulmonary arterial pressure as well as an increase in lung lymph flow following thermal injury.

359

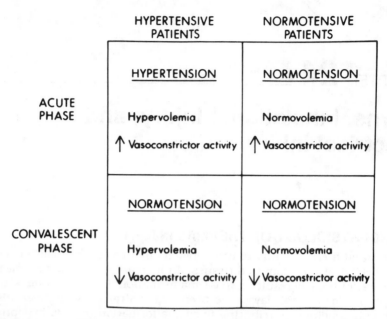

FIGURE 24.1. Correlation of hypertension with abnormalities in circulating blood volume and vasoconstrictor activity in burned children. (From Popp MB, Silberstein EB, Laxmi SS, et al: A pathophysiologic study of the hypertension associated with burn injury in children. *Ann Surg* 193:823, 1981.)

Renal

Renal failure following thermal injury is uncommon but can result from the following: (*a*) prolonged systemic hypotension secondary to inadequate or delayed fluid resuscitation, (*b*) myoglobin released from damaged muscle tissue, or rarely, (*c*) hemoglobin released as a result of heat-induced hemolysis. Renal blood flow is decreased immediately following thermal injury. Later, the glomerular filtration rate may increase dramatically, coinciding with the onset of the postburn hypermetabolic state and hyperdynamic circulation. This alteration in renal blood flow becomes important when achieving therapeutic serum concentrations of antibiotics that are excreted by the kidneys is attempted.

Hepatic

Hepatic dysfunction is common following burn injury. Failure of active ion transport or changes in relative cell membrane permeability are implicated in the etiology of hepatic dysfunction. Patients with hepatic injury had a larger surface area burn and greater mortality than patients without evidence of hepatic dysfunction. Clinical jaundice was associated with 90% mortality. The etiology of hepatic dysfunction remains speculative, although early hemodynamic alterations, hypoxia, and sepsis may be related.

Hematologic
Platelets

Mild thrombocytopenia occurs during the first several days following burn injury and is followed by thrombocytosis (2–4 times normal) by the end of the first week.

Clotting Factors

Prothrombin, partial thromboplastin, and thrombin times show little change following burn injury. There are, however, significant increases in fibrinogen as well as factors V and VIII. Fibrin-fibrinogen split products are usually elevated and tend to parallel fibrinogen levels.

Bleeding and thrombotic complications following thermal injury are usually related to local tissue disease (e.g., Curling's ulcer, thrombophlebitis from venous catheters) rather than to systemic hypocoagulation or hypercoagulation.

Disseminated intravascular coagulation with generalized bleeding can occur following thermal injury. Disseminated intravascular coagulation is suggested by occurrence of thrombocytopenia, hypofibrinogenemia, prolongation of prothrombin time and partial thromboplastic time, and elevation of fibrin-fibrinogen split products.

Red Blood Cells

After burn injury, there is a decrease in red cell mass associated with fragmented red cells. Red cell pigment may appear in the plasma and urine. A low hemoglobin is masked in the early stages by hemoconcentration as fluid is lost from the intravascular compartment.

Central Nervous System

Central nervous system dysfunction is frequently present in pediatric burn patients. Hypoxia occurring in the first 48 hours is the most common cause of encephalopathy and is related to smoke and carbon monoxide inhalation sustained in enclosed area fires. Hypovolemia, hyponatremia, sepsis, cortical vein thrombosis, and gliosis secondary to "water shed" infarct are other entities that produced encephalopathy. Seizures, obtundation, coma, or hallucinations are presenting neurologic manifestations of the central nervous system dysfunction in these patients.

Gastrointestinal

Stress ulceration (Curling's ulcer) of the stomach or duodenum is a life-threatening but preventable complication in the burned patient. In patients with severe burns, gastric mucosal abnormalities are found in 90% of patients. Antacid prophylaxis and cimetidine are efficacious, and combined therapy can be utilized when bleeding occurs during antacid therapy.

ESTIMATION OF BURN SIZE AND DEPTH

Burn size is expressed as a percentage of the total body surface area (BSA) and changes according to the age of the child, from 1 year until adult proportions are reached at 15 years of age. This percentage may be estimated by the "rule of nines" in children age 15 (Fig. 24.2) but requires a more exact estimate in younger children (Fig. 24.3). For small burns, the size of the child's hand is approximately equal to 1% of the BSA.

First-Degree Burn

First-degree burn is a superficial injury characterized by erythemia and pain and perhaps by minor blistering; sunburn is an example. Tissue loss is restricted to epithelial cells. No treatment is required except for pain

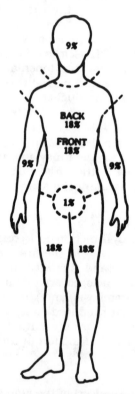

FIGURE 24.2. An estimate of the percentage of total body surface skin that is burned can be obtained by use of the "rule of nines" whereby the total surface area of skin is divided into areas equaling 9% of the total. (From Demling RH: Fluid and electrolyte management. *Crit Care Clin* 1:34, 1985.)

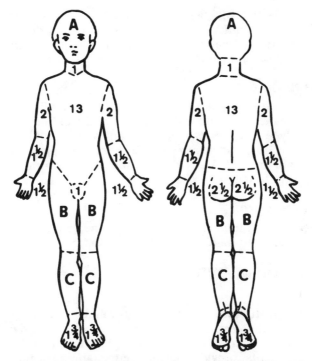

PERCENTAGE OF SURFACE AREA OF HEAD AND LEGS AT VARIOUS AGES.

	AGE IN YEARS				
AREA IN DIAGRAM	0	1	5	10	15
A = ½ of head	9½	8½	6½	5½	4½
B = ½ of one thigh	2¾	3¼	4	4¼	4½
C = ½ of one lower leg	2½	2½	2¾	3	3¼

FIGURE 24.3. This chart of body areas, together with the table showing the percentage of surface area of the head and legs at various ages, can be used to estimate the surface area burned in a child. (From Solomon JR: Pediatric burns. *Crit Care Clin* 1:161, 1985.)

relief. Very rarely, an extensive first-degree burn may require intravenous fluid therapy.

Second-Degree Burn

In second-degree burn, tissue death occurs through the epidermis and into a variable portion of the dermis. When damage is superficial partial-thickness burn, the extent of the damage to the dermis is slight. Healing will take place with little or no scarring within 10–12 days; if the patient is black, pigment will return to the injured area. The clinical appearance of a superficial partial-thickness burn is moist, red, and tender. Within a few days the color becomes pale as a superficial eschar develops, but vary often the viable dermal papillae can be seen through the thin eschar as tiny red dots separated by intervals of no more than 1 mm.

Third-Degree Burn

In third-degree burn, which is also referred to as a full-thickness injury, the necrotic area extends through all layers of the skin into the hypodermic fat. This type of burn may heal by contracture if it is very small in size, but usually surgical closure is indicated. The appearance of such a burn varies from dry and charred to red and nonblanching with pressure. It is not sensitive to touch.

Fourth-Degree Burn

Fourth-degree burn implies deep injury to bone, joint, or muscle, usually occurring secondary to high-voltage electrical injury.

CLASSIFICATION OF BURNS

Minor Burn

In minor burn, the total surface area involved is <5%. No significant involvement of hands, feet, face, or perineum is present. No full-thickness component and no other complications are present. These children may be treated as outpatients, provided social circumstances permit.

Moderate Burn

Moderate burn is characterized by involvement of 5–15% BSA or by the presence of any full-thickness component. Involvement of the hands, feet, face, or perineum or the presence of any complicating factor such as chemical or electrical injury also constitutes moderate burn. These patients should be admitted to the hospital.

Severe Burn

Severe burns are characterized by a total burn size of >15% BSA, by a full-thickness component in excess of 5% BSA, or by the presence of smoke inhalation or carbon monoxide poisoning. The child should be admitted to a special burn treatment facility or pediatric intensive care unit following stabilization.

TRANSPORTING THE BURNED CHILD

If a burned child is to be transported to a facility specializing in burn therapy, the accepting hospital should request the following from the referring hospital:

1. Intravenous access should be obtained prior to transport, and initial volume resuscitation should be begun. A Foley catheter and nasogastric

tube should also be inserted. Resuscitation should be initiated according to the Parkland formula.

2. Airway management should include endotracheal intubation prior to transport if indications of airway burns or respiratory distress are present.

3. Monitoring of the patient should include vital signs and urinary output measurements.

4. If the patient is hemodynamically stable, the patient should be transported with the head elevated to minimize airway edema. Burned extremities should also be elevated.

5. Copies of all medical records, including laboratory data and X-rays, should accompany the patient.

PHYSIOLOGY OF FLUID RESUSCITATION

The most useful index of adequate intravascular replacement is urine output. A urine output of 0.5–1.0 ml/kg/hr is optimal. With rare exceptions, a urine output of <0.5 ml/kg/hr is indicative of insufficient intravascular volume. Diuretics are rarely indicated in burn patients, and the induced diuresis obscures the most useful gauge of intravascular volume. Measurements of central venous pressure and pulmonary capillary wedge pressure must be interpreted cautiously in the burn patient, as cardiac output is restored prior to blood and plasma volumes. Arbitrary attempts to elevate filling pressures may result in administration of massive volumes of fluid, leading to increased morbidity from edema formation without evidence of clinical improvement related to the higher filling pressures.

Children with burns exceeding 15% BSA will require intravenous resuscitation. If the burn size exceeds 30% BSA, placement of a central venous catheter is recommended. If the burn is >50% BSA, two central venous catheters may be required. It is our practice in children with large burns (>30% BSA), in whom the need for prolonged intravenous therapy can be anticipated, to place the initial intravenous catheter through a burned area while it is still relatively sterile, preserving unburned sites for later use.

Crystalloid resuscitation provides the principal element necessary to restore circulating plasma volume, namely, the sodium ion. There are few areas in the management of critically ill patients laden with more controversy than the inclusion or exclusion of colloid from burn resuscitation in the first 24 hours. The most popular formula in use today is the Parkland formula.

First 24 Hours. Lactated Ringer's solution (4 ml/kg/BSA burned (in percent)) is given during the first 24 hours. In infants, maintenance fluid volume (500 mg) per square meter per day, given as lactated Ringer's solution, must be added to the Parkland formula. One-half of this volume is given in the initial 8 hours postburn, and the other half is given during the next 16 hours. The rate of resuscitation should be adjusted to maintain a urine output of 0.5–1.0 ml/kg/hr.

Second 24 Hours. Maintenance fluid (1500 ml/m²/day) is begun with glucose-containing hypotonic fluid. Colloid may be used to improve urinary output and treat hypoalbuminemia. After the completion of the second postburn day, intravenous fluid should be chosen to maintain normal sodium, phosphate, calcium, and potassium homeostasis. Because of the intense adrenal response to burn stress, potassium wasting in the urine is common and may reach 200 mEq/l.

AIRWAY MANAGEMENT

Within days following thermal injury, it is imperative that nondepolarizing muscle relaxants be used in place of succinylcholine if a muscle relaxant is necessary to facilitate endotracheal intubation. Hyperkalemia associated with cardiac arrest is a potential complication of succinylcholine in the postburn period. The period of risk for succinylcholine-induced hyperkalemia begins 5–15 days postburn and lasts for 3–16 months.

WOUND MANAGEMENT

The burn wound should be gently cleansed with saline, and blisters should be debrided. This may be done in the hydrotherapy tub or in bed. After a brief period of drying, a suitable topical agent should be applied to the wound, and the wound should be dressed. Escharotomy or fasciotomy may become necessary within hours of admission in order to relieve peripheral vascular or nerve compression. Occasionally, thoracic escharotomy is necessary to facilitate chest expansion.

Medications

Providing appropriate tetanus prophylaxis is mandatory. In addition, it is our practice to administer penicillin for 3 days to patients with major burns as antistreptococcal prophylaxis. Penicillin may be given intravenously in doses appropriate for age.

Topical Chemotherapy

The most commonly available agents and their advantages and disadvantages are illustrated in Table 24.1

Biologic Dressings

Allograft, amnion, and artificial dressings are useful when the eschar has separated completely and the wound is clean and awaiting surgical closure. They are also useful for the protection of donor sites after surgery and on fresh partial-thickness burns for pain relief, provided the area involved is not large enough to need thorough protection from infection (which biologic dressings do not provide). Of the materials available, allograft is preferred by most burn surgeons, with fresh, fresh frozen, and lyophilized being the order of priority.

TABLE 24.1.
Commonly Used Topical Antibacterial Agents

Name	Advantages and Disadvantages	Side Effects	Dressing Orders
Silver sulfadiazine (Silvadene)	Broad antibacterial action; painless; fair penetration of eschar	Sulfonamide sensitivity (rash); absorption into fetal circulation is unknown; is contraindicated in pregnancy; occasional leukopenia (reversible upon discontinuation)	Apply twice daily; cover with a light layer of dressings on extremities; leave face and chest open
Mafenide (Sulfamylon)	Excellent antibacterial action, particularly against Gram-positives and clostridia; also Gram-negatives; rapid eschar penetration	Painful; sulfonamide sensitivity (rash); carbonic anhydrase inhibition leading to acidosis	Apply twice daily; leave face, chest, and abdomen open; one light layer of dressings elsewhere
Aqueous silver nitrate solution	Universal antibacterial action; poor penetration of eschar	Leaking of chloride into the dressings with potential hypochloremic alkalosis; strong staining of tissues	Apply twice daily; dress with a light layer of gauze dressings
Iodophors (e.g., Efodine)	Universal antibacterial action; poor penetration of eschar	Strong staining of tissues; iodine absorption	Apply twice daily; dress with a light layer of gauze dressings
Topical bacitracin cream	Limited antibacterial action; poor eschar penetration; cosmetically acceptable; easy to apply; transparent	Rapid development of resistance; conjunctivitis if contacts the conjunctiva	Should only be applied to small areas of cosmetic importance, e.g., second-degree burns of the face; leave open: apply twice daily

NUTRITION

We currently use the following formula:

Carlories required per day = (25 × kg of body weight) + (40 × %BSA burn)

In addition to the absolute caloric intake, the calorie-to-nitrogen ratio is also important, with a currently recommended ratio of approximately 100:1 to 150:1. Trace elements and vitamin supplements are given according to recommended daily requirements for age.

PAIN MANAGEMENT

Intravenous morphine (0.1–0.2 mg/kg) given slowly is recommended for controlling pain in the acute phase of burn injury. The dose required to relieve pain will vary from patient to patient, and frequent small doses (e.g., 0.02–0.03 mg morphine per kilogram every 10–15 minutes) can be titrated to achieve adequate analgesia without rigid adherence to a standard dose. Continuous infusion of narcotics has been utilized by some. Tolerance may occur during therapy, and narcotic dose should be increased, with discontinuation of narcotics anticipated as the wound heals. Fear of inducing addiction is unfounded.

Ketamine has been used successfully in alleviating pain associated with short procedures in burn units. Its popularity stems from several factors including its properties as a profound analgesic and cardiovascular and respiratory stimulant and because of preservation of airway reflexes. Side effects include hypertension, emergence dilirium and hallucinations, and, rarely, aspiration of gastric contents and laryngospasm. Suction equipment, oxygen, and AMBU bag and mask, as well as emergency supplies for intubation and resuscitation, should be available.

INHALATIONAL INJURY, AIRWAY BURNS, AND CARBON MONOXIDE POISONING

Thermal Injury

Thermal injury of the airway is largely limited to the upper airway, as the efficient heat-dissipating mechanism of the upper airway cools the air prior to its reaching the lungs. Direct thermal injury to the lungs is rare except when steam is inhaled, as it has 4000 times the heat-carrying capacity of dry air. Early recognition of upper airway burns is extremely important, as massive edema can develop rapidly, either before or during fluid resuscitation. This can result in total airway obstruction and difficult or impossible conditions for endotracheal intubation. Relative indications for endotracheal intubation include a history of enclosed space fire, burns to the lips and nose, visible edema of the oral cavity or posterior pharynx, wheezing, air hunger, hoarse cry, croupy cough, stridor, the presence of soot in the mouth or nares, or circumferential burns of the neck. It is important to realize that arterial P_aO_2, as well as the chest X-ray, may be normal in the face of impending airway obstruction

Airway Management of the Patient with Airway Burns

Intubating the trachea of a child who has sustained thermal airway injury presents special problems. As mentioned earlier, thermal injury involving the face, lips, pharynx, and upper airway can lead to massive upper airway edema, making tracheal intubation extremely difficult or impossible. Endotracheal intubation prior to the onset of edema allows for a standard approach, namely, the use of intravenous anesthetic and muscle relaxant. A "rapid-sequence" technique utilizing cricoid pressure is suggested, as aspiration of gastric contents is a significant risk. Other acceptable methods of securing the airway include fiberoptic-guided endotracheal intubation or endotracheal intubation without anesthetic or muscle relaxant (awake intubation). The topic of risks of succinylcholine in burned patients has already been discussed.

Carbon Monoxide Poisoning

Pathophysiology of Carbon Monoxide Poisoning

The mechanism of CO poisoning, resulting in reversible combination with hemoglobin, leading to tissue hypoxia, was described by Bernard in 1857. Haldane in 1895 described the equilibrium reactions pertaining to CO and hemoglobin. CO toxicity is, in part, due to its tremendous affinity for hemoglobin, binding to hemoglobin with an affinity 240 times greater than oxygen. Haldane's first law states that

$$(COHb)/O_2Hb) = MPCO/PO_2$$

where M is the affinity constant of 240, COHb and O_2Hb are concentrations of CO and oxygen bound to hemoglobin, and PCO and PO_2 are partial pressures of CO and oxygen to which the hemoglobin is exposed. The hemoglobin molecule is 50% saturated with CO at a partial pressure of only 0.10 mm Hg. In contrast, the hemoglobin molecule is 50% saturated with oxygen (P_{50}) at a partial pressure of 27 mm Hg. CO also caused a leftward shift in the oxyhemoglobin dissociation curve (Fig. 24.4), thereby enhancing oxygen affinity for hemoglobin and impeding oxygen delivery from blood to tissue.

CO also binds to myoglobin and to the intracellular oxygen transport system (cytochrome oxidases), thereby blocking cellular oxidation, resulting in cellular anoxia. The importance of the cytochrome oxidase system in CO poisoning is that inhalation of CO likely results in high concentrations of dissolved CO in the blood leaving the lungs. Dissolved CO can then cross into the tissues and combine with the cytochrome oxidase system.

Diagnosis of Carbon Monoxide Poisoning

The diagnosis of CO poisoning is made from history of exposure, physical signs and symptoms, and laboratory data including measurement of COHb concentration in the blood. COHb in the blood can be measured spectrophotometrically or can be measured from the patient's exhaled air in parts per million by using a CO analyzer and then converting the value

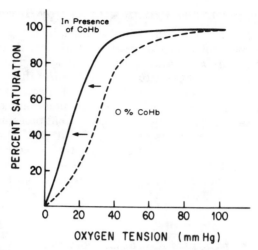

FIGURE 24.4. Oxygen saturation in carbon monoxide poisoning. (Reproduced by permission of Zimmerman SS, Truxal B: Carbon monoxide poisoning. *Pediatrics* 68:218, 1981.)

to COHb concentration by use of equations. The spectrophotometric method is most accurate. A COHb value within normal limits does not rule out recent CO poisoning. If significant time has elapsed since exposure to CO or if supplemental oxygen has been given, the COHb values may have declined by the time the first blood sample was analyzed for COHb concentration. Gross error occurs in calculating oxyhemoglobin from partial pressures of oxygen in the presence of a significant COHb concentration. Pulse oximetry is not useful in carbon monoxide poisoning because it measures the percentage of saturation of available binding sites (not including sites bound by CO) and thus is inaccurate in CO poisoning.

Organ System Response to Carbon Monoxide Poisoning

Cardiovascular

The heart is especially vulnerable to the anoxic effects of CO poisoning in the child or adult with pre-existing cardiac disease. Exposure to CO results in abnormalities of S-T segment of T wave abnormalities, atrial fibrillation, intraventricular block, extrasystoles, ischemia, and infarction.

Pulmonary

Pulmonary injury frequently accompanies CO poisoning, with pulmonary edema occurring in 10–30% of cases. The mechanism of pulmonary edema associated with CO poisoning remains speculative.

Neurologic

The neurologic manifestations of CO poisoning are protean, and some are listed in Table 24.2. Disorientation, slurred speech, dizziness, weak-

TABLE 24.2.
Clinical Neurologic Symptoms of CO Poisoning

Headache	Akinetic mutism
Dizziness	Amnesia
Disorientation	Dysphagia
Lethargy	Unilateral/bilateral
Delirium	pyramidal signs
Altered level of	Extrapyramidal signs
consciousness	Hemiplegia
Seizures	Cortical blindness
Depression	Delayed neurologic
Irritabilitity	changes

ness, seizures, and decreased levels of consciousness are common in acute poisoning and can be grossly correlated with COHb concentrations. Facial spasms and trismus, mimicking tetanus, have been reported in CO poisoning. Cerebral edema may complicate severe CO poisoning, and aggressive therapy is recommended if evidence of cerebral edema is present.

Muscular and Renal

Muscle necrosis leading to myoglobinuria and subsequent acute renal failure may complicate CO poisoning. The mechanisms of myonecrosis include: (a) the patient falling unconscious in a position that occludes venous drainage, resulting in swelling and compression of arterial circulation; (b) anoxia as the direct effect of CO poisoning; and (c) associated crush or electrical injury.

Cutaneous

Erythema, edema, and blistering are cutaneous manifestations of CO poisoning and can be mistaken for burns. Histologically, skin necrosis is present. The frequently mentioned cherry-red color of skin and mucous membranes is uncommon in CO poisoning.

Ophthalmologic

Blindness (temporary and permanent), visual field deficits secondary to cortical lesions, and retinal findings including venous congestion, papilledema, retinal hemorrhages, and red retinal veins may occur with CO poisoning.

Signs, Symptoms, and Presentation of Carbon Monoxide Poisoning

The signs and symptoms of CO poisoning in the pediatric patient may be subtle and nonspecific, making the diagnosis of CO poisoning difficult when a typical history of exposure is lacking. With COHb concentrations of <10%, only shortness of breath with vigorous exertion is seen. With levels of 20%, tightness across the forehead and headache are common.

With higher levels (30–50%), irritability, nausea, vomiting, weakness, dizziness, dimness of vision, confusion, and fainting of exertion may be present. With COHb concentrations above 50%, loss of consciousness and convulsions may appear, with fatalities commonly occurring when COHb concentrations of 60–80% are reached. These correlates are only useful as guidelines, as overlap can occur with incongruence existing between signs and symptoms and COHb concentrations.

Therapy in Carbon Monoxide Poisoning

Oxygen therapy (including hyperbaric oxygen), intensive supportive care, and specific therapy of complications are the mainstays in the therapeusis of the child poisoned with CO. The comatose or hypercapneic child should be intubated. Cerebral edema, if present, should be treated with hyperventilation, hyperosmolar agents (mannitol), diuretics and fluid restriction.

The definitive therapy for CO poisoning is oxygen. Oxygen (100%) by tight-fitting, nonrebreathing mask should be given as soon as CO poisoning is suspected, and it should be maintained until the COHb concentration falls below 5%. It is inappropriate to withhold oxygen therapy until laboratory confirmation of CO poisoning is obtained.

The effects of oxygen on the patient poisoned by CO are twofold. The immediate goal is to reverse arterial hypoxemia. Oxygen also accelerates the dissociation of CO from the hemoglobin molecule. During breathing of room air, small quantities of oxygen are dissolved in plasma. Breathing 100% oxygen at atmospheric pressure results in a dissolved oxygen content of 2.1 vol% in the plasma, thus supplying one-third of the arterial-to-venous oxygen content difference.

Oxygen is critical in eliminating CO by mass action, significantly reducing the half-life of CO. The half-life of CO is 5–6 hours with breathing of room air, 1½ hours with breathing of 100% oxygen, and <30 minutes with breathing of 100% oxygen at 2.5 atm.

Hyperbaric Oxygen Therapy

Some authors consider hyperbaric oxygen to be the mainstay of therapy for CO poisoning, while others suggest cautious skepticism until randomized controlled trials are completed. Little argument can be offered against instituting hyperbaric oxygen therapy when a patient has a COHb concentration of >25% and signs and symptoms of CO poisoning and a hyperbaric oxygen facility is readily available.

ELECTRICAL INJURY

Pathophysiology of Electrical Injury

Electrical injury is thought to be primarily a burn resulting from heat produced as current flows through the resistance of tissues. Joule's law states that power (heat) equals amperage squared times resistance ($P = I^2R$).

In the past, emphasis on varying tissue resistances underscored the belief that once skin resistance was overcome, current traveled preferentially through tissues of low resistance. In high-tension electrical injury, this is not the case. Tissue resistance in decreasing order is as follows: bone, fat, tendon, skin muscle, blood vessels, and nerves.

Types of Electrical Injury

Three types of injury are found in high-tension electrical injury. These are entry and exit wounds, arc burns, and surface burns. Surface burns result from ignition of clothing or from the heat of the current traveling close to the skin. The entry wound is usually charred and depressed, with swelling occurring proximal to the wound. At the site of grounding, a collection of energy results in extensive tissue necrosis as the current explodes through the skin, creating an exit wound that is usually charred, dry, and circumscribed. Arc burns are produced by a current that travels external to the body, as an electric arc forms between two objects of opposite charge (usually a highly charged source and the ground).

Type of Current

At low voltages, alternating current is more dangerous than direct current because of its ability to "freeze" the extremity to the source of electricity. The slowly alternating current of household sources (60 Hz) results in tetanic muscle contractions. If the victim's hand makes contact with the source, he or she may be unable to release the grasp, owing to the fact that the forearm flexors are more powerful than the extensors. Resistance and heat production are increased until carbonization of tissue occurs and the point of contact is broken. At high frequencies, alternating and direct current have a similar effect, as the sensitivity of the individual muscle fiber to electrical stimulus is exceeded.

Clinical and Pathologic Findings in Electrical Injury

The hallmark of electrical injury is a deep burn, frequently involving muscle and other structures. This type of injury, compared to that of surface burns, necessitates a different therapeutic approach, as clinical course, complications, and sequelae are unique to this type of injury.

Cardiovascular

Cardiac arrest is common in electrical injury and is precipitated by a variety of mechanisms. The conducting system of the heart is particularly sensitive to the common frequency of 60 Hz, with ventricular fibrillation caused by a current of 100 mA passing through the chest. Asphyxiation can result from tetanic spasm of the respiratory muscles at a current density of 30 mA. Respiratory arrest without cardiac arrest may occur following electrical injury and rapidly leads to cardiac arrest if artificial ventilation is not instituted.

Neurologic

Neurologic complications are particularly frequent following electrical injury and include loss of consciousness, seizures, spinal cord lesions, deafness, and mood disturbances, Peripheral nerve injury may occur secondary to vascular injury or thermal injury or by a direct effect of the electrical current. After electrical injury, peripheral nerve injury is usually transient, unless the injury is a direct result of the burn.

Renal

Acute renal failure is more common in electrical than surface burns, in part occurring from the massive release of myoglobin from damaged muscle. Renal injury can also result from direct damage by the electrical current.

Vascular

Vascular complications include delayed hemorrhage from underlying vessels and thrombosis resulting from progressive tissue edema.

Treatment of Electrical Injury

Prompt cardiopulmonary resuscitation results in a favorable prognosis in patients suffering cardiac arrest from electrical injury. Vigorous and prolonged resuscitation of such victims is indicated.

Fluid therapy is similar to that for burn injury, although larger volumes are usually necessary for a given percentage of surface burn, owing to the large "hidden" component of electrical injury. Mannitol and sodium bicarbonate are advocated by some to prevent acute tubular necrosis from pigment precipitation in the renal tubules. Intravenous fluids are adjusted following gross clearing of pigmenturia to maintain a urine output of 0.5–1.5 ml/kg/hr.

Fasciotomy is frequently necessary following electrical injury. Indications for immediate surgical decompression include extensive limb burns, marked limb edema, decreased distal nerve function, and absent pulses. Persistent severe pain is also a common indication for fasciotomy.

Appendix:
Comprehensive Formulary

The following is a compendium of drugs used in the pediatric intensive care unit. The dosages and indications are intended to be helpful suggestions. Some of these are controversial, however, and should be applied with appropriate caution.

Drug	Dose[a]	Pharmacokinetics and Pharmacotherapeutics	Metabolism[a, b]	Side Effects/Interactions[a, b]	Pharmacology[a, b]
Acetaminophen	• 5–15 mg/kg/dose 4–6 times/day p.o., p.r. • adult dose: 300–1000 mg q. 4 hr • maximum adult dose: 4000 mg/day	• $t_{1/2}$ = 2 hr • 0% protein bound (nontoxic) • effective concentrations: 10–20 μg/ml	• 3% urinary excretion with mostly hepatic microsomal metabolism	• in usual therapeutic dosages well tolerated with few, if any, side effects; contraindicated in G6PD deficiency • skin rash, drug fever, hematologic disturbances • hepatic necrosis after 200–250 mg/kg • 90% of patients will have severe hepatic damage if 4 hr after ingestion the level is >45 μg/ml • if the concentration 4 hr after ingestion is <120 μg/ml or 12 hr after ingestion the level is <30 μg/ml, then little hepatic damage will occur • toxic ingestions are treated with stomach evacuation, charcoal administration, and acetylcysteine	• antipyretic and analgesic • little anti-inflammatory action
Acetazolamide (Diamox)	• diuretic and urine alkalinization: 5 mg/kg/dose p.o., i.v. i.m. q.d. • glaucoma: 8–30 mg/kg/	• $t_{1/2}$ = 4–10 hr	• renal excretion complete within 24 hr	• causes an alkaline urine because of bicarbonate sodium and potassium wasting	• reversible inhibition of carbonic anhydrase which is found in RBC, renal cortex, gastric

Drug	Dose	Pharmacokinetics	Side Effects	Comments
	day, divided q. 6 hr • elevated ICP: 25 mg/kg/day, increased by 25 mg/kg/day, maximum: 100 mg/kg/day, divided t.i.d. p.o., i.v.; maximum: 2000 mg/day • seizures: 8–30 mg/kg/day, divided q. 6–12 hr		• systemic metabolic acidosis • drowsiness, paresthesias • treatment for absence of seizures limited by development of tolerance	mucosa, pancreas, eye, and CNS • inhibits the following reaction: $H_2O + H_2CO_3$; subsequently dissociates into HCO_3^- and H^+ • decreases the rate of CSF production
Acetylcysteine (Mucomyst)	• acetaminophen toxicity enteral load: 140 mg/kg p.o., diluted 1:4 in carbonated beverage NG, then 70 mg/kg q. 4 hr × 17 doses p.o., NG i.v. load: 150 mg/kg in 200 ml NS over 15 min, then 50 mg/kg in 500 ml NS over 4 hr, then 100 mg/kg in 1000 ml NS over 16 hr • nebulized: 3–5 ml of 20% solution diluted with equal volume of water t.i.d. to q.i.d.	• $t_{1/2} = 2.1$ hr • excreted in urine	• inhalation: bronchial pain (use with caution in asthmatics) • stomatitis rhinorrhea, bronchorrhea, nausea, vomiting • if charcoal used, give i.v.	• liquifies mucus and DNA by opening disulfide bonds • for use in acetaminophen toxicity (>200 mg/kg) administered within 24 hr of ingestion • replenishes hepatic stores of glutathione
Acyclovir	• HSV in newborns: 10 mg/kg/dose q. 8 hr i.v. • in children <12 yr old: 250 mg/m²/dose q. 8 hr i.v. • in adults: 5 mg/kg/dose q. 8 hr i.v. given over 1 hr	• 15% protein bound • $t_{1/2} = 2.5$ hr (3.8 hr in neonates) • 75% urinary excretion	• resistance • few side effects • renal dysfunction • CNS effects	• synthetic purine nucleoside analog • activity against HSV I greater than HSV II • interacts with viral thymidine kinase

Drug	Dose[a]	Pharmacokinetics and Pharmacotherapeutics	Metabolism[a, b]	Side Effects/Interactions[a, b]	Pharmacology[a, b]
Albuterol (Proventil)	· 2–90 μg inhalations q. 4–6 hr · nebulized: 2.5–5 mg in 3 ml NS		· hepatic COMT · hepatic MAO	· tachycardia, nausea, vomiting, hypertension	· β_2 agonist—relax bronchial uterine and skeletal vascular smooth muscle · activation of adenylate cyclase · increased 3′:5′-monophosphate
Allopurinol (Zyloprim)	· <6 yr old: 50 mg/kg/ dose q. 8 hr p.o. · 6–10 yr old: 100 mg/kg/ dose q. 8 hr p.o. · >10 yr old: 33–65 mg/ kg/dose q. 8 hr p.o.	· $t_{1/2}$ = 2–3 hr (alloxanthine: $t_{1/2}$ = 18–30 hr) · 0% protein bound	· 20% excreted in feces · 30% excreted unchanged in urine	· enhances theophylline toxicity · rash · hematologic abnormalities, hepatomegaly, nausea, vomiting	· for use in hyperuricemic states (gout, antineoplastic therapy) · inhibits xanthine oxidase · slightly alkaline urine enhances uric acid clearance
Aluminum hydroxide (Amphojel, AlternaGel)	· Hyperphosphatemia: 50–150 mg/kg/day, divided q. 4–6 hr · GI prophylaxis: 1 ml/kg (320 mg/5 ml) q. 1–2 hr		· aluminum is eliminated in urine	· constipation · hypophosphatemia · hyperaluminumemia · delay gastric emptying · bioavailability affected with hypotension, bradycardia	· enhances mucus secretion · alkalinization of GI contents
Amikacin sulfate (Amikin)	· 2.5 mg/kg/dose; frequency of dose depends on age/maturity · <7 days (<28 wk: q. 24 hr, 28–34 wk: q. 24 hr, q. 18 hr, term: q. 12 hr)	· 4% plasma bound · $t_{1/2}$ = 2–3 hr · levels: 8–16 μg/ml (peak)	· 98% urinary excretion; peritoneal and hemodialysis effective	· cochlear and vestibular toxicity occurs with high peaks in the absence of low troughs · renal cortex toxicity · can exacerbate neuromuscular blockade	· inhibits protein synthesis at the 30S mRNA · for use in Gram-negative infections · polar cations, so poor levels attained in the CSF

Drug	Dose	Metabolism/Pharmacokinetics	Side Effects	Mechanism/Actions
Aminocaproic acid (Amicar)	• >7 days (<28 wk: q. 18 hr; 28–34 wk: q. 12 hr; term: q. 8 hr) • children: q. 8 hr • 100 mg/kg (or 3 g/m²) × 1 hr), then 1 g/m²/hr i.v. • maximum: 18 g/m²/day • p.o.: 100 mg/kg/dose, divided q. 6–8 hr • adults: 5 g p.o., i.v., then 1 g/hr		• rapid administration associated with hypotension, bradycardia	• antidote for an overdose of fibrinolytic agents • prevents hyperfibrinolysis activators
Aminophylline	• maximum: 30 gzyh • Load: 3–6 mg/kg/20 min • maintenance dose differs by age • neonates: 0.2 mg/kg/hr • 1 mo–1 yr: 0.2–0.9 mg/kg/hr • 1–9 yr old: 0.8 mg/kg/hr • adults: 0.5 mg/kg/hr	• levels: 10–20 mg/l • $t_{1/2}$ = 20–36 hr • hepatic • increased metabolism by smoking, Dilantin • slowed metabolism by cimetidine, macrolide antibiotics • converted to caffeine • slowed metabolism in neonates	• tachycardia, nausea, vomiting, seizures	• inhibition of cyclic nucleotide phosphodiesterase • antagonism of receptor-mediated actions of adenosine • sensitizes mechanism for release of calcium from terminal cisternae of the sarcoplasmic reticulum
Amiodarone (Cordarone)	• adults load: 800–1600 mg/day for 1–3 wk • maintenance: 600–800 mg/day × 4 wk, then 200–400 g/day • maximum dose: 15 mg/kg/day for 3–4 wk p.o.	• $t_{1/2}$ = 25 days • 96% protein bound • levels: 0.5–2.5 mg/ml • 0% urinary excretion metabolized in liver	• corneal microdeposits • peripheral neuropathy • thyroid dysfunction • levels >2.5 µg/ml • ?increases digoxin and quinidine levels • pulmonary disturbances	• increases ventricular fibrillation threshold • slows repolarization • suppresses ventricular tachycardia • slows AV conduction

Drug	Dose[a]	Pharmacokinetics and Pharmacotherapeutics	Metabolism[a,b]	Side Effects/Interactions[a,b]	Pharmacology[a,b]
Amphotericin B	• test dose: 0.1 mg/kg/dose up to 1 mg/dose i.v. in D5W • initial dose: 0.25 mg/kg/day, increased to 1 mg/kg/day over 4 days • maximum dose: 1.5 mg/kg/day, infused over 6 hr	• 90% protein bound • $t_{1/2} = 15$ days	• small urinary excretion; bile excretion hemodialysis ineffective	• ?Candida resistance • fever and chills, hypotension, dyspnea, vomiting • hydrocortisone (0.7 mg/kg), meperidine, and diphenhydramine can ameliorate symptoms • renal toxicity, thrombocytopenia convulsions, anemia, anaphylaxis, electrolyte disturbances	• binds to the steroid moiety on fungal cell membranes • poor penetration into CSF
Ampicillin	• neonates of <7 days: 50–100 mg/kg/day, divided q. 12 hr i.m., i.v. • of >7 days: 100–200 mg/kg/day, divided q. 8 hr i.m., i.v. • children: 50–400 mg/kg/day, divided q. 4–6 hr, depending on severity of infection			• see penicillin	• see penicillin
Amrinone (Inocor)	• load: 0.75 mg/kg/3 min • maintenance: 5–10 µg/kg/min • maximum: 10 mg/kg/day	• duration of action, 4–6 hr • 35–49% protein bound • $t_{1/2} = 4$ hr	• 25% excreted in urine	• relaxes vascular and tracheal smooth muscle • increase HR and SV • decrease SVR, LVEDP • GI intolerance • thrombocytopenia at levels of >2.5 µg/ml	• positive inotrope • inhibits cyclic nucleotide phosphodiesterase

Drug	Dosage	Pharmacokinetics	Effects/Cautions	Mechanism
Aspirin	• 10–15 mg/kg/dose q. 4 hr up to antirheumatic 100 mg/kg/day, divided q. 4 hr	• $t_{1/2}$ = 15 min (salicylate: $t_{1/2}$ = 2–3 hr) • excreted in urine	• irreversible platelet dysfunction • acute renal failure • vasomotor rhinitis and angioneurotic edema and bronchospasm in susceptible individuals • respiratory alkalosis and metabolic acidosis	• inhibits cyclo-oxygenase • inhibits the conversion of arachidonic acid to PGG_2
Atenolol (Tenormin)	• 1 mg/kg p.o. q. 24 hr • maximum: 100 mg/day	• $t_{1/2}$ = 6.3 hr • <5% protein bound • 85% urinary excretion	• see propranolol	• β blocker, $β_1$ selective • see propranolol
Atracurium	• intubation: 0.6 mg/kg i.v.	• lasts 45–60 min • ester hydrolysis • Hoffman degradation	• hypotension	• nondepolarizing neuromuscular blocker • minimal ganglionic blockade • causes histamine release
Atropine	• 0.01–0.04 mg/kg i.v., s.c. i.m., intratracheal • minimum: 0.15 mg • maximum: 1 mg • can also be administered nebulized (0.05 mg/kg)	• lasts 2.5 hr • renal excretion	• tachycardia, dilated pupils, dry mouth, urinary retention, mental status changes	• blocks the vagal-tonic effects of laryngoscopy • to use with neostigmine for reversal of nondepolarizing neuromuscular blockers • muscarinic ACh blocker
Bretylium (Bretylol)	• arrest dose: 5–10 mg/kg q. 15–30 min • maximum: 30 mg/kg • chronic: 5–10 mg/kg over 10–30 min q. 6 hr i.v.; may be given undiluted i.m.	• 0–8% protein bound • $t_{1/2}$ = 9 hr • 77% urinary excretion	• postural hypotension • hypotension • nausea • tricyclics may inhibit uptake of drug to site of action preventing hypotensive but not antidysrhythmic effect	• inhibits the release of norepinephrine from the nerve terminals, although it may release norepinephrine • inhibits uptake of adrenergic nerve terminals • increases duration of action potention • increases refractory period

Drug	Dose[a]	Pharmacokinetics and Pharmacotherapeutics / Metabolism[a,b]	Side Effects/Interactions[a,b]	Pharmacology[a,b]
(Bretylium—*continued*)				• increases PR and QT intervals
Calcium	• chloride salt (27% elemental calcium) • arrest and hyperkalemia: 20 mg/kg/dose i.v. q. 10 min • gluconate salt (10% elemental calcium) • arrest and hyperkalemia: 80 mg/kg/dose i.v. q. 10 min • tetany adult: 5–20 ml 10% calcium gluconate by slow i.v.	• urinary excretion	• subcutaneous injection (infiltrate) can cause slough • vasodilation upon rapid injection • bradycardia, arrhythmias	• affects cardiac contractility by its effect on the plateau phase of the action potential • hypercalcemia: weakness, lethargy, and coma • hypocalcemia: seizures
Captopril (Capoten)	• neonates: 0.1–0.4 mg/kg/dose p.o. q. 6–24 hr • infants: 0.5–0.6 mg/kg/day, divided q. 6–12 hr p.o. • adults: 25–50 mg p.o. b.i.d. to t.i.d.; increase weekly by 25 mg/dose in up to a maximum of 450 mg/day	• $t_{1/2} = 2$ hr • 50% urinary excretion • 30% protein bound	• rare side effects • rashes, hypotension • rare potassium retention • reduction of aldosterone production • coronary and cerebral blood flow preserved • pulmonary artery pressure decreased • increased renin production	• inhibits the conversion of inactive angiotensin I to angiotensin II • useful in the treatment of CHF

Drug	Dosage	Pharmacokinetics	Comments
Carbamazepine (Tegretol)	· load: 10 mg/kg/day p.o., divided q. 8–12 hr · maximum: 200 mg b.i.d. · maintenance: 20–30 mg/kg/day, divided q. 8–12 hr · maximum: 1200 mg/day	· 75% protein-bound hepatic oxidative enzymes · levels: 6–12 mg/l · $t_{1/2}$ = 10–20 hr	· reduces levels of ADH · clonidine may inhibit antiseizure activity · coma, convulsions, respiratory depression, ataxia, diplopia, nausea, vomiting, aplastic anemia, leukopenia, thrombocytopenia, agranulocytosis, dermatitis, lymphadenopathy, splenomegaly · for generalized tonic-clonic, simple, complex, and partial seizures · facilitate inhibitory inputs · ?partial adenosine agonist
Cefamandole (Mandol)	· 50–150 mg/kg/day, divided q. 4–8 hr i.m. or i.v. · maximum dose: 12 g/day	· 74% protein bound · $t_{1/2}$ = 0.8 hr · 96% urinary excretion	· see comments on cephalosporins · second-generation cephalosporin · see comments on cephalosporins
Cefazolin (Ancef, Kefzol)	· 25–100 mg/kg/day, divided q. 6–8 hr i.v., i.m. · maximum dose: 12 g/day	· $t_{1/2}$ = 1.8 hr · 80% urinary excretion	· development of resistance · see comments on cephalosporins · first-generation cephalosporin · inhibition of cell wall synthesis · activity against *Escherichia coli, Klebsiella* · see comments on cephalosporins
Cefoperazone (Cefobid)	· 25–100 mg/kg/day, divided q. 12 hr i.m., i.v. · maximum dose: 12 g/day	· 90% protein bound · $t_{1/2}$ = 2 hr · predominantly excreted in bile (75%)	· hypoprothrombinemia causes bleeding · diarrhea · see comments on cephalosporins · third-generation cephalosporin · activity against *Pseudomonas aeruginosa* · good for biliary infections · see comments on cephalosporins

Drug	Dose[a]	Pharmacokinetics and Pharmacotherapeutics	Metabolism[a, b]	Side Effects/Interactions[a, b]	Pharmacology[a, b]
Cefotaxime (Claforan)	• 0–1 wk: 50–100 mg/kg/day, divided q. 12 hr i.m., i.v. • 1–4 wk: 75–150 mg/kg/day, divided q. 8 hr i.m., i.v. • >4 wk: 50–180 mg/kg/day, divided q. 4–6 hr i.m., i.v. • maximum: 12 g/day	• $t_{1/2} = 1$ hr	• see comments on cephalosporins	• see comments on cephalosporins	• third-generation cephalosporin • good CSF penetration • see comments on cephalosporins
Cefoxitin (Mefoxin)	• 80–160 mg/kg/day, divided q. 4–6 hr i.m., i.v. • maximum: 12 g/day	• $t_{1/2} = 0.65$ hr • 73% protein bound	• see comments on cephalosporins • 78% urinary excretion	• see comments on cephalosporins	• see comments on cephalosporins • best Gram-negative coverage of the second generations • good for mixed anaerobic and aerobic infections (e.g., pelvic inflammatory disease and lung abscess)
Ceftazidime (Fortraz)	• neonate: 60 mg/kg/day, divided q. 12 hr i.v. • children: 90–150 mg/kg/day, divided q. 8 hr i.v. • maximum: 6 g/day	• $t_{1/2} = 1.5$ hr • 17% protein bound	• see comments on cephalosporins • 84% urinary excretion	• see comments on cephalosporins	• third-generation cephalosporin • good activity against Pseudomonas • see comments on cephalosporins
Ceftizoxime (Cefizox)	• 150–200 mg/kg/day, divided q. 6–8 hr i.v., i.m. • maximum: 12 g/day	• $t_{1/2} = 1.8$ hr • 28% protein bound	• 93% excreted in urine	• see comments on cephalosporins	• third-generation cephalosporin • good CSF penetration • see comments on cephalosporins

Drug	Dose	Pharmacokinetics	Comments
Ceftriaxone (Rocephin)	• infant and child: 50 mg/kg/day q.d. i.m., i.v. • meningitis: 75 mg/kg/dose ×1, then 100 mg/kg/day, divided q. 12 hr i.v. • maximum dose: 4 g/day	• $t_{1/2} = 8$ hr • 60% urinary excretion • 40% biliary excretion	• third-generation cephalosporin • see comments on cephalosporins
Cefuroxime (Zinacef)	• neonates: 10 mg/kg/day, divided q. 12 hr i.m, i.v. • children: 50–100 mg/kg/day, divided q. 6–8 hr i.m., i.v. • meningitis: 200–400 mg/kg/day, divided q. 6–8 hr i.v. • maximum: 9 g/day	• $t_{1/2} = 1.7$ hr • see comments on cephalosporins • 96% urinary excretion	• second-generation cephalosporin • adequate CSF penetration • see comments on cephalosporins
Cephalothin (Keflin)	• 80–160 mg/kg/day, divided q. 4–6 hr i.v., i.m. • maximum dose: 12 g/day	• $t_{1/2} = 30$–40 min • 71% protein bound • see comments on cephalosporins • 52% urinary excretion	• first-generation cephalosporin • the most resistant cephalosporin to β-lactamase, producing staphylococcal infections • see comments on cephalosporins
Charcoal (activated)	• 1 g/kg p.o. or NG in 70% sorbitol solution	• not absorbed	• should not be given simultaneously with ipecac • if depressed mental status, secure the airway first • diarrhea can cause electrolyte disturbances • absorbs drugs and is lost in the feces • especially useful in drugs with enterohepatic circulation: theophylline, phenobarbital, tricyclics, digoxin, Tegretol

Drug	Dose[a]	Pharmacokinetics and Pharmacotherapeutics	Metabolism[a, b]	Side Effects/Interactions[a, b]	Pharmacology[a, b]
Chloral hydrate (Noctec, Aquachloral)	· 25–75 mg/kg/dose · maximum: 2 g rectally	· $t_{1/2}$ = 4–12 hr	· reduced in liver	· little effect on respirations or blood pressure at therapeutic levels · gastric necrosis after p.o. · hypotension and apnea in combination with furosemide and porphyrias	· little analgesic effect · for sedation
Chloramphenicol (Chloromycetin)	· loading: 20 mg/kg/day i.v., p.o. · maintenance dose in infant of <7 days: 10 mg/kg/day, divided q. 12–24 hr i.v. · 1–3 wk: 20 mg/kg/day, divided q. 8–12 hr i.v. · 3–5 wk: 30 mg/kg/day, divided q. 6–12 hr i.v. · >5 wk: 50–100 mg/kg/day, divided q. 6 hr i.v. · maximum dose: 2 g/day	· levels: 15–20 mg/l · $t_{1/2}$ = 4 hr · hemodialysis ineffective · 53% protein bound	· ester hydrolysis in many organs · 20–50% excreted by kidney · mostly hepatic metabolism	· dermatitis · resistance · rash, bone marrow toxicity · pancytopenia (reversible and irreversible) · nausea, vomiting · gray baby syndrome in neonates	· 50S ribosomal binding, inhibiting protein synthesis · activity against chlamydia, mycoplasma, rickettsial organisms, and Gram-negatives · 45–99% of plasma concentrations in CSF · irreversibly inhibits hepatic cytochrome P-450
Chlorothiazide (Diuril)	· <6 mo: 20–30 mg/kg/day, divided q. 12 hr p.o. · >6 mo: 20 mg/kg/day, divided q. 12 hr p.o. · maximum dose: 2 g/day	· $t_{1/2}$ = 1.5 hr · duration of action: 6–12 hr · 95% protein bound	· secreted by proximal tubule · 92% urinary excretion	· urate crystal formation · decrease renal excretion of calcium · CNS depression · use with caution in hepatic and renal dysfunction	· acts directly on the distal tubule to increase sodium chloride and water loss · some carbonic anhydrase inhibition which causes wasting

Drug	Dosage	Pharmacokinetics		
				• may decrease urine volume in DI
Cholestyramine (Questran, Cumid)	• 80 mg/kg t.i.d. p.o. • maximum: 4 g/day t.i.d. p.o.	• not absorbed from GI tract	• hyperglycemia by diminished insulin secretion, enhanced glycogenolysis, and diminished glycogenesis • increased serum triglycerides and cholesterol • GI discomfort • elevated liver function tests • hyperchloremic acidosis • diarrhea can cause vitamin loss (A,D,E,K) • absorbs other oral medications given within 1 hr	• decreases cholesterol and LDL by binding bile acids • good for pruritis caused by bile salts
Cimetidine (Tagamet)	• 5–10 mg/kg q. 6 hr p.o. or i.v. • maximum dose: 2400 mg/day	• 19% protein bound • $t_{1/2} = 2$ hr • levels: 0.78–3.9 μg/ml	• 62% urinary excretion	• rare and minor reactions • does not cross the normal blood-brain barrier compared with ranitidine, cimetidine lacks the antiandrogenic activity, binds less avidly to P-450, decreases hepatic blood flow less dramatically, has less incidence of CNS side effects (re: seizures) • rapid i.v. administration may result in bradycardia	• reversible competitive antagonists at the histamine-2 receptor • decreases both volume and acidity of gastric secretion • enhances cell-mediated immune response (not ranitidine) • mostly, ranitidine has supplanted cimetidine

Drug	Dose[a]	Pharmacokinetics and Pharmacotherapeutics	Metabolism[a, b]	Side Effects/Interactions[a, b]	Pharmacology[a, b]
Clindamycin (Cleocin)	• 15–40 mg/kg/day, divided 6–8 hr i.m., i.v. • maximum: 4.8 g/day	• $t_{1/2}$ = 2.7 hr • 90% protein bound	• 10% excreted in urine, mostly hepatic metabolism	• resistance • antibiotic-associated colitis can occur with oral or parenteral administration • rashes, reversible transaminitis • potentiation of neuromuscular blockers	• binds to the 50S subunit of the ribosome suppressing protein synthesis • excellent anaerobic activity • poor CSF penetration • accumulates in PMNs and macrophages
Clonazepam (Clonopin)	• initial: 0.01–0.03 mg/kg/day, divided q. 8 hr p.o. • increments: not >0.5 mg q. 3 days • maximum: 0.2 mg/kg/day, divided q. 8 hr	• 85% protein bound • $t_{1/2}$ = 23 hr • levels: 5–7 ng/ml	• <1% renal excretion • see diazepam	• see diazepam	• see diazepam • for absence and myoclonic seizures
Clonidine (Catapres)	• adults: 0.2–0.8 mg/day, divided b.i.d. p.o.	• $t_{1/2}$ = 9 hr • levels: 1.5–2 ng/ml	• 50% metabolized in liver • 50% excreted in urine	• sedation drowsiness • increased potency of anesthetics • nausea • fluid retention • sudden withdrawl associated with hypertensive crisis • respiratory depression at toxic doses	• α_2 agonist • reduces SVR, SV, and HR • intrathecal analgesic
Codeine	• 0.5–1.0 mg/kg/dose q. 4–6 hr • maximum: 60 mg/dose	• lasts 2.5–3 hr	• metabolized in the liver; inactive metabolites excreted in urine	• very active orally • see morphine	• see morphine

Drug	Dose	Pharmacokinetics	Excretion	Side effects	Notes
	• p.o.: sulfate and phosphate salt				
Cromolyn (Intal)	• s.c. and i.v.: phosphate salt only • inhalation: 20 mg q. 6 hr for >5 yr old • nebulization: 1 ampule (2 cc) q. 6–8 hr (for >2 yr old) • aerosol: 2 puffs (800 μg/spray) q.i.d.		• 50% excreted in bile • 50% excreted in urine	• rare side effects	• inhibits the release of histamines and leukotrienes • not for acute asthma
Cyclosporin (Sandimmune)	• 5–10 mg/kg i.v. over 2–6 hr q.d. (p.o. dose 3 times i.v. dose)	• $t_{1/2} = 14$ hr • 95% protein bound • levels: 100–400 ng/ml	• 4% urinary excretion	• nephrotoxicity at levels of >400 ng/ml • slow i.v. infusions necessary • hepatotoxicity • increased susceptibility to infection and ?lymphomas	• suppressed T-cell-mediated immunity by blocking interleukin II • ?role in diabetes mellitus treatment
Dantrolene (Dantrium)	• spasticity in children: 0.5 mg/kg b.i.d., then t.i.d. after 1 day, increase by 0.5 mg/kg/day up to 3 mg/kg q.i.d. • adult: 25 mg p.o. q.d., then 25 mg p.o. b.i.d. to q.i.d., increased by 25-mg increments up to 100 mg p.o. q.i.d. • malignant hyperthermia: 1 mg/kg i.v.; repeat p.r.n. up to maximum of 10 mg/kg, then p.o. 1–2 mg/kg q.i.d.	• $t_{1/2} = 9$ hr	• urinary excretion • hepatic metabolism	• hepatotoxicity, especially fulminant hepatitis • CNS changes • enhances the action of neuromuscular blocker	• decreases calcium release from the sarcoplasmic reticulum • does not alter neuromuscular transmission • relaxes muscle contractions associated with upper motor lesions

Drug	Dose[a]	Pharmacokinetics and Pharmacotherapeutics	Metabolism[a, b]	Side Effects/Interactions[a, b]	Pharmacology[a, b]
Deferoxamine (Desferal)	• iron overdose • i.m. challenge: 1 g i.m.; presence of vin rosé color to urine indicates significant ingestion; then 500 mg q. 4 hr × 2 • i.v. (in shock states): 15 mg/kg/hr until level of <300 μg/dl, no greater than 6 g/day; continue therapy 24 hr after patient has produced normal color and quantity of urine • chronic overdose in transfusions: 2.0 g/unit of blood not given in the same i.v. as the transfusion		• metabolized by plasma enzymes, then excreted in urine	• pruritis, wheals, rash anaphylaxis • dysuria GI discomfort • tachycardia	• chelates of iron • for iron levels of >500 μg/dl, chelation therapy should commence
Desmopressin (DDAVP)	• 0.3–0.4 μg/kg/day i.v. over 15–30 min, divided b.i.d. • intranasal: 10 times the above dose • maximum adult dose: 40 μg/day • minimum dose: 2–5 μg	• $t_{1/2}$ (α) = 8 min • $t_{1/2}$ (β) = 75 min		• hypertension • dose must be titrated to the minimum quantity to obtain desired endpoint • tachyphylaxis	• smooth muscle constriction • analog of ADH • increases factor VIII activity in von Willebrand's disease type I and hemophilia
Dexamethasone (Decadron)	• for ICP elevation, load: 0.5–1.5 mg/kg i.v., i m	• $t_{1/2}$ = 3 hr	• 2.6% urinary excretion; see hydrocortisone	• see hydrocortisone	• see hydrocortisone • compared with hydrocortisone: 25 × the antiinflammatory action

Drug	Dosing	Pharmacokinetics	Clinical effects / toxicity	Mechanism / notes
Diazepam (Valium)	mg/kg/day, divided by q. 6 hr • airway edema: 0.25–0.5 mg/kg/dose q. 6 hr • sedation: 0.04–0.2 mg/kg/dose i.v.; 0.2–0.8 mg/kg/day p.o. • seizures: 0.2–0.5 mg/kg/dose	• 85–95% protein bound • $t_{1/2}$ (α) = 1 hr • $t_{1/2}$ (β) = 1.5 days • $t_{1/2}$ for desmethyldiazepam: 70–100 hr • effective concentration: 300–400 ng/ml	• glucuronization in liver	• slight decrease in respiration, BP, CO and LVSW	• antianxiety • potentiation of neural inhibition mediated by GABA • in antiseizure doses, can suppress respirations requiring intubation • enhanced GABA-induced increases in chloride conductance
Diazoxide (Hyperstat, Proglycem)	• 1–5 mg/kg i.v. q. 30 min up to 300 mg	• $t_{1/2}$ = 20–60 hr • 90% protein bound	• 33% eliminated in urine • 67% metabolized in liver	• severe hypotension associated especially with conditions of depressed serum proteins (e.g., renal failure) • hyperglycemia • fluid retention	• related to the thiazides • antidiuretic action as well as arteriolar smooth muscle relaxation • no sodium retaining activity
Digoxin	• digitalizing dose in premature: 20 μg/kg p.o.; maintenance: 5 μg/kg/day p.o. • in full-term: 30 μg/kg p.o.; maintenance: 8–10 μg/kg/day p.o. • in children: 30–40 μg/kg p.o.; maintenance: 8–12 μg/kg/day p.o. • digitalization: give half the dose, then a quarter of the dose q. 8 hr × 2	• 25% protein bound • $t_{1/2}$ = 39 hr • level: >0.8 ng/ml • toxic: >1.7 ng/ml (10% likely) • >3.3 ng/ml (90% likely)	• eliminated by kidney	• nausea, diarrhea and vomiting, change in mental status • virtually any dysrhythmia • toxicity is exacerbated by hypokalemia so any drug that can change potassium equilibrium can cause digitalis toxicity (i.e., diuretics, amphotericin B, succinylcholine)	• directly inhibits Na-K$^+$ ATPase increasing intracellular calcium and increases slow inward current • positive inotrope • negative chronotrope • prolonged refractory period in the atria

Drug	Dose[a]	Pharmacokinetics and Pharmacotherapeutics	Metabolism[a, b]	Side Effects/Interactions[a, b]	Pharmacology[a, b]
(Digoxin—*continued*)	• i.v. or i.m. dose is equal to p.o. dose in >10 yr old but is 75% of the p.o. dose in <10 yr old				
Diltiazem	• adults: 30 mg p.o. q.i.d. up to 60 mg t.i.d. to q.i.d. p.o.	• $t_{1/2}$ = 3.2 hr • 78% protein bound	• 4% urinary excretion	• excessive vasodilation • negative inotrope • depression of sinus node rate • AV conduction disturbances • use with caution in conjunction with β-adrenergic blockers	• calcium channel blocker activity on smooth muscle (especially vascular) and cardiac muscle
Dimercaprol (British anti-lewisite)	• lead poisoning: 4 mg/kg q. 4 hr × 48 hr i.m., then 4 mg/kg q. 6 hr × 48 hr	• lasts 4 hr	• hepatic metabolism and urinary excretion	• fever, pain at injection site • hypertension, tachycardia • nausea, headache, burning sensations, pain in throat, chest and hands, conjunctivitis • contraindicated in organic mercury poisoning, G6PD deficiency, and hepatic insufficiency (except as a result of metal poisoning)	• forms sulfhydryl bonds • lead levels of 50–60 µg/dl should warrant chelation • alkaline urine ensures excretion of chelated metal • for lead, arsenic, gold, and mercury poisoning • calcium EDTA should be given at a separate site

Drug	Dose	Pharmacokinetics	Side effects	Comments
Diphenhydramine (Benadryl)	• sedation and antihistamine: 5 mg/kg/day, divided q. 6 hr; maximum: 50 mg/dose • for dystonic reactions: 1–2 mg/kg i.v.; maximum dose: 300 mg/day	• 78% protein bound • $t_{1/2} = 4$ hr • toxic: >100 ng/ml	• hepatic metabolism	• dizziness, tinnitus, diplopia, nausea, vomiting, anorexia • anticholinergic effects: dry mouth and throat, urinary retention, tachycardia changes in mental status • paradoxical excitation in infants	• used for sedation • histamine-1 receptor antagonist • central antitussive
Disopyramide (Norpace)	• <1 yr: 10–30 mg/kg/day, divided q. 6 hr p.o. • 1–4 yr old: 10–20 mg/kg/day, divided q. 6 hr p.o. • 4–12 yr old: 10–15 mg/kg/day, divided q. 6 hr p.o. • 12–18 yr old: 6–15 mg/kg/day, divided q. 6 hr p.o. • adults: 400–800 mg/day, divided q.i.d. p.o.	• 28–68% protein bound • $t_{1/2} = 6$ hr • level: >3 µg/ml	• 55% urinary excretion	• cholinergic blockade (10% as potent as atropine; see atropine) • reduces CO directly and increases SVR • hypoglycemia • prolongation of PR interval • apnea	• type I antiarrhythmic • slows sinus rate • decreases slope of phase 4 depolarization in Purkinje fibers • prolongs action potential • increases refractory period • increased QRS and QT_c complex • oral treatment of ventricular dysrhythmias
Dobutamine (Dobutrex)	• 2 µg/kg/min • titrate up to effect • maximum: 40 µg/kg/min	• $t_{1/2} = 2.5$ min		• metabolized in liver • positive dromotrophy, inotropy • no effect on dopaminergic receptors • tachycardia, especially when >20 µg/kg/min • dysrhythmias • contraindicated in IHSS	• β_1 activity increases inotropy • some α_1 agonism at very high doses • lower LVEDP • reduction in myocardial oxygen demand while increasing oxygen supply

Drug	Dose[a]	Pharmacokinetics and Pharmacotherapeutics	Metabolism[a, b]	Side Effects/Interactions[a, b]	Pharmacology[a, b]
Dopamine (Intropin, Depastat)	• 2–50 µg/kg/min titrated up from the lower dose	• $t_{1/2}$ = 3 min	• MAO and COMT	• no CNS effect because it does not cross the blood-brain barrier • tricyclics and MAO inhibitors exaggerate the action • higher rates cause α_1 effects and vascular insufficiency (>20 µg/kg/min)	• metabolic precursor of norepinephrine • β_1 agonism directly releases norepinephrine • dopaminergic agonism at 2–5 µg/kg/min causes increased blood flow to renal and mesenteric vasculature
Doxycycline (Vibramycin)	• initial: 4.4 mg/kg/day, divided q. 12 hr p.o., i.v. up to 200 mg/day • maintenance: 2.2 mg/kg/day, divided q. 12–24 hr p.o., i.v. up to 100 mg/day • adult maximum: 300 mg/day; infuse over 1–4 hr not in concentration of >5 mg/ml	• $t_{1/2}$ = 16 hr	• excreted in feces not effected by renal dysfunction	• resistance • hepatic toxic • ?renal toxicity • brown discoloration of teeth and bones in <7 yr old • thrombophlebitis • hematologic abnormalities • antibiotic-associated colitis • pseudotumor cerebri • see neostigmine	• 30S subunit of the ribosome inhibiting protein synthesis • some CSF penetration
Edrophonium (Tensilon)	• test for myasthenia gravis: 0.2 mg/kg/dose i.v.; range: 0.1–10 mg • for SVT: 0.1–0.2 mg/kg/dose i.v. • give 20% of dose slowly	• $t_{1/2}$ = 1.8 hr			• works faster than any other reversal agent • see neostigmine

Drug	Dose	Metabolism/Kinetics	Comments
EDTA	muscular blockade: 1 mg/kg i.v. given after a dose of atropine of 0.02 mg/kg i.v. • 1–1.5 g/m² day, divided q. 4–12 hr • maximum: 75 mg/kg/day i.m., divided b.i.d. to t.i.d. • i.m. is preferable to i.v.	• $t_{1/2}$ = 20–60 min • excreted in urine	• rapid administration causes hypocalcemic seizures • nephrotoxic • thrombophlebitis • rapid i.v. administration in patients with cerebral edema may increase intracranial pressure • chelates divalent and trivalent metals • adequate urine output must be maintained
Epinephrine (Adrenalin)	• bolus: 5–20 µg/kg i.v. • drip: 0.05 µg/kg/min i.v. titrated up	• hepatic COMT and MAO	• increases coagulation, increases total leukocyte counts, but decreases eosinophils transient hyperkalemia, hyperglycemia, fear, anxiety, tension, dizziness, palpitations, tachydysrhythmias, pallor, cerebral hemorrhage • high doses can cause vascular insufficiency • α effects (hypertension) as well as β effects (tachycardia); activation of adenylate cyclase increases 3':5'-monophosphate • β_2 agonist relaxes uterine and bronchial smooth muscle • positive inotrope, chronotrope, and dromotrope
Epinephrine (racemic) (Vaponefrine, Micronetrin, Asthmanefrin solution 2.25%)	• 0.05 ml/kg/dose diluted to 3 ml NS • maximum: 1.5 ml	• hepatic COMT and MAO	• for use in croup (also postextubation croup) • has a risk of rebound

Drug	Dose[a]	Pharmacokinetics and Pharmacotherapeutics	Metabolism[a, b]	Side Effects/Interactions[a, b]	Pharmacology[a, b]
Erythromycin	· 10–20 mg/kg/day, divided q. 6 hr i.v. · 30–50 mg/kg/day, divided q.i.d. p.o. · p.o.: stearate estolate ethylsuccinate · i.v.: lactobionate gluceptate · adult maximum: 8 g/day p.o.	· $t_{1/2} = 1.6$ hr · levels: 0.3–1.9 μg/ml p.o.; up to 10 μg/ml i.v.	· 12–15% excreted in urine, demethylation in liver not removed by dialysis	· rare side effects · fever, eosinophilia, rashes · hepatitis · thrombophlebitis · increases levels of theophylline	· macrolide antibiotic · activity against Gram-positives, mycoplasma, *Legionella*, chlamydia, pertussis · binds to the 50S subunit of the ribosome · poor CSF penetration
Esmolol	· load: 500 μg/kg/min × 5 min · infusion: 25–100 μg/kg/min titrated to effect	· $t_{1/2} = 8$ min	· metabolized by red cell esterases	· see propranolol	· relatively selective β_1 antagonist · see propranolol
Ethosuximide (Zarontin)	· maintenance: 20–40 mg/kg/day · maximum: 1.5 g/day	· not bound to proteins · $t_{1/2} = 30$–50 hr · levels: 40–100 μg/ml	· 25% excreted in urine · 75% hepatic microsomal enzymes	· GI: nausea, vomiting · SLE pancytopenia, dermatitis aplastic anemia, ataxia	· for absence seizures
Fentanyl (Sublimaze)	· 1–2 μg/kg/dose	· $t_{1/2} = 3.7$ hr · 80% protein bound	· termination of action by redistribution, metabolized in liver	· muscle rigidity due to dopaminergic transmission in the striatum · see morphine · levels of >1 ng/ml, associated with respiratory depression	· μ agonist more specific than morphine · see morphine
Flecainide (Tambocor)	· adults: 100 mg p.o. q. 12 hr; increase dose by 50 mg q. 12 hr every 4 days to maximum of 400 mg/day	· $t_{1/2} = 7$–24 hr	· urinary excretion	· worsen ventricular function · sinus bradycardia · wider QRS, prolong PR	· depress fast sodium channels · decrease Vmax action potential in most cardiac tissue · suppresses PVCs

Drug	Dose	Pharmacokinetics	Excretion	Notes
Furosemide (Lasix)	• 2 mg/kg/dose q. 6–8 hr p.o.; maximum: 600 mg/day • 1 mg/kg/dose q. 6–12 hr i.v., i.m.; maximum: 6 mg/kg single dose	• 98% protein bound • $t_{1/2}$ = 92 min • toxicity: >25 µg/ml	• 67% excreted in urine	• enhances calcium excretion • increases the excretion of titratable acid and ammonia • enhances renal blood flow • increased pulmonary venous capacitance decreasing LV filling pressures • metabolic alkalosis • hyperuricemia • deafness • nephrotoxicity (increased in the presence of cephalosporins and renal-toxic drugs • acts on the thick ascending loop of Henle by inhibiting electrolyte reabsorption • mild carbonic anhydrase inhibition • redistributes renal blood flow from medulla to cortex
Gentamicin	• 2.5 mg/kg/dose i.v. or i.m.; frequency of dose depends on age/maturity • <7 days (<28 wk: q. 24 hr; 28–34 wks: q. 18 hr; term: q. 12 hr) • >7 days (<28 wk: q. 18 hr; 28–34 wk: q. 12 hr; term: q. 8 hr) • children: q. 8 hr	• $t_{1/2}$ = 2–3 hr • levels: 6–10 mg/l (peak) • <2 mg/l (trough)	• >90% urinary excretion • <10% protein bound	• cochlear and vestibular toxicity occurs with high peaks in the absence of low troughs • renal cortex toxicity • can exacerbate neuromuscular blockade • inhibits protein synthesis at the 30S mRNA • for use with Gram-negative infections • polar cations, so poor levels attained in CSF
Glucagon	• 0.1 mg/kg up to 1 mg i.m., s.c. (1 mg = 1 unit)	• $t_{1/2}$ = 3–6 min	• degraded in liver, kidney, and plasma	• acts only on liver glycogen stores converting them to glucose • increases serum glucose • stimulates adenylate cyclase • positive inotrope and chronotrope • treats insulin-induced hypoglycemia

Drug	Dose[a]	Pharmacokinetics and Pharmacotherapeutics	Metabolism[a,b]	Side Effects/Interactions[a,b]	Pharmacology[a,b]
(Glucagon—*continued*)					• relaxes the intestinal tract
Glycopyrrolate (Robinul)	• 0.015 mg/kg/dose q. 4–8 hr i.v., i.m.			• see atropine	• muscarinic blocker with minimal associated tachycardia or mental status changes • see atropine
Haloperidol (Haldol)	• age 3–12 yr; sedation: 0.5–1 mg p.o.; psychosis: 0.05–0.15 mg/kg/day, divided b.i.d. to t.i.d. p.o. • age >12 yr; agitation: 2–5 mg i.m., p.o.	• $t_{1/2} = 17.9$ hr • level: 1 ng/ml	• no urinary excretion • 92% protein bound • hepatic microsomal metabolism	• extrapyramidal side effects, see promethazine • toxic levels of 15 ng/ml • sedation • hypotension • lower seizure threshold	• dopaminergic blocker • α_1 blocker
Heparin	• (120 international units = 1 mg) • bolus: 50–100 units/kg q. 4 hr i.v. up to 500 units/kg/day continuous heparinization • initial: 50 units/kg i.v.; maintenance: 10–25 units/kg/hr	• 99% protein bound • $t_{1/2} = 26 + (0.323 \times \text{dose}$ in i.v./kg/min)	• metabolized in liver by heparinase metabolites excreted in urine	• lines flushed with heparinized saline have higher fatty acid concentrations that inhibit protein binding of lipophilic drugs, thus interfering with quantification of some drugs (digoxin, propranolol, phenytoin) • chills, fever, anaphylactic shock, hemorrhage, osteoporosis, thrombocytopenia	• reduces serum triglycerides by releasing tissue lipoprotein lipase antithrombin III and heparin cofactor II form complexes with thrombin • heparin accelerates the velocity of this reaction, also inactivates factor X • reversal with protamine 1 mg for every 100 units heparin • adjust dose following clotting time (20–30 min) or PTT 1½–2½ times control

Drug	Dose	Metabolism	Side effects	Mechanism
Hydralazine (Apresoline)	• acute: 0.1–0.5 mg/kg/dose i.m., i.v. • chronic: 0.75–3 mg/kg/day, divided q. 6–12 hr p.o.	• $t_{1/2} = 1$ hr • duration of action: 2–4 hr	• metabolized in liver: fast and slow acetylators have different bioavailabilities after oral but not parenteral administration	• tachycardia, increased contractility and renin activity, fluid retention • increased coronary renal and cerebral blood flow • postural hypotension, headache • lupus-like syndrome in slow acetylators in summer, 2 months after administration	• directly relaxes arterial vascular smooth muscle by activation of guanylate cyclase and accumulation of GMP
Hydrocortisone (Solu-Cortef)	• loading: 4–8 mg/kg/dose; maximum: 250 mg; maintenance: 8 mg/kg/day, divided q. 6 hr	• $t_{1/2} = 1.5$ hr • physiologic level: 16 μg/dl at 8 a.m. and 4 μg/dl at 4 p.m.	• 90% protein bound • 70% hepatic metabolism; some kidney metabolism	• Cushing's habitus, psychiatric changes, cataracts, osteoporosis, myopathy, susceptibility to disease, hyperglycemia, peptic ulcers, sodium retention, suppression of adrenal-pituitary axis (9 months after cessation) • abrupt withdrawal: fever, myalgias and arthralgias, pseudotumor cerebri	• physiologically 20 mg/day secreted • steroids react with receptor proteins in cytoplasm • block the effect of MIF on macrophages
Imipenem-cilastatin (Primaxin)	• 50 mg/kg/day, divided q. 6–8 hr i.v. • maximum dose: 4 g/day	• $t_{1/2} = 1$ hr	• metabolized in renal brush border by dehydropeptidase • 70% excreted in urine	• nausea, vomiting, pruritis • ? penicillin allergies	• β-lactam ring resistant to β-lactamase • good anaerobic and aerobic activity, including Listeria, Pseudomonas • cilastatin inhibits dehydropeptidase

Drug	Dose[a]	Pharmacokinetics and Pharmacotherapeutics	Metabolism[a, b]	Side Effects/Interactions[a, b]	Pharmacology[a, b]
Indomethacin (Indocin)	• ductus closure: 3 doses separated by 12–24 hr • first dose: 0.2 mg/kg • second and third doses depend on age: • <48 hr: 0.1 mg/kg • 2–7 days: 0.2 mg/kg • >7 days: 0.25 mg/kg • anti-inflammatory (>14 yr old): 1–3 mg/kg/day, divided t.i.d. or q.i.d.; maximum dose: 100 mg/day	• 90% protein bound • $t_{1/2}$ = 2.4 hr • levels: 0.3–3 μg/ml	• 15% urinary excretion	• GI side effects • hematopoietic side effects • renal dysfunction • platelet dysfunction • cross reactions between aspirin and indomethacin	• inhibits cyclo-oxygenase • anti-inflammatory, analgesic and antipyretic • antipyretic effects in Hodgkin's disease
Insulin	• regular i.v. onset $\frac{1}{2}$–1 hr: lasts 5–8 hr • semi-lente s.c. onset $\frac{1}{2}$–1 hr: lasts 12–16 hr • NPH s.c. onset 1–2 hr: lasts 18–24 hr • in diabetic ketoacidosis: 0.1 unit/kg i.v. regular insulin, followed by 0.1 unit/kg/hr • hyperkalemia: 0.15 unit/kg/hr i.v. of regular insulin with 0.5 g/kg of glucose		• kidney metabolism • liver metabolism	• allergic reactions: rash • hypoglycemia • insulin binds to plastic i.v. administration materials	• stimulates transport of metabolites (especially glucose) and ions (especially potassium and magnesium) through membranes • stimulates glycogen and fat synthesis • inhibits glycogenolysis and lipolysis
Isoetharine (Bronkosol)	• 1–2 puffs q. 3 hr • nebulization: 0.25–0.5 ml 1% solution diluted to 2 ml in NS q. 4 hr			• nausea, tachycardia, hypertension, anxiety, headache • see isoproterenol	• β_2 agonist • see isoproterenol

Drug	Dose/Use	Pharmacokinetics	Side Effects	Comments
Isoniazid (INH)	• treatment in children: 10–20 mg/kg/day, divided q. 12–24 hr p.o., i.m.; maximum dose: 500 mg/day • adults: 5 mg/kg/day q.d.; maximum dose: 300 mg/day	• 0% protein bound • $t_{1/2} = 1.1–3.1$ hr	• slow and rapid (hepatic) acetylators affect the plasma concentrations; 7–29% excreted in urine • resistance • most common to least common: rash, jaundice, peripheral neuritis • other: hematologic vasculitis, arthritis, seizures, CNS effects • peripheral neuritis (very common especially if pyridoxine not administered • decreases metabolism of phenytoin • severe hepatic injury rare in <20 yr old	• mechanism of action unknown, but tubercle bacilli take up the drug preferentially • CSF concentrations 20% of plasma concentrations
Isoproterenol (Isuprel)	• 0.05 μg/kg/min i.v. • increase q. 4 min by 0.05 μg/kg/min and titrate to effect and side effect		• hepatic COMT • poor substrate for MAO • palpitation, tachycardia, flushing of skin, angina, nausea, tachyarrhythmias	• practically no α effects, some β_1 effects • lowers SVR by β_2 agonism • see epinephrine • inhibits antigen-induced release of histamine • relaxes bronchial smooth muscle by β_2 agonism
Kanamycin	• bacterial overgrowth in adults: 50–100 mg/kg/day, divided q. 6 hr p.o.; maximum dose: 12 g/day • in infants and children: 15–30 mg/kg/day, divided q. 8–12 hr i.m., i.v.; maximum dose: 1.5 g/day i.v.	• $t_{1/2} = 2.1$ hr • levels: peak 25–30 mg/l through <6 mg/l	• partly absorbed p.o. • 97% eliminated in urine • 0% protein bound • drug-induced malabsorption • administer over 30 min	• see gentamicin • main use is as an oral adjunct to treating hepatic coma • also used for "bowel prep" prior to surgery

Drug	Dose[a]	Pharmacokinetics and Pharmacotherapeutics	Metabolism[a, b]	Side Effects/Interactions[a, b]	Pharmacology[a, b]
Ketamine	• intubation: 1–2 mg/kg i.v., 6–13 mg/kg i.m. • sedation: one-sixth of the above doses	• 45–50% protein bound • $t_{1/2}\ (\alpha) = 7$–17 min • $t_{1/2}\ (\beta) = 2$–3 hr	• ?hepatic metabolism	• releases endogenous catecholamines, increasing BP and HR • direct myocardial depressant • in the absence of benzodiazepines, emergent psychosis possible • increases cerebral blood flow and metabolism, and intraocular and intracranial pressures increases • lowers seizure threshold • stimulates salivary secretions (atropine should be given concomitantly)	• site of actions(?): cortex and limbic systems • reduces polysynaptic spinal reflexes • provides cardiovascular stability
Ketoconazole (Nizord)	• children of >2 yr old: 3.3–6.6 mg/kg q.d. p.o. • maximum: 400 mg/kg q.d. p.o.	• 90% protein bound • $t_{1/2} = 1.5$–4 hr (higher doses are associated with longer $t_{1/2}$	• hepatic metabolism	• reduction of gastric activity (e.g., H_2 blockers) decrease absorption • nausea, vomiting, thrombocytopenia • transaminitis to hepatic toxicity • ?antagonism with amphotericin B	• useful for many nonmeningeal fungal infections • minimal CSF penetration
Labetolol (Trandate)	• adults: 5–10 mg i.v. bolus, titrated to effect	• $t_{1/2} = 5$ hr	• 5% excreted unchanged in urine; the remainder is metabolized in the liver	• α to β activity ratio: 1:3 to 1:7 • rashes • see propranolol	• selective α_1 antagonism • nonselective β antagonism • inhibits reuptake of nor-

Drug	Dose	Kinetics	Metabolism	Effects/Toxicity	Mechanism/Notes
					· epinephrine into nerve terminals
Lactulose (Cephulac)	· infant: 2.5–10 ml/day, divided t.i.d. to q.i.d. p.o. · children: 40–90 ml/day, divided t.i.d. to q.i.d. · adults: 30–45 ml/dose t.i.d. to q.i.d. p.o.	· latency of 1–7 days to reduce serum ammonia levels	· minimal absorption metabolized by gut flora to monosaccharides and lactate	· diarrhea with electrolyte and water disturbance	· semisynthetic nonabsorbable disaccharide · osmotic laxative · adjust to effect: 2–3 soft stools/day with a fecal pH of 5–5.5
Lidocaine	· 1–1.5 mg/kg i.v. or intratracheal i.v. drip of 20–50 µg/kg/min	· 70% plasma bound to α_1-glycoprotein · levels: 1.5–6 mg/l · $t_{1/2}$ = 100 min · toxicity: >7 mg/l	· hepatic de-ethylation	· can suppress a diseased SA node · agitation (5µg/ml) · hearing disturbances · convulsions (>7 µg/ml)	· blocks some of the stimulation of laryngoscopy and tracheal intubation · decrease slope of phase 4 depolarization of Purkinje fibers · increased diastolic electrical threshold by increasing potassium conductance without changing resting Vmax · treats ventricular dysrhythmias
Lorazepam (Ativan)	· 0.03–0.1 mg/kg/dose p.o., i.v., i.m.	· $t_{1/2}$ = 10–20 hr	· diazepam is metabolized to lorazepam · see diazepam	· see diazepam	· see diazepam
Mannitol	· diuretic: 0.2 g/kg i.v. · cerebral edema: 0.25 g/kg i.v.		· not metabolized · filtered and excreted in urine · urine unchanged	· fluid overload by expansion of the extracellular space, especially in heart failure and anuria · can accumulate and raise the serum osmolarity to dangerous levels of >340 mOsm/kg	· osmotically active agent · ?free radical scavenger

Drug	Dose[a]	Pharmacokinetics and Pharmacotherapeutics	Metabolism[a, b]	Side Effects/Interactions[a, b]	Pharmacology[a, b]
Meperidine (Demerol)	• p.o., i.m., i.v., s.c.: 1–1.5 mg/kg/dose q. 3 hr • maximum: 100 mg q. 3 hr	• lasts 3 hr	• metabolized in the liver to form normeperidine	• see morphine • CNS convulsant side effects, blocked by naloxone, are mediated by normeperidine • neonates do not clear the drug well	• see morphine • interacts with the κ receptors more than does morphine • unique among the opioids because of its local anesthetic effects and its effect in increasing heart rate
Metaproterenol (Metaprel, Alupent)	• nebulized: 0.2–0.3 ml 5% solution in 2.5 ml NS • aerosol: 1–3 puffs q. 3 hr (650 μg/puff) • oral: 1.3–2.6 mg/kg/day, divided t.i.d. to q.i.d.		• not metabolized by COMT; excreted in urine conjugated with glucuronic acid	• see isoproterenol	• β_2 agonist selective with relatively less β_1 than isoproterenol • see isoproterenol
Methadone (Dolphine)	• 0.7 mg/kg/day, divided q. 4–6 hr p.o. or s.c.	• $t_{1/2}$ = 1–1.5 days • level: 35 μg/ml	• 90% protein bound • biotransformed in the liver	• constipation, sedation, miosis, biliary spasm	• antitussive • little addiction potential • little respiratory depression
α-Methyldopa	• adults: 250 mg p.o. b.i.d., increased to a maximum of 3 g/day p.o., divided b.i.d. to q.i.d. or to a maximum of 65 mg/kg/day p.o. 250–1000 mg i.v. q. 6 hr • children: 10 mg/kg/divided b.i.d. to q.i.d. or 20–40 mg/kg divided q. 6 hr i.v.	• $t_{1/2}$ = 1.8 hr • 1–16% protein bound	• 66% clearance is renal	• sedation, postural hypotension, dizziness, dry mouth, headache • hematologic abnormalities • lupus-like syndrome • liver function abnormalities	• central α_2 agonist • reduces SVR

Drug	Dosage	Pharmacokinetics	Comments	
Methylprednisone (Medrol, Solu-Medrol)	• anti-inflammatory: 0.4–1.6 mg/kg/day, divided q. 6–12 hr i.v. • asthma load: 1–2 mg/kg/dose; maintenance: 0.5–4 mg/kg/dose q. 4–6 hr i.v.; maximum: 250 mg/dose q. 4 hr	• $t_{1/2} = 12$–36 hr	• see hydrocortisone	• see hydrocortisone • 5 times the anti-inflammatory and half the sodium-retaining potency of hydrocortisone • dosages are controversial
Metoprolol (Lopressor)	• adults: 5 mg i.v. q. 2 min × 3, then after 15 min 50 mg p.o. q. 6 hr, then after 2 days 100 mg p.o. b.i.d. • maximum: 450 mg/day p.o.	• 10% excreted in urine • 90% hydroxylated in the liver (slow hydroxylations have higher plasma levels)	• reduction in FEV₁ in asthmatics • see propranolol	• selective β_1 antagonist • see propranolol
Metronidazole (Flagyl)	• anaerobic infections load: 15 mg/kg i.v., then 7.5 mg/kg/dose q. 6 hr • maximum: 4 g/day (less frequent in neonate)	• 10% protein bound • levels: 3–6 μg/ml • $t_{1/2} = 8$–10 hr	• GI (nausea, diarrhea, etc. • neurotoxicity (especially CNS) • thrombophlebitis • red urine	• good CSF penetration • activity against Trichomonas, Giardia and amebae
Miconazole (Monistat)	• >1 yr: 15–40 mg/kg/day, divided q. 8 hr • adult maximum: 1200 mg/dose q. 8 hr	• $t_{1/2} = 24$ hr • 90% protein bound	• hepatic metabolism	• frequent adverse effects include: nausea, vomiting, anemia, thrombocytosis, hyponatremia, anaphylactoid reactions, CNS toxicity, anthralgias • cardiorespiratory arrest when given faster than 2 hr and dilated in more than 200 ml (adult dose) • inhibits metabolism of phenytoin and warfarin	• no good indications as a first drug; due to toxicity • poor CSF penetration • used only when first-line drugs not tolerated • available as a 2% cream or lotion

Drug	Dose[a]	Pharmacokinetics and Pharmacotherapeutics	Metabolism[a, b]	Side Effects/Interactions[a, b]	Pharmacology[a, b]
Midazolam (Versed)	• 0.05–0.2 mg/kg i.m., i.v.	• $t_{1/2} (\alpha) = 1$ hr	• hepatic metabolism	• see diazepam	• water soluble • see diazepam
Minoxidil (Loniten)	• adults: 5 mg q.d., increased up to 20 mg b.i.d. p.o.	• $t_{1/2} = 3.1$ hr	• 12% urinary excretion	• prompt withdrawal causes hypertension • toxicity: fluid retention and hypertrichosis • reflex tachycardia	• direct vascular smooth muscle relaxation similar to that produced by hydralazine
Morphine sulfate	• 0.1–0.2 mg/kg/dose s.c., i.v., or i.m.	• 2.5–3 hr	• 33% protein bound • hepatic conjunction	• sedation, nausea vomiting, respiratory depression, miosis, constipation, biliary spasm, muscular rigidity in high doses • suppresses the cough reflex, vasodilation • histamine release causing hypotension and bronchospasm • withdrawal symptoms after prolonged use • may exacerbate spinal cord brain injury by direct effects and by increasing P_aCO_2 and increasing ICP	• μ and κ agonist, little effect on σ • μ: supraspinal, analgesia, respiratory depression, euphoria, physical dependence • κ: spinal analgesia, sedation miosis • σ: dysphoric hallucinations
Nafcillin (Staphcillin)	• newborn of <7 days: 40 mg/kg/day, divided q. 12 hr i.v., i.m. • newborn of >7 days: 60 mg/kg/day, divided q. 6–8 hr	• 90% protein bound • $t_{1/2} = 1$ hr	• 27% urinary excretion (higher in extrahepatic biliary obstruction)	• see penicillin	• see penicillin • resistant to penicillinase • active against staphylococcal infections • good bile and spinal fluid concentrations

Drug	Dosage	Pharmacokinetics	Elimination	Adverse effects	Notes
Naloxone (Narcan)	kg/day, divided q. 4 hr i.v. • adults: 4–12 g/day, divided q. 4 hr i.v. • 5–10 μg/kg/dose i.m. or i.v. q. 3–5 min, titrated to effect	• 45–60 min	• hepatic	• can acutely precipitate a withdrawal syndrome • can acutely cause loss of analgesia • narcotic can outlast naloxone	• μ receptor antagonist • ?effect in reversal of shock and ameliorating the damage associated with CSN trauma (in large doses) • some antagonism to κ and σ receptors
Neomycin	• acute hepatic encephalopathy: 2.5–7 g/m^2/day, divided q. 6 hr p.o. × 5–7 days • chronic: 2.5 g/m^2/day • bowel preparation: 90 mg/kg/day, divided q. 4 hr	• 0% protein bound	• partially absorbed p.o. • 97% eliminated in feces	• see gentamicin • drug-induced malabsorption	• see gentamicin • main use is as an oral adjunct to treating hepatic coma • also used for "bowel prep" prior to surgery
Neostigmine	• 0.06–0.07 mg/kg i.v. • maximum: 3 mg	• lasts 3–4 hr	• plasma esterases excreted in urine	• salivation, lacrimation, diarrhea, vomiting, bradycardia, bronchiolar and ureteral contractions, to be given with atropine • inhibits the action of cholinesterase	• inhibits acetylcholinesterase • to be given with an anticholinergic (muscarinic) such as atropine
Nifedipine	• 0.15–0.5 mg/kg/dose q. 6–8 hr p.o. or sublingual • maximum: 30 mg/dose (or 180 mg/day)	• 98% protein bound • $t_{1/2}$ = 3.5 hr	• 0% urinary excretion; metabolites excreted in urine	• hypotension, tachycardia, headaches, dizziness, palpitations	• calcium entry blocker • more potent of a vasodilator than verapamil and diltiazem • arterial dilator causes reflex changes to increased HR and CO slightly

Drug	Dose[a]	Pharmacokinetics and Pharmacotherapeutics	Metabolism[a,b]	Side Effects/Interactions[a,b]	Pharmacology[a,b]
Nitroglycerin	• drip: 0.1 µg/kg/min, titrated up to effect	• $t_{1/2}$ = 1–3 min • levels: 1.2–11 ng/ml	• hepatic reductive hydrolysis	• venodilation reduces LVEDP and RVEDP • headaches, postural hypotension • few side effects • absorbed onto the plastic of many i.v. administration sets	• increase cGMP in smooth muscle • improves both myocardial oxygen supply and demand • less effective hypotensive agent than nitroprusside
Nitroprusside (Nipride, Nitropres)	• 0.5–8 µg/kg/min	• toxic level of thiocyanate: >10 mg/ml • toxicity: >8 µg/kg/min	• cyanide ion is formed in the RBCs and then reduced in the liver to thiocyanate which is excreted in the urine with a $t_{1/2}$ = 3–4 days	• hypotension, sweating, headache • reflex tachycardia • methemoglobinemia • acute withdrawal can cause hypertensive crisis • cyanide toxicity with metabolic acidosis	• decrease both preload and afterload • direct vascular smooth muscle vasodilator
Norepinephrine (Levarterenol)	• test dose: 0.1–0.2 µg/kg • infusion: 0.05 µg/kg/min, titrated up		• metabolized in the liver	• hypertension • α agonism can cause vascular insufficiency • cardiac arrhythmias • reflex bradycardia	• β_1 agonism • little β_2 agonism • α agonist
Pancuronium	• intubation: 0.1–0.15 mg/kg i.v. or 0.2 mg/kg i.m.	• lasts 1 hr	• renal with some hepatic	• tachycardia	• accentuated by respiratory acidosis, myasthenic syndromes, metabolic alkalosis, local anesthetics, many antibiotics, magnesium, hypothermia, dantrolene, furosemide, nitroglycerin

Drug	Dosage	Pharmacokinetics	Adverse effects	Comments
Paraldehyde	• anticonvulsant: 150 mg/kg/dose i.m.; 300 mg/kg/dose in oil p.r. q. 4–6 hr • i.v. drip: 0.1–0.15 ml/kg/hr (dilute with NS to 5% solution; maximum: 1 ml/min)		• 70–80% metabolized in liver	• avoid plastic containers • acidosis, bleeding, gastritis, azotemia, pulmonary hemorrhages	• the use of paraldehyde is largely supplanted by other drugs (especially benzodiazepines)
Penicillin G (potassium or sodium)	• <7 days: 50,000–150,000 units/kg/day, divided q. 12 hr • >7 days: 75,000–250,000 units/kg/day, divided q. 6–8 hr • children: 40,000–300,000 units/kg/day, divided q. 4–6 hr	• 65% protein bound • $t_{1/2}$ = 30 min • $t_{1/2}$ (<1 wk) = 3 hr	• 60–90% renal excretion • 10% by filtration • 90% by tubular secretion	• resistance • from most to least likely: rash, fever, bronchospasm, vasculitis, serum sickness, exfoliative dermatitis, Stevens-Johnson syndrome, anaphylaxis • less common: eosinophilia, interstitial nephritis • CNS effects (with procaine)	• interferes with cell wall synthesis • 1 mg = 1600 units • potassium: 1,000,000 units = 1.68 mEq • sodium: 1,000,000 units = 1.68 mEq • activity against Gram-positive cocci, anaerobes, some Gram-negatives • 5% of plasma concentrations found in CSF in meningitis • probenecid blocks tubular secretion
Pentamidine (Isethionate, Pentam)	• 4 mg/kg/dose q.d. i.m. or i.v. × 12–14 days • i.m. is preferable to i.v. • maximum total dose: 56 mg/kg		• slowly excreted unchanged in urine	• protect from light to avoid hepatotoxic compounds • i.m. better than i.v. • breathlessness, tachycardia, dizziness, fainting, headache, vomiting, hypotension, histamine release, disruption of glucose homeostasis, renal dysfunction	• little CNS penetration • second-line drug after TMP-SMX for *Pneumocystis carinii* • antiprotozoan activity

Drug	Dose[a]	Pharmacokinetics and Pharmacotherapeutics	Metabolism[a, b]	Side Effects/Interactions[a, b]	Pharmacology[a, b]
Pentobarbital (Nembutal)	• sedation: 2–6 mg/kg/dose p.o. • i.v. coma induction: 10 mg/kg, then 1–4 mg/kg/hr	• toxic levels: >1 mg/l • $t_{1/2}$ = 15–48 hr	• hepatic cytochrome P-450; termination of action by redistribution	• apnea • hypotension • decreases cardiac output, renal plasma flow, CBF, ICP • increase in SVR • contraindicated in porphyrias • intra-arterial injection can cause loss of limb	• antianalgesic in sub-anesthetic doses • site of action: reticular activating system • suppresses polysynaptic responses • inhibits synapses that are GABAergic • enhances GABA-induced increases in chloride conductance • autonomic ganglionic blocker
Phenobarbital (Luminal)	• sedation: 2–3 mg/kg/dose p.o., i.m., i.v. q. 8 hr • seizure control: 15–25 mg/kg/dose i.v. • maximum: 600 mg/day • chronic: 4–6 mg/kg/day p.o., divided q. 12 hrs	• $t_{1/2}$ = 80–120 hr • levels: 15–40 mg/l	• see pentobarbital	• see pentobarbital	• see pentobarbital
Phentolamine	• in diagnosis of pheochromocytoma: 10 µg/kg/min i.v., titrated up		• 10% excreted in urine	• muscarinic agonist: salivation, lacrimation, diarrhea • tachycardias and GI side effects	• α_1 and α_2 blocker • cardiac stimulation as well as vasodilation
Phenylephrine (Neo-Synephrine)	• hypotension: 1 µg/kg i.v., repeat and titrate p.r.n., then start with 0.01 µg/kg/min i.v. drip and increase	• duration of action: <20 min	• hepatic	• decrease CO • increase SVR venous pressure, pulmonary artery pressure • bradycardia (reflex)	• α_1 stimulation • may release norepinephrine

Drug	Dose	Pharmacokinetics	Metabolism/Excretion	Side Effects	Comments
	...titrated to effect				· α agonism may cause vascular insufficiency in high doses
Phenytoin (Dilantin)	· seizures: 15–20 mg/kg i.v. · antiarrhythmic: 2–4 mg/kg i.v.; maximum: 500 mg not given faster than 1 mg/kg/min · maintenance: 4–7 mg/kg/day, divided b.i.d. i.v., p.o.	· 90% protein bound · $t_{1/2}$ = 6–24 hr · levels: 10–20 μg/ml	· hepatic microsomal enzymes	· cardiac arrhythmias · hypotension megaloblastic anemia, gingival hyperplasia nystagmus, ataxia diplopia, vertigo, inhibition of ADH release, neutropenia leukopenia, dermatitis, lymphadenopathy, hypoprothrombinemia	· for treatment of all seizures except absence · stabilizes neural membranes · below toxic levels, there are no CNS effects · follow QT_c interval on ECG while loading
Physostigmine (Antilirium)	· children of <5 yr: 0.5 mg i.v. q. 5 min; maximum: 2.0 mg · >5 yr: 1–2 mg i.v.; maximum: 4 mg/30 min	· lasts 2 hr	· plasma esterases	· atropine will reverse toxic side effects of physostigmine that include salivation, lacrimation, seizures	· inhibits the action of cholinesterase · physostigmine crosses the blood-brain barrier
Piperacillin (Pipracil)	· 75–300 mg/kg/day, divided q. 4–6 hr · maximum: 24 g/day	· 16–48% protein bound · $t_{1/2}$ = 0.93 hr	· 71% urinary excretion	· see penicillin	· see penicillin · activity against *Klebsiella* and *Pseudomonas* · sodium: 2 mEq per gram of piperacillin
Prazosin (Minipress)	· adults: initially 1 mg b.i.d. to t.i.d. p.o., then increased · maximum: 40 mg/day (though rarely >10 mg/day)	· $t_{1/2}$ = 3.1 hr	· <1% urinary excretion	· hypotension especially with first dose	· α₁ antagonist · decrease in SVR and MAP without change in HR
Prednisolone	· anti-inflammatory and asthma: 0.5–2 mg/kg/day, divided q. 6 hr · physiologic replacement: 4–5 mg/m²/day, divided b.i.d.	· $t_{1/2}$ = 2.2 hr · 90–95% protein bound	· converted in liver to methylprednisolone · 15% urinary excretion	· supersensitivity to catecholamines · requires 3 weeks for full hypotensive effect · change in mental status · contraindicated in de-	· decreased HR and BP · see hydrocortisone · 4 times the anti-inflam-

Drug	Dose[a]	Pharmacokinetics and Pharmacotherapeutics	Metabolism[a, b]	Side Effects/Interactions[a, b]	Pharmacology[a, b]
(Prednisolone—*continued*)				· pressed patients, peptic ulcer disease · see hydrocortisone	matory effects and 0.8 times the sodium-retaining effects as hydrocortisone
Primidone (Mysoline)	· initial dose for <8 yr old: 125 mg/day q.d.; · for >8 yr old: 250 mg/ day q.d.; · maintenance: 10–25 mg/kg/day, divided b.i.d. to t.i.d. · maximum: 2000 mg/ day	· therapeutic levels: 8–12 mg/l of primidone or 15–40 mg/l of phenobarbital · $t_{1/2} = 7–14$ hr	· converted to phenobarbital and PEMA	· see pentobarbital	· see pentobarbital
Procainamide (Pronestyl)	· i.m.: 20–30 mg/kg/day, divided q. 4–6 hr (adults: 1 g/dose ×1, then 250 mg q. 3 hr; maximum: 4 g/day) · i.v. load: 2 mg/kg/dose over 5 min, repeated q. 10–30 min (adult i.v. load: 100 mg over 2–4 min q. 5 min, titrated to control of dysrhythmia; maintenance: 20–80 μg/kg/min; adult maximum: 8 g/day) · nausea and vomiting;	· $t_{1/2} = 3$ hr · 16% protein bound · levels: 3–14 μg/ml	· 67% urinary excretion; hepatic metabolism forms N-acetylprocainamide (fast and slow acetylators metabolize a different percentage of the drug)	· hypotension especially when dose is >600 mg · toxicity: >14 μg/ml · less vagolytic side effects than quinidine · discontinuation—same criteria as in quinidine · GI disturbances, CNS disturbances, agranulocytosis, SLE syndrome	· used for PVCs, also moderate activity on atrial flutter/fibrillation · decreases automaticity, Vmax, action potential amplitude · prolonged action potential and effective refractory period · prolongs QRS, QT · usually digitalization should commence prior to quinidine initiation
Promethazine (Phenergan, Provigan)	· antihistamine: 0.1 mg/ kg/dose q. 6 hr; maximum: 12.5 mg q.i.d. · nausea and vomiting:	· $t_{1/2} = 20–40$ hr	· hepatic microsomes, oxidation and glucuronidation	· anticholinergic side effects: tachycardia, dry mouth, change in mental status	· phenothiazine · antihistaminic properties · central dopaminergic

Propranolol (Inderal)

Dosing:
- 0.25–0.5 mg/kg/dose i.m. p.o., i.v., p.r.
- sedative: 0.5–1 mg/kg/dose; maximum: 50 mg i.m., i.v.
- arrhythmias: 0.01 mg/kg/dose i.v., titrated up to 5 mg to effect
- tetralogy spells: 0.15–0.25 mg/kg/dose i.v. q. 15 min, then 1–2 mg/kg/dose q. 6 hr p.o.; maximum single dose: 10 mg i.v.
- thyrotoxicosis for neonatal: 2 mg/kg/day p.o., divided q. 6 hr; for adults: 1–3 mg/dose i.v. over 10 min, then 10–40 mg p.o. q. 6 hr
- hypertension: 0.5–1 mg/kg/day, divided q. 6–12 hr p.o.; in adults, increase 10–20 mg/dose q. 3 days; maximum dose: 480 mg p.o.

Pharmacokinetics:
- 93% protein bound
- $t_{1/2} = 4$ hr
- level: 20 ng/ml

Metabolism:
- hepatic metabolism

Adverse effects:
- CV system: orthostatic hypotension by α blockade
- CNS extrapyramidal signs: Parkinsonism, acute dystonia, neuroleptic malignant syndrome, akathisia, tardive dyskinesia, and perioral tremor
- blood dyscrasias
- may decrease seizure threshold
- bronchospasm
- withdrawal phenomenon
- augments the hypoglycemic actions of insulin by reducing the compensatory effect of sympathetic adrenal activation
- bradycardia
- nausea, vomiting

Mechanism:
- blocker including the CTZ
- blocks reuptake of amines
- prolongs barbiturate sleeping time
- nonspecific β antagonist
- local anesthetic effect
- decreases inward sodium currents, so reduces the height and rate of rise of depolarization
- decreases HR, CO
- blocks renin release from juxtaglomerular sites
- decreases spontaneous firing in atria and ectopic sites
- increase AV conduction time

Drug	Dose[a]	Pharmacokinetics and Pharmacotherapeutics	Metabolism[a, b]	Side Effects/Interactions[a, b]	Pharmacology[a, b]
Prostaglandin E₁ (PGE₁) (alprostadil) (Prostin VR)	· initial: 0.05 μg/kg/min i.v., titrated up to 0.4 μg/kg/min	· 95% inactivated through one pass in the lungs		· apnea, seizures, fever, flushing, bradycardia, hypotension, diarrhea · decreases platelet aggregation	· stimulates smooth muscle in low doses but relaxes at higher doses · activates adenylate cyclase · pulmonary and ductal tissue relaxation · new synthetic analog used for treatment of peptic ulcer disease caused by nonsteroidal anti-inflammatory drugs
Protamine sulfate	· must be titrated to effect (e.g., against ACT) · maximum dose: 50 mg			· dyspnea, flushing, bradycardia, hypotension avoided by central venous administration of <20 mg/min in adults · ?histamine release · hypersensitivity, especially to fish allergic individuals	· combines with heparin ionically · 1 mg protomine antagonizes 100 units of heparin
Quinidine	· p.o. is preferable to i.m. which is preferable to i.v. · test dose: 2 mg/kg p.o. · in children: 15–60 mg/kg/day, divided q. 6 hr p.o. · in adults: 200–400 mg/dose q. 4–6 hr i.v.; 400 mg/dose q. 4–6 hr	· 90% protein bound · $t_{1/2}$ = 6.2 hr · effective levels: 2–6 mg/l	· metabolized in the liver · 20% excreted in urine	· at 6 μg/ml, 10% of patients will demonstrate toxic effects · at 14 μg/ml, 50% of patients will demonstrate toxic effects · syncope, sudden death · paradoxical increased ventricular rate when treating atrial fibrilla-	· decrease action potential, Vmax automaticity · prolongs action potential and refractory · prolongs QRS, QT_c · activity for atrial fibrillation and flutter, APCs, VPC and re-entry tachycardias · some activity as an an-

Drug	Dose	Pharmacokinetics	Side Effects	Comments
(continued)	i.v.; 200–300 mg/dose q. 6–8 hr p.o., titrated to effect (ECG changes)		• tion, so oftentimes AV block is indicated prior to initiating therapy • hypotension, tachycardia, tinnitus hearing loss, GI disturbances, fever, anaphylaxis, thrombocytopenia	• timalacide, antipyretic and oxytocic • vagolytic and α-blocking properties
Ranitidine	• children: 2–4 mg/kg/day, divided q. 12 hr p.o.; 1–3 mg/kg/day, divided q. 6–8 hr i.v. • adults: 150 mg p.o. b.i.d.; 50 mg i.v., i.m. q. 6–8 hr	• 69% urinary excretion • 15% protein bound • $t_{1/2}$ = 2 hr • ineffective level: 100 ng/ml (50% inhibition of gastric secretion)	• rare and minor side effects • ranitidine crosses the blood-brain barrier and binds less avidly to the hepatic P-450 system so that there are much fewer CNS and hepatic (i.e., drug interaction) side effects compared with those from cimetidine • small hepatic blood flow reductions causing accumulation of drugs that are metabolized in the liver	• histamine-2 blocker inhibits gastric secretion, reducing gastric volume and increasing gastric pH
Reserpine	• adults: 0.1–1 mg p.o. q.d., divided b.i.d. • test dose: 0.005 mg/kg i.m., then 0.06 mg/kg i.m. q. 8–12 hr		• sensitivity to catecholamines • requires 3 weeks for full hypotensive effect • changes in mental status • contraindicated in depressed patients, peptic ulcer disease	• inhibits uptake of catechols, depleting catecholamines • decreased HR and BP • newer agents have supplanted its common use

Drug	Dose[a]	Pharmacokinetics and Pharmacotherapeutics	Metabolism[a,b]	Side Effects/Interactions[a,b]	Pharmacology[a,b]
Ribavirin (Varazole)	• aerosol (20 mg/ml of sterile water)	• 12–18 hr/day		• can interfere with respirator function	• for RSV treatment
Spironolactone (Aldactone)	• children: 3.3 mg/kg/day, divided q.i.d. to b.i.d. • adults: 15–200 mg/day, divided q.i.d. to b.i.d. p.o. 100–400 mg/day for primary aldosteronism (especially in preparation for surgery)	• highly protein bound	• metabolized in liver	• hypercalcemia (especially in renal failure) • gynecomastia • GI disturbances	• antagonist of aldosterone • increases urinary Na/K ratio • sites of action include salivary glands, colon, and nephron • increases renal calcium excretion
Succinylcholine	• intubation: 1–1.5 mg/kg i.v. or 4 mg/kg i.m.	• 3–5 min	• plasma pseudocholinesterase	• hyperkalemia associated with burns, trauma, and nerve damage >24 hr after injury • increases intraocular and intracranial?	• atypical or absent pseudocholinesterase documented by a high dibucaine number associated with prolongation of action • must have airway
Sucralfate (Carafate)	• adults: 1 g p.o. q.i.d.	• lasts 6 hr	• poorly absorbed systemically	• rare side effects • constipation • dry mouth • in uremic patients, increases serum aluminum and decreases serum phosphate levels	• sulfated sucrose and aluminum compound polymerizing below a pH of 4 • adheres to ulcer craters for 6 hr • more adherent to duodenal than gastric ulcers • no acid-neutralizing action and requires an acid environment to

Drug	Dose	Pharmacokinetics		Side effects	Notes
Terbutaline (Brethine, Bricanyl)	• s.c.: 0.005–0.01 mg/kg/dose; maximum: 0.25 mg q. 15–20 min ×2 • inhalation: 2 inhalations q. 4 hr		• not metabolized by COMT	• see metaproterenol	• work, so antacids should be withheld 30 min prior to its administration • see metaproterenol
Tetracycline	• 25–50 mg/kg/day, divided q. 6 hr p.o. • 10–20 mg/kg/day, divided q. 12 hr i.v. • 15–25 mg/kg/day, divided q. 8 hr i.m. • maximum: 2 g/day	• 65% protein bound • $t_{1/2} = 10.6$ hr	• 58% urinary excretion	• resistance • hepatic toxicity • ?renal toxicity • brown discoloration of teeth and bones in <7-yr-olds • thrombophlebitis • hematologic abnormalities • antibiotic-associated colitis	• 30S subunit of the ribosome-inhibiting protein synthesis • some CSF penetration
Thiopental	• 1–6 mg/kg i.v.	• $t_{1/2}$ (α) = 3 min • $t_{1/2}$ (β) = 9 hr	• termination of action is by redistribution • $t_{1/2}$ (α) is 3 min, then metabolism by P-450 in the liver ($t_{1/2}$ (β)) is 9 hr	• pseudotumor cerebri • hypotension: direct myocardial depression, ganglionic blockade • not to be used in porphyrias • histamine release: hypotension, bronchospasm • intra-arterial injection can cause loss of limbs • see pentobarbital	• potentiates both GABA and non-GABA-induced chloride conductance • decreases calcium release of neurotransmitters • decreases cerebral metabolic rate and cerebral blood flow and volume, thus decreasing intracranial hypertension • see pentobarbital

Drug	Dose[a]	Pharmacokinetics and Pharmacotherapeutics	Metabolism[a, b]	Side Effects/Interactions[a, b]	Pharmacology[a, b]
Ticarcillin	• neonates of <2 kg and of age 0–7 days: 150 mg/kg/day, divided q. 8 hr i.v. • >7 days: 225 mg/kg/day, divided q. 8 hr i.v. • >2 kg: 225–300 mg/kg/day, divided q. 8 hr i.v. • children: 200–300 mg/kg/day, divided q. 4–6 hr i.v.	• 65% protein bound • $t_{1/2}$ = 1.3 hr	• 92% urinary excretion	• see penicillin	• see penicillin • each gram contains 5 mEq sodium • enhanced activity against *Pseudomonas*
Tobramycin (Nebcin)	• 2.5 mg/kg/dose i.v., i.m.; frequency of dose depends upon age/maturity • at <7 days (<28 wk: q. 24 hr; 28–34 wk: q. 18 hr; term: q. 12 hr) • at >7 days (<28 wk: q. 18 hr; 28–34 wk: q. 12 hr; term: q. 8 hr) • for children: q 8 hr	• levels peak 6–10 mg/l through <2 mg/l • <10% protein bound • $t_{1/2}$ = 2.2 hr a very long terminal half-life (β) ($t_{1/2}$=100 hr) due to tissue binding	• 90% urinary excretion	• see gentamicin	• see gentamicin • enhanced activity against enterococci and mycobacteria
Trimethaphan (Arfonad)	• 5–150 µg/kg/min		• predominantly excreted by kidney	• mydriasis and cycloplegia, constipation, xerostomia, anhidrosis, urinary retention • histamine release • ?respiratory depression	• ganglionic blockade, vasodilation and hypotension, decreased cardiac output • blocks postsynaptic blockade of acetylcholine in ganglia

Drug	Dose/Indication	Pharmacokinetics	Toxicity	Comments
Trimethoprim-sulfamethoxazole (TMP-SMX) (Bartrim, Septra)	• severe infections and *Pneumocystis carinii* pneumonia; TMP dose: 20 mg/kg/day, divided q. 6–8 hr p.o., i.v.; • *Pneumocystis* prophylaxis: 10 mg/kg/day, divided q. 12 hr p.o., i.v.	• TMP: $t_{1/1}$ = 11 hr; • SMX: $t_{1/2}$ = 10 hr; • 60% TMP and 25–50% SMX excreted in urine	• resistance; • blood dyscrasias (especially megaloblastic anemia); rashes very common, renal toxicity	• can be used to treat autonomic hyperreflexia; • inhibits folic acid metabolism in bacteria (especially dihydrofolate reductase); • TMP has good CSF penetration
d-Tubocurarine	• intubation; • in newborn: 0.2 mg/kg; • in >6 wk old: 0.6 mg/kg	• 60 min	• hypotension	• histamine release; • ganglionic blockade; • myocardial depression; • see pancuronium (except nitroglycerin) precautions
Valproic Acid (Depakene, Depakote)	• initial: 10–15 mg/kg/day, divided b.i.d.; • maintenance: 30–60 mg/kg/day, divided q.d. to t.i.d. (increase by weekly intervals)	• 90% protein bound; • levels: 50–100 µg/ml; • <3% excreted in urine	• minimum sedation; • nausea, vomiting; • fulminant hepatitis; • phenobarbital levels increase 40% in the presence of valproic acid	• antiseizure activity for all types of seizures (?use in partial seizure)
Vancomycin (Vancocin)	• neonates of <7 days: 10 mg/kg (<1000 g: q. 24 hr; 1–2 kg: q. 18 hr; >2 kg: q. 12hr) • >7 days: 10 mg/kg (<1000 g: q. 18 hr; 1–2 kg: q. 12 hr; >2 kg q. 8 hr) • children, for CNS infections: 45 mg/kg/day, divided q. 8 hr i.v.; for other infections: 30–40 mg/kg/day, di-	• 55% protein bound; • $t_{1/2}$ (α) = 5.6 hr; • levels: 10–25 mg/l; • 90% urinary excretion	• ototoxicity (especially at levels of >30 µg/ml), nephrotoxicity phlebitis; • red neck syndrome	• Gram-positive activity; • cell wall synthesis inhibition

Drug	Dose[a]	Pharmacokinetics and Pharmacotherapeutics	Metabolism[a,b]	Side Effects/Interactions[a,b]	Pharmacology[a,b]
Vancomycin (Vancocin) —continued	vided q. 8 hr i.v.; maximum: 2 g/day; • for antibiotic-associated colitis: 2 g/1.73 m²/ day, divided q. 6 hr p.o.				
Vasopressin (Pitressin)	• 0.5 mU/kg/hr or 22 pg/ kg/min, titrated up to 2 maximum of 10 mU/kg/ Hr	• $t_{1/2} = 17$–35 min	• 10% dependent on renal function; the remainder metabolized by the lvier	• vasoconstriction at high doses, causing tissue ischemia, especially myocardial ischemia	• no histamine release, no ganglionic blockade, no effect on muscarinic cardiac receptors
Vecuronium	• intubation: 0.07–0.1 mg/kg i.v.	• 60 min		• void of cardiovascular effects	
Verapamil (Isoptin, Calan)	• 1–15 yr of age: 0.1– 0.3 mg/kg i.v.; maximum: 5 mg • adult: 5–10 mg q. 30 min, administer over 2–3 min	• $t_{1/2} = 5$ hr • level: 100 ng/ml • 90% protein bound	• <3% urinary excretion	• cardiovascular collapse when given in conjunction with a β blocker • hypotension • bradydysrhythmias • controversial indications for infants <6 mo old	• negative: dromotropy, chronotropy, inotropy • calcium channel blocker • vascular smooth muscle relaxation
Vidarabine (ara-A, Vira A)	• HSV encephalitis: 15 mg/kg/day i.v. given over a 12–24-hr period		• dependent on renal function for elimination	• few side effects • nausea, vomiting, diarrhea, rash, weakness, thrombophlebitis • CNS manifestations at high doses (20 mg/kg)	• inhibits viral DNA polymerase, especially HSV • no activity against other DNA viruses (adenoviruses, papovaviruses, or RNA viruses)

[a] Abbreviations: ACh, acetylcholine; ACT, activated clotting time; ADH, antidiuretic hormone; APC, atrial premature contraction; ATPase, adenosine triphosphate; AV, atrioventricular; BP, blood pressure; cGMP, cyclic guanosine monophosphate; CBF, cerebral blood flow; CHF, congestive heart failure; CNS, central nervous system; CO cardiac output; COMT, catechol-o-methyl transferase; CSF, cerebrospinal fluid; CTZ, chemoreceptor trigger zone; CV, cardiovascular; DI, diabetes insipidus;

..., .. dextrose in water; DNA, deoxyribonucleic acid; DT, diphtheria toxoid; ECG, electrocardiogram; FEV_1, forced expiratory volume; GABA, γ-aminobutyric acid; G6PD, glucose-6-phosphate dehydrogenase; GI, gastrointestinal; GMP, guanosine monophosphate; HR, heart rate; HSV, herpes simplex virus; ICP, intracranial pressure; IHSS, idiopathic hypertrophic subaortic stenosis; INH, isoniazid; LDL, low-density lipoprotein; LV, left ventricle; LVEDP, left ventricular end-diastolic pressure; LVSW, left ventricular stroke work; MAO, monoamine oxidase; MAP, mean arterial pressure; MIF, migration inhibitory factor; mRNA, messenger ribonucleic acid; NG, nasogastric; NPH, a type of insulin; NS, normal saline; PEMA, phenylethylmalonamide; PGG_2, prostaglandin G_2; PMNs, polymorphonuclear leukocytes; PTT, partial thromboplastin time; PVC, premature ventricular contraction; RBC, red blood cell; RSV, respiratory syncytial virus; RVEDP, right ventricular end-diastolic pressure; SA, sinoatrial; SLE, systemic lupus erythematosus; SV, stroke volume; SVR, supraventricular rhythm; SVT, supraventricular tachycardia; TMP-SMX, trimethoprim-sulfamethoxazole; Vmax, maximum velocity of cardiac contraction; and VPC, ventricular premature contractions.

b Comments on cephalosporins:
(1) mechanism of action—inhibition of cell wall synthesis;
(2) first-generation drugs (cephalothin, cefazolin)—good activity against Gram-positives, modest activity against Gram-negative; second-generation drugs (cefoxitin, cefuroxime)—increased activity against Gram-negatives; and third-generation drugs (cefotaxine, ceftazidime)—good activity against Gram-negatives at the expense of Gram-positive coverage;
(3) adverse reactions 5–20% of patients reacting to penicillin will cross-react with cephalosporins, decreasing the likelihood of rash, fever, bronchospasm, vasculitis, serum sickness, exfoliative dermatitis, Stevens-Johnson syndrome, anaphylaxis, nausea, vomiting, eosinophilia, interstitial nephritis and of other reactions, such as phlebitis, bone marrow depression, hepatitis;
(4) virtually all of the cephalosporins (except cefoperazone) are excreted in the urine, and doses must be adjusted in renal failure; virtually are all removed by dialysis in variable amounts.

Index

Page numbers in *italics* denote figures; those followed by "t" denote tables.